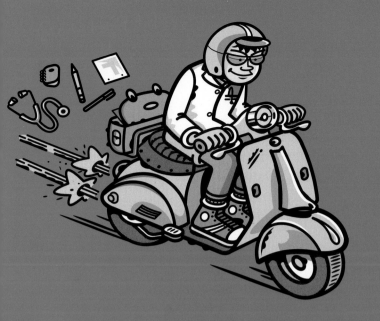

Series editor
Daniel Horton-Szar
BSc (Hons) MBBS (Hons)
GP Registrar
Northgate Medical Practice
Canterbury
Kent

Faculty advisor
Paul M Smith
MD, FRCP
Retired Consultant Gastroenterologist
Llandough and University Hospital of
Wales, Cardiff

Gastrointestinal system

SECOND EDITION

Melanie Sarah Long

BSc (Hons) Biochemistry and Immunology
4th year Medical Student
St. George's Hospital Medical School
Tooting, London

First Edition Author
Elizabeth Cheshire

D1380143

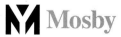 Mosby

Edinburgh • London • New York • Oxford • Philadelphia • St Louis • Sydney • Toronto 2002

MOSBY
An affiliate of Elsevier Science Limited

Commissioning Editor	**Alex Stibbe**
Project Manager	**Colin Arthur**
Project Development Manager	**Ruth Swan**
Designer	**Andy Chapman**
Illustration Management	**Mick Ruddy**

First edition 1998
Second edition 2002
Reprinted 2003

ISBN 0723432511

British Library Cataloguing in Publication Data
A catalogue record for this book is available from the British Library

Library of Congress Cataloging in Publication Data
A catalog record for this book is available from the Library of Congress

Note
Medical knowledge is constantly changing. As new information becomes available, changes in treatment, procedures, equipment and the use of drugs become necessary. The author, editors and the publisher have taken care to ensure that the information given in this text is accurate and up to date. However, readers are strongly advised to confirm that the information, especially with regard to drug usage, complies with the latest legislation and standards of practice.

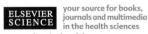 your source for books,
journals and multimedia
in the health sciences
www.elsevierhealth.com

The
publisher's
policy is to use
**paper manufactured
from sustainable forests**

Typeset by Kolam, Pondicherry, India
Printed in Spain by Graphycems

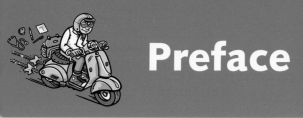

Preface

Medical students are expected to take in, digest and regurgitate an awful lot of information! Medical training is now split into discrete systems, each containing anatomy, embryology, histology, physiology, pathology, pharmacology and clinical knowledge on that particular system. Traditional textbooks tend to cover only a particular subject, such as anatomy, but encompass all systems.

So, with this book, I aim to provide a good broad knowledge of the gastrointestinal system, which will be useful on the wards and fare the student well for exams, particularly for those who like to 'cram' the week before!

Hopefully, this book will lessen your exam stress!

Melanie Sarah Long

The gastrointestinal system includes the gut, the liver, the biliary system and the pancreas, and has profited by being the subject of many diagnostic and scientific advances in the last forty years. This book brings together all the relevant knowledge necessary to pass the final MB or the MRCP in a concise and simple format.

Paul M Smith
Faculty Advisor

In the six years since the First Editions were published, there have been many changes in medicine, and in the way it is taught. These Second Editions have been largely rewritten to take these changes into account, and keep Crash Course up to date for the twenty-first century. New material has been added to include recent research and all pharmacological and disease management information has been updated in line with current best practice. We have listened to feedback from hundreds of students who have been using Crash Course and have improved the structure and layout of the books accordingly: pathology material has been closely integrated with the relevant basic medical science; there are more multiple-choice questions and the clarity of text and figures is better than ever.

The principles on which we developed the series remain the same, however. Medicine is a huge subject, and the last thing a student needs when exams are looming is to waste time assembling information from different sources, and wading through pages of irrelevant detail. As before, Crash Course brings you all the information you need, in compact, manageable volumes that integrate basic medical science with clinical practice. We still tread the fine line between producing clear, concise text and providing enough detail for those aiming at distinction. The series is still written by medical students with recent exam experience, and checked for accuracy by senior faculty members from across the UK.

I wish you the best of luck in your future careers!

Dr Dan Horton-Szar
Series Editor (Basic Medical Sciences)

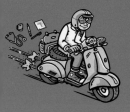

Acknowledgements

I would like to thank Dr Paul Smith and Dr Dan Horton-Szar for their invaluable suggestions, guidance and patience when going through the text. I would also like to thank Prof Paul Andrews, for his advice and brilliant lectures, which provided me with such a good basis for knowledge on this topic. Many thanks to Dr Alan Grundy and Dr James Pilcher, both at St. George's Hospital, for kindly providing images for the book (Figs 11.6, 11.7 and 11.8).

Finally, thank you Abi, for putting up with my complaining!

Figure acknowledgements
Figs 3.5 and 6.4 reproduced with permission from A Stevens and J Lowe. Human Histology, 2nd edition. Mosby, 1997
Figs 3.6, 3.9A, 3.11, 3.12, 6.5 and 7.27 adapted with permission from L Johnson. Gastrointestinal Physiology, 6th edition. Mosby, 2000
Fig. 3.13 redrawn with permission from General and Systematic Pathology, edited by JCE Underwood. Churchill Livingstone, 1992
Fig. 4.13 redrawn with permission from A Gaw, R Cowan, D O'Reilly, M Stewart and J Sheperd. Clinical Biochemistry, 2nd edition. Churchill Livingstone, 1999
Fig. 4.16 adapted with permission from HP Rang, M Dale, JM Ritter. Pharmacology, 4th edition. Churchill Livingstone, 1999
Fig. 5.1 redrawn with permission from General and Systematic Pathology, 2nd edition, edited by JCE Underwood. Churchill Livingstone, 1996
Fig. 5.8 redrawn with permission from PJ Kumar and ML Clarke. Clinical Medicine, 3rd edition. Bailliere Tindall, 1994
Figs 5.11 and 5.12 reproduced with permission from L Friedman and EB Keefe. Handbook of Liver Disease. Churchill Livingstone, 1997
Fig. 7.19 redrawn with permission from RM Berne, MN Levy. Principles of Physiology, 3rd edition. Mosby, 2000
Figs 9.15, 11.1A, and 11.2A redrawn with permission from Davidson's Principles and Practice of Medicine, 18th edition, edited by C Haslett. Churchill Livingstone, 1999
Figs 11.6 and 11.7 reproduced courtesy of Dr A Grundy
Fig. 11.8 reproduced courtesy of Dr J Pilcher

Figs 9.1–5, 9.7–14, 9.16, 9.17 and 9.20 redrawn courtesy of Dr HL Greene II, from Clinical Medicine, 2nd edition. Mosby

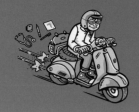

Dedication

For my family.

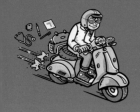

Contents

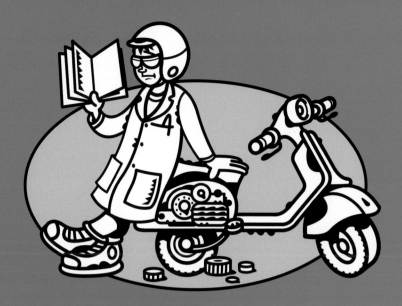

BASIC MEDICAL SCIENCE OF THE GASTROINTESTINAL SYSTEM

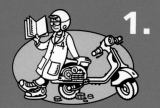

1. Overview of the Gastrointestinal System

Anatomical overview

The gastrointestinal (GI) system (Fig. 1.1) develops entirely from the endoderm in the embryo. It maintains a basic structure throughout its length (Fig. 1.2), with a mucosal layer, submucosa, muscular layer, and adventitia or serosa. There are also intrinsic submucosal and mucosal nerve plexuses (Meissner's plexus and Auerbach's plexus), the activity of which is moderated by extrinsic innervation.

The gastrointestinal tract takes in, breaks down, and absorbs food and fluids. The system has different specialized regions to perform these functions. Food is moved through the tract by gravity and peristalsis.

Peristalsis is a wavelike movement that propels food along the gut by the coordinated contraction of muscle in one area and relaxation in the next. A series of sphincters prevent any backflow of food (reflux) (Fig. 1.3).

Reflexes occurring in different parts of the tract act with hormonal and neuronal factors to control the speed of food movement through the tract. The contents move through the tract at a rate at which they can be processed.

Functions of the gastrointestinal tract

The functions of the GI tract are given in Fig. 1.4. Other functions involved in food digestion are:
- Storage of waste material in the sigmoid colon and rectum.

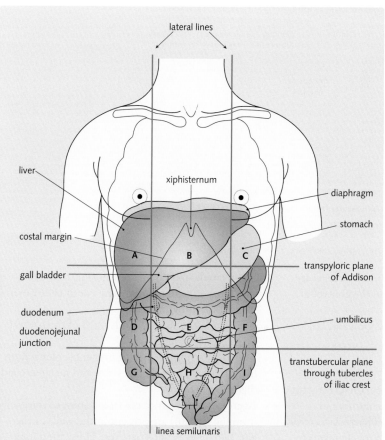

lateral lines

liver

xiphisternum

diaphragm

stomach

costal margin

gall bladder

duodenum

duodenojejunal junction

transpyloric plane of Addison

umbilicus

transtubercular plane through tubercles of iliac crest

linea semilunaris

Fig. 1.1 Anatomy of the gastrointestinal tract, showing its surface markings. The transpyloric plane of Addison passes midway between the jugular notch and the symphysis pubis, and midway between the xiphisternum and the umbilicus. It passes through the pylorus, the neck of the pancreas, the duodenojejunal flexure, and the hila of the kidneys. Surface regions: A right hypochondriac; B epigastric; C left hypochondriac; D right lumbar; E umbilical; F left lumbar; G right iliac fossa; H hypogastric; I left iliac fossa.

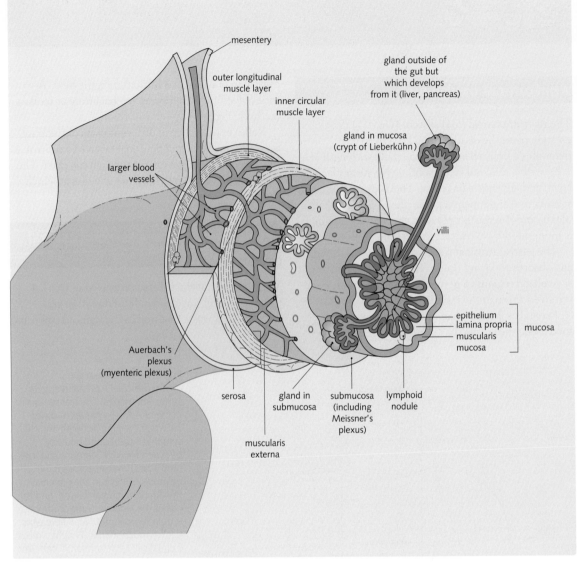

Fig. 1.2 The basic structure of the gastrointestinal tract.

- Exocrine, endocrine, and paracrine secretions are all involved in active digestion and the control of digestion and motility in the gut.
- Some GI peptide hormones have local and systemic effects (see Fig. 5.11).
- Excretion of waste products.

Although it is an internal structure, the GI tract is not sterile, and it is presented with a number of insults on a daily basis, from harmful bacteria to toxic substances. It requires good defence mechanisms to deal with these:

- Sight, smell, and taste often alert us to the fact that food is contaminated. The vomit reflex exists to eject harmful material.
- The acid in the stomach kills most of the bacteria ingested with food.
- The natural flora of the gut prevents colonization by potentially harmful bacteria, and it can also aid digestion of food.
- Aggregations of lymphoid tissue (part of the immune system) are present in the walls of the gut, known as Peyer's patches. These mount an immune response to antigen found in the diet.

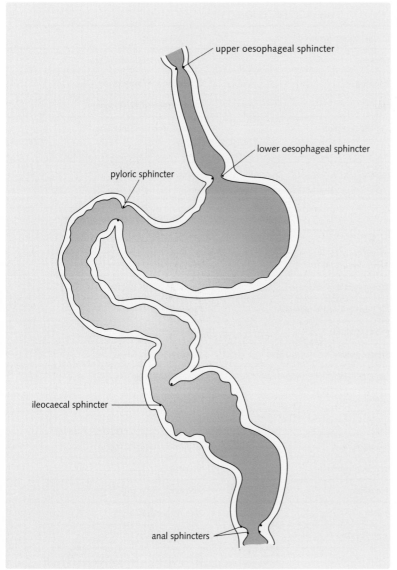

Fig. 1.3 Sphincters of the gastrointestinal tract.

upper oesophageal sphincter

lower oesophageal sphincter

pyloric sphincter

ileocaecal sphincter

anal sphincters

Constituents of food

The body requires food as a source of energy, minerals, and vitamins. These are essential for growth, maintenance, and repair. The main food groups are carbohydrates, fat, and protein. These are oxidized to generate high energy bonds in ATP (adenosine triphosphate) and to provide materials for building new tissues.

Excess food, stored as fat, leads to obesity and associated diseases such as ischaemic heart disease and non-insulin-dependent diabetes. Men and women have different patterns of fat distribution in the body. When deprived of food, an average 70 kg man may survive for 5–6 weeks on body fat stores provided he is able to drink water. Blood glucose levels drop during the initial few days, then rise and stabilize (the brain needs a constant supply of glucose, although other organs are better able to utilize other forms of energy). During prolonged fasting, the body will also break down muscle, including heart muscle, to provide energy. This may lead to death from cardiac failure. Most patients do not die from starvation directly, but from the inability to fight off infectious disease.

Fat

Dietary fat is chiefly composed of triglycerides (esters of free fatty acids and glycerol, which may be

Functions of the GI tract		
Function	**Mechanism/process involved**	**Where it occurs**
Digestion of food	i) Mastication	Mouth: with teeth and tongue
	ii) Swallowing	Oropharynx: relaxation of UOS
	iii) Mixing	Stomach and small intestine
	iv) Enzymatic digestion	Stomach and small intestine
	v) Absorption	Stomach, small intestine and large intestine
Motility	i) Peristalsis	Throughout gut
	ii) Mass movement	Throughout gut
Storage of food waste		Stomach, sigmoid colon, and rectum
Excretion	Defecation	Rectum and anus
Exocrine secretions	i) Mucus/saliva secretion	Salivary gland
	ii) HCl/pepsin/mucus secretion	Gastric glands of stomach
	iii) HCO_3/amylase/lipase secretion	Pancreas
	iv) Bile salt secretion	Liver
Endocrine secretions	i) Gastrin secretion	Stomach
	ii) Secretin secretion	Duodenal mucosa
	iii) Insulin secretion	Pancreas
Paracrine secretions	Somatostatin secretion	Mucosa
Defence	i) Smell, sight, taste	Oral cavity, cephalic region
	ii) Gastric acid secretion	Stomach
	iii) Vomit reflex	Stomach up to mouth
	iv) Gut flora	Throughout gut
	v) Mucus secretion	Throughout gut
	vi) Immune response	Peyer's patches, macrophages in mucosa
	vii) Secretion of IgA	Mucosal secretions

Fig. 1.4 A summary of the functions of the gastrointestinal (GI) tract. (UOS, upper oesophageal sphincter.)

saturated, monounsaturated, or polyunsaturated). The essential fatty acids are linoleic acid and α-linoleic acid, which cannot be manufactured and so must be obtained from our diet.

The body is efficient at manufacturing fats (triglycerides, sterols, and phospholipids), and it will lay down subcutaneous fat stores even on low-fat diets.

Dietary fat provides 37 kJ (9 kcal) of energy per gram. Fat intake should be less than 35% of the total energy intake.

Carbohydrate

Dietary carbohydrates comprise the polysaccharides, starch, disaccharides (mainly sucrose and lactose), monosaccharides (glucose, fructose and galactose), and non-starch polysaccharides (previously called fibre).

Carbohydrates are a cheap form of food, and they can be taken in excess, often limiting the intake of other food constituents. Carbohydrates provide 17 kJ (4 kcal) of energy per gram.

Protein

Protein is composed of amino acids, nine of which are essential for protein synthesis and nitrogen balance.

We need 0.75 g protein per kilogram of body weight per day, but in developed countries most people exceed this.

In developing countries, where protein is less readily available, combinations of certain foods can provide enough of the essential amino acids even though those foods, on their own, are low in some amino acids.

Examples of good combinations are maize and legumes, or baked beans on toast!

Water

Fluid intake and oxidation of food provides water for the body. About 1 L of water is needed per day to balance insensible losses such as sweating, metabolism, and exhalation of water vapour (more water is required in hot climates).

Excess water is excreted in the urine by the kidneys; inadequate intake leads to dehydration.

Minerals

Minerals are chemicals that must be present in the diet to maintain good health; over 20 have so far been identified (e.g. iron and calcium).

Trace elements (e.g. zinc, copper, and iodine) are substances that, by definition, are present in the body in low concentrations (less than 100 parts per million) and include some minerals. It is not yet known whether all trace elements are essential for health.

Vitamins

Vitamins are classified as fat soluble or water soluble; vitamins A, D, E, and K are fat soluble, the other vitamins are water soluble.

Fat soluble vitamins are stored in fatty tissue in the body (mainly in the liver), and they are not usually excreted in the urine.

The absorption of fat soluble vitamins is dependent upon the absorption of dietary fat: deficiency can occur in cases of fat malabsorption.

Body stores of water soluble vitamins (other than vitamin B_{12}) are smaller than stores of fat soluble vitamins. They are excreted in the urine and deficiencies of water soluble vitamins are more common.

A summary of the nutrient groups is given in Fig. 1.5.

For further information, see the companion volume on *Metabolism and Nutrition* in the *Crash Course* series.

Summary of nutrients in the diet				
Food group		**Source**	**Digested**	**Absorbed**
Fats		Meats, oil, butter, etc.	Small intestine	Small intestine
Carbohydrates	Polysaccharides, starch, etc.	Sugary food, potatoes, pasta, etc.	Mouth and small intestine	Small intestine
	Non-starch polysaccharides (NSPs i.e. fibre)	Plant foods	Usually undigestable, some colonic bacteria can digest NSPs	Not absorbed
Protein		Meat, pulses, etc.	Stomach and small intestine	Small intestine
Minerals		Meat, milk, vegetables, cereals	Not digested	Small intestine
Vitamins	Fat soluble (A,D,E and K)	Meat, fish, and vegetable oils	Not digested	With fat
	Water soluble	Milk, meat, fruit, and vegetables	Not digested	Small intestine

Fig. 1.5 A summary of the nutrient groups obtained from the diet. (NSPs, non-starch polysaccharides.)

Development of the gastrointestinal tract

The GI tract is the main organ system derived from the endodermal germ layer. The formation of the tube is largely passive; it depends on the cephalocaudal and lateral folding of the embryo.

The yolk sac produces blood cells and vessels, and it is the site of haematopoiesis for the first 2 months from conception. Later, it becomes inverted and incorporated into the body cavity. The folding of the embryo constricts the initial communication between the embryo and the yolk sac.

The remnant of this communication is the vitelline duct, which normally disappears *in utero*. Where it persists (as it does in about 2% of the population), it is known as a Meckel's diverticulum.

The gut tube divides into foregut, midgut, and hindgut, each of which has its own blood supply (Fig. 1.6). The superior mesenteric artery is in the umbilicus. The gut tube starts straight but twists during development and the midgut grows rapidly, with the developing liver occupying most of the space.

There is not enough room in the fetal abdomen to accommodate the rapidly developing gut. The gut herniates between weeks 7–11 of gestation, continuing its development outside the abdominal cavity.

It undergoes a clockwise rotation of 180° and what was the inferior limb becomes the superior limb (and vice versa). It then undergoes a 270° turn anticlockwise so that the caecum lies under the liver. The tube then elongates again so that the caecum points downwards. Sometimes the caecum remains pointing up instead of down, which makes diagnosis of appendicitis difficult!

The falciform ligament lies in front of the liver, and the lesser omentum lies behind the liver. The liver and pancreas develop from endodermal diverticula that bud off the duodenum in weeks 4–6 (see Fig. 4.5).

Much of the mouth (including the muscles of mastication and tongue) and the oesophagus develop from the branchial arches.

The muscles of mastication, mylohyoid, and anterior belly of digastric develop from the first (mandibular) arch, supplied by the trigeminal nerve (V).

The anterior two thirds of the tongue develop from three mesenchymal buds from the first pair of branchial arches. The posterior belly of digastric develops from the second arch, supplied by the facial nerve (VII).

Stylopharyngeus develops from the third arch, supplied by the glossopharyngeal nerve (IX).

Cricothyroid, the constrictors of the pharynx, and the striated muscles of oesophagus develop from the fourth and sixth arches, supplied by branches of the vagus nerve (X). The fifth arch is often absent. The developmental stages are shown in Fig. 1.7.

Divisions of the primitive gut tube			
Divisions of gut	Blood supply	Nerve supply	Components
Foregut	Coeliac artery	Vagus	Pharynx Oesophagus Stomach Proximal half of duodenum Gives rise to: liver gall bladder pancreas
Midgut	Superior mesenteric artery	Vagus	Distal half of duodenum Jejunum Ileum Caecum Ascending colon Proximal two thirds of transverse colon
Hindgut	Inferior mesenteric artery	Pelvic splanchnic	Distal one third of transverse colon Descending colon Sigmoid colon Proximal two thirds of anorectal canal

Fig. 1.6 Divisions of the primitive gut tube.

A

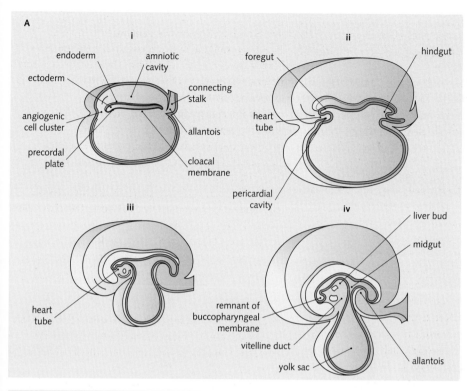

i

ectoderm
endoderm
amniotic cavity
connecting stalk
angiogenic cell cluster
allantois
precordal plate
cloacal membrane

ii

foregut
hindgut
heart tube
pericardial cavity

iii

heart tube

iv

liver bud
midgut
remnant of buccopharyngeal membrane
vitelline duct
yolk sac
allantois

B

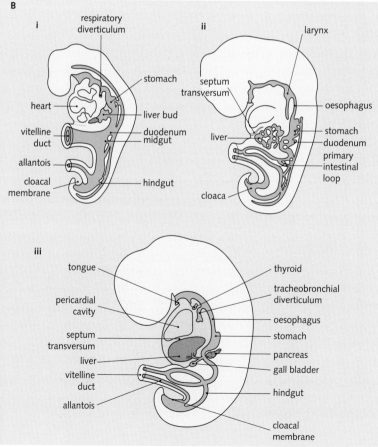

i

respiratory diverticulum
stomach
heart
liver bud
vitelline duct
duodenum midgut
allantois
cloacal membrane
hindgut

ii

larynx
septum transversum
oesophagus
liver
stomach
duodenum
primary intestinal loop
cloaca

iii

tongue
thyroid
pericardial cavity
tracheobronchial diverticulum
oesophagus
septum transversum
stomach
liver
pancreas
vitelline duct
gall bladder
allantois
hindgut
cloacal membrane

Fig. 1.7 Stages of embryonic development of the gastrointestinal tract. (A) Schematic drawings of sagittal sections through embryos at various stages of development, showing the development of the foregut, midgut, and hindgut. **i** Presomite embryo. **ii** 7-somite embryo. **iii** 14-somite embryo. **iv** Embryo at 1 month. (B) Schematic drawings showing the primitive gastrointestinal tract and formation of the liver. **i** Diagram showing a 3 mm embryo (approx 25 days). **ii** Embryo at 32 days (5 mm). **iii** Diagram of a 9 mm embryo (36 days) showing caudal expansion of the liver.

- Draw a labelled diagram of the basic organization of the gut wall.
- What are the main functions of the GI tract? Where do the main functions occur?
- How does the GI tract defend itself from bacteria?
- What are the major food constituents and where are they absorbed?
- How many kcal of energy do a gram of fat and carbohydrate provide?
- Briefly describe the embryological development of the gut.
- What are the main divisions of the primitive gut tube? What components do these divisions encompass and what are the major nerve and blood supplies to these divisions?

2. The Upper Gastrointestinal Tract

Organization of the mouth and oropharynx

Regional anatomy

The oral cavity extends from the lips to the pillars of the fauces, which is the opening to the pharynx. It contains the tongue, alveolar arches (which anchor the teeth), gums, teeth, and the openings of the salivary ducts (Fig. 2.1).

The oral cavity is divided into the vestibule (anterior to the teeth) and the oral cavity proper (posterior to the incisors).

The blood supply of the oral cavity and oropharynx comes from branches of the external carotid artery, such as the facial artery and lingual artery. Innervation comes from branches of the cranial nerves.

Tongue

The tongue is a muscular structure and its dorsum (upper surface) is divided into the anterior (two thirds) and posterior (one third) by a V-shaped borderline—the sulcus terminalis.

The dorsal surface is covered with small fungiform (tip of tongue) and filiform (middle of tongue) papillae. Circumvallate papillae are found just anterior to the sulcus terminalis and taste buds are located in the circular trenches surrounding these papillae (Fig. 2.2). The posterior third contains the lingual tonsil.

The tongue consists of four pairs of intrinsic muscles (superior and inferior longitudinal, transverse, and vertical), which have no attachments outside the tongue itself. These muscles are involved with changing the shape of the tongue.

Paralysis or total relaxation of the genioglossus muscle, such as with general anaesthesia, allows the tongue to fall posteriorly and obstruct the airways, causing suffocation. Anaesthetized patients are always intubated to prevent this happening.

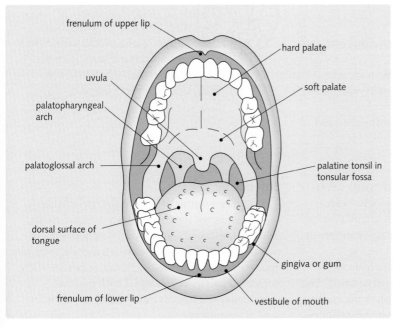

Fig. 2.1 The oral cavity. The lateral walls of the pillars of the fauces are composed of the palatoglossal arches (anterior) and the palatopharyngeal arches (posterior). The palatine tonsils lie between the two arches, covered with mucous membrane.

frenulum of upper lip
hard palate
uvula
soft palate
palatopharyngeal arch
palatoglossal arch
palatine tonsil in tonsular fossa
dorsal surface of tongue
gingiva or gum
frenulum of lower lip
vestibule of mouth

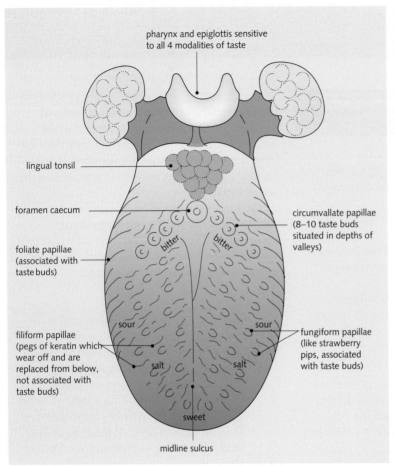

Fig. 2.2 The tongue and taste buds. The filiform papillae are numerous and arranged in rows parallel to the sulcus terminalis. They are sensitive to touch and facilitate licking. The circumvallate, foliate, and fungiform papillae are all associated with taste buds. The underlying serous glands secrete a watery fluid that flushes out debris and lingering tastes.

The extrinsic muscles originate outside the tongue and attach to it. They act to control movement of the tongue.

The extrinsic muscles are:

- Genioglossus—a fan shaped muscle that attaches to the mandible in the midline.
- Hyoglossus—attaches to the hyoid bone.
- Styloglossus—attaches to the styloid process and its fibres interdigitate with the hyoglossus.
- Palatoglossus—originates in the soft palate and enters the lateral part of the tongue.

The palatoglossus muscle is innervated by the fibres from the cranial root of the accessory nerve (XI), through the pharyngeal branch of the vagus nerve (X). The other lingual muscles are innervated by the hypoglossal nerve (XII). The nerve supply of the tongue is summarized in Fig. 2.3.

The arterial supply to the tongue is from the lingual artery (a branch of the external carotid). The lingual vein drains the tongue. Lymph drains to the deep cervical, submandibular and submental nodes.

Asking a patient to stick out their tongue is a good test of function of the hypoglossal nerve. If one of the hypoglossal nerves has a lesion, then the tongue will deviate to the side of paralysis when the tongue is protruded.

Soft palate

The hard and soft palates form the roof of the mouth, and they separate it from the nasal cavity. The oral surface of the soft palate contains many mucous glands. The soft palate is a mobile, muscular aponeurosis attached to the posterior border of the bony hard palate. It is covered with mucous membrane, and it is continuous laterally with the wall of the pharynx.

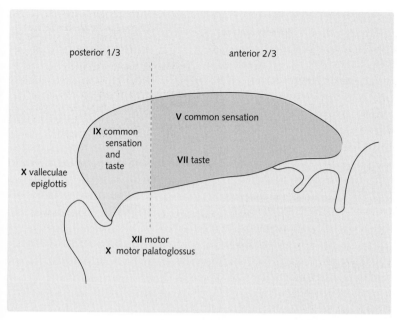

Fig. 2.3 Nerve supply to tongue and epiglottis, in median section. (V, lingual nerve—from mandibular division of trigeminal; VII, chorda tympani—joins the lingual nerve to be distributed.)

The palatoglossal and palatopharyngeal arches join the tongue and the pharynx, respectively, to the soft palate. The curved free border of the soft palate lies between the oropharynx and the nasopharynx. From this hangs the uvula, in the midline, which is seen to move when a patient says 'ahh'.

The muscles of the soft palate are:

- Levator veli palatini.
- Tensor veli palatini.
- Palatoglossus.
- Palatopharyngeus.
- Musculus uvulae.

All are supplied by the pharyngeal motor fibres of the vagus (X) via the pharyngeal plexus, except the tensor veli palatini, which is supplied by the mandibular nerve, a branch of the trigeminal (V).

Muscles of mastication

The muscles of mastication are:

- The masseter.
- The temporalis.
- The lateral pterygoid muscles.
- The medial pterygoid muscles.

These develop from the mesoderm of the first pharyngeal (branchial) arch. Their motor nerve supply is from the mandibular branch of the trigeminal nerve (V). They all arise from the skull and insert into the mandible, causing movement of

the mandible and the temporomandibular joint (Fig. 2.4). The muscles are summarized in Fig. 2.5.

Salivary glands

There are three pairs of large salivary glands (the parotid, submandibular, and sublingual glands) and numerous smaller glands, scattered throughout the mouth (Fig. 2.6).

Parotid gland

This is the largest salivary gland and it produces serous saliva. It lies between the ramus of the mandible and the mastoid and coronoid processes, and its anterior border overlies the masseter. An accessory lobe may be found above this muscle. The parotid gland is covered with a fibrous capsule that is continuous with the deep investing fascia of the neck. The facial nerve (VII) passes through the parotid gland.

The parotid duct is about 5 cm long. It pierces the buccinator muscle and opens into the mouth opposite the second upper molar tooth. This opening can be felt with the tongue.

The parotid gland is supplied by branches of the external carotid artery; venous blood drains to the retromandibular vein. It is innervated by both the sympathetic and parasympathetic systems. Parasympathetic innervation is secretomotor (causing production of saliva); sympathetic innervation is vasoconstrictor (causing a dry mouth).

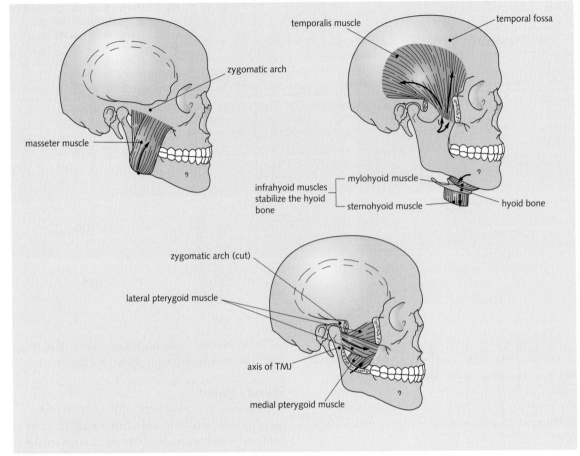

Fig. 2.4 The muscles of mastication and infrahyoid muscles. (TMJ, the temporomandibular joint).

Parasympathetic fibres are carried from the glossopharyngeal nerve (IX) through the otic ganglion and auriculotemporal nerve.

Sympathetic fibres from the superior cervical ganglion pass along the external carotid artery.

Lymph from the superficial part of the gland drains to the parotid nodes and from the deep part to the retropharyngeal nodes.

Submandibular gland

The submandibular gland lies in the floor of the mouth, covered by a fibrous capsule, and it produces mixed serous and mucous secretions. Both its superficial and deep parts communicate around the posterior border of the mylohyoid muscle.

Its duct passes forwards between the mylohyoid and hyoglossus muscles to open onto sublingual papillae at the base of the frenulum. The lingual nerve crosses the duct.

The gland is supplied by the facial and lingual arteries (branches of the external carotid arteries); venous drainage is by the facial and lingual veins.

It is innervated by both the parasympathetic and sympathetic systems.

Parasympathetic fibres are conveyed from the facial nerve through the chorda tympani and submandibular ganglion.

Sympathetic innervation is from the superior cervical ganglion, with fibres passing along the arteries of the gland.

Lymphatic drainage is to the submandibular lymph nodes, which are partly embedded in the gland and partly lie between it and the mandible.

Sublingual gland

This is the smallest of the paired salivary glands, and it is also the most deeply situated. It is almond shaped and found below the mucous membrane of the floor of the mouth. It produces mainly mucous secretions, which either pass into numerous small ducts (10–20) that open into the floor of the mouth,

The muscles of mastication			
Muscle (Nerve supply)	**Origin**	**Insertion**	**Action**
Masseter (V^3)	Inferior border + medial surface of zygomatic arch	Lateral surface of ramus of mandible	Elevates and protrudes jaw, closing it. Retrusion of chin
Temporalis (V^3)	Temporal fossa, overlying temporal fascia	Tip and medial surface of coronoid plexus	Elevates mandible (closes jaw) + retrudes mandible after protrusion
Lateral pterygoid (V^3)	**Superior head** Infratemporal surface and crest of greater wing of sphenoid **Inferior head** Lateral surface of lateral pterygoid plate	**Superior and inferior heads** Neck of mandible + capsule + articular disc of temporomandibular joint	**Together** Protrude mandible **Alone** Acting alternatively, they produce side to side movement
Medial pterygoid (V^3)	**Deep head** Medial surface of lateral pterygoid plate **Superficial head** Tuberosity of maxilla	**Superficial and deep heads** Medial surface of ramus of mandible, inferior to mandibular foramen	**Together** Help elevate mandible, closing jaw. Also help protrude mandible **Alone** Acting alternate, they produce a grinding motion

Fig. 2.5 The muscles of mastication.

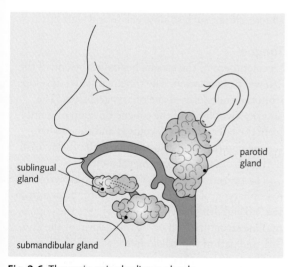

Fig. 2.6 The main paired salivary glands.

or they pass into the submandibular duct. The innervation, blood supply, and venous and lymphatic drainage are similar to the submandibular gland.

Pharynx

The pharynx is a fibromuscular tube, approximately 15 cm long, that extends from the base of the skull to the inferior border of the cricoid cartilage anteriorly, and to the inferior border of the C6 vertebra posteriorly. It communicates with the nose, middle ear (by the auditory tube), mouth, and larynx.

It conducts food and fluids to the oesophagus and air to the larynx and lungs (however, some air is swallowed with food).

The pharynx can be split into three functional parts: the nasopharynx, the oropharynx, and laryngopharynx. Its walls have mucous, submucous, and muscular layers.

The muscular layer of the pharynx consists of:
- Superior, middle, and inferior constrictors.
- Salpingopharyngeus.
- Stylopharyngeus.
- Palatopharyngeus.

The cricopharyngeus muscle forms the upper oesophageal sphincter (Fig. 2.7). Stylopharyngeus is supplied by the glossopharyngeal nerve (IX), but all the other muscles of the pharynx (Fig. 2.8) are supplied by the vagus (X) through the pharyngeal plexus on the outer surface of the middle constrictor.

Superior to the superior constrictor muscle, the submucosa thickens to form the pharyngobasilar membrane, which blends with buccopharyngeal fascia to form the pharyngeal recess.

15

The superior, middle, and inferior pharyngeal constrictor muscles are arranged so that the superior one is innermost and the inferior one is outermost; like three flowerpots stacked inside each other.

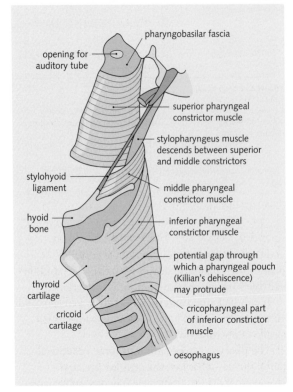

Fig. 2.7 The muscles of the pharynx.

The pharyngeal tonsils, or adenoids, lie submucosally in the nasopharynx. The palatine tonsils lie between the pillars of the fauces in the oropharynx (Fig. 2.1).

The epiglottis, a flap of cartilage covered with mucous membrane, lies posterior to the tongue in the laryngopharynx, and it closes the entrance to the larynx during swallowing. On either side of the epiglottis lie the piriform fossae—a common site for fish bones to lodge!

The pharynx is supplied by branches of the ascending pharyngeal, superior thyroid, maxillary, lingual, and facial arteries. Venous drainage is to the internal jugular vein, via the pharyngeal venous plexus. Lymph from the nasopharynx drains to the retropharyngeal lymph nodes. The rest of the pharyngeal lymph drains to the deep cervical nodes.

Development of the mouth and oropharynx

The head and neck derive primarily from the pharyngeal (branchial) arches, which are bars of mesenchymal tissue with an outer covering of ectoderm and inner covering of endoderm, separated by pharyngeal clefts and outpocketings called pharyngeal pouches.

Each pharyngeal arch contains neural crest cells to contribute to skeletal components. Each also contains an arterial, cranial nerve, and muscular component. Initially there are six arches, but the fifth disappears (Fig. 2.9).

At about four and a half weeks of embryological development, the 1st and 2nd arches form the mesenchymal prominences. The 1st pharyngeal arch consists of a dorsal and ventral portion called the maxillary and mandibular prominences, respectively.

These fuse and develop with the frontonasal prominence to give rise to the mandible, upper lip, palate, and nose. Failure to fuse results in abnormalities, such as cleft palate and cleft lip.

Tongue

Development of the tongue begins at the end of the 4th week of gestation. The tongue mucosa develops from the endoderm of the pharyngeal floor. The anterior two thirds of the tongue develop primarily from the lateral lingual swellings and the median tongue bud (or tuberculum impar), all of which are derived from the 1st pharyngeal arch.

The posterior third is formed by the growth of the hypopharyngeal eminence (a structure formed from the 3rd and 4th pharyngeal arches) over the copula, a midline structure formed by mesoderm of the 2nd, 3rd, and part of the 4th arches.

The muscles of the tongue, except palatoglossus, are formed from mesoderm derived from the myotomes of the occipital somites. The muscles (except palatoglossus) are supplied by the hypoglossal nerve, which is consistent with their origin.

The parotid gland is formed from a tubular ectodermal outgrowth at the inner surface of the cheek. The submandibular and sublingual glands are formed in a similar fashion from invaginations of the endoderm of the floor of the mouth.

Muscles of the pharynx			
Name of muscle (nerve supply)	Origin	Insertion	Action
Superior constrictor (pharyngeal plexus)	Medial pterygoid plate, pterygoid hamulus, pterygomandibular ligament, mylohyoid line of mandible	Pharyngeal tubercle of occipital bone, midline raphe	Assists in separating oro- and nasopharynx and propels food bolus downward
Middle constrictor (pharyngeal plexus)	Stylohyoid ligament, lesser and greater horns of hyoid bone	Pharyngeal raphe	Propels food bolus downward
Inferior constrictor (pharyngeal plexus)	Lamina of thyroid cartilage, cricoid cartilage	Pharyngeal raphe	Propels food bolus downward
Cricopharyngeus (pharyngeal plexus)	Fibres of inferior constrictor muscle attached to cricoid cartilage	Pharyngeal raphe	Sphincter at lower end of pharynx
Palatopharyngeus (pharyngeal plexus)	Palatine aponeurosis	Thyroid cartilage	Elevates pharyngeal wall and pulls palatopharyngeal folds medially
Salpingopharyngeus (pharyngeal plexus)	Auditory tube	Merges with palatopharyngeus	Elevates pharynx and larynx
Stylopharyngeus (IX)	Styloid process of temporal bone	Thyroid cartilage	Elevates larynx during swallowing

Fig. 2.8 Summary of the muscles of the pharynx.

Tissues
Mucosal surface
The mouth is lined with stratifed squamous epithelium with an underlying submucosa containing collagen, elastin, and salivary glands. The inner surface of the lips, cheeks, floor of the mouth, and undersurface of the tongue are all covered with non-keratinizing squamous epithelium. The submucosa of the cheeks contain minor salivary glands and some sebaceous glands with skeletal muscle fibres (buccinator muscles) deep to these structures.

The pharyngeal mucosa is continuous with that of the nose, oral cavity, auditory tube, larynx, and oesophagus. The nasopharynx is lined with respiratory epithelium (ciliated mucous membrane with goblet cells).

The oropharynx and laryngopharynx are lined with stratified squamous epithelium to withstand abrasion from the passage of food.

Taste receptors
The four basic tastes detected by taste buds are sweet, sour, salty, and bitter. Taste receptors (buds) are found in different areas of the tongue (Fig. 2.3). They can provide early warning that food may be bad. The majority of our 'taste' is actually smell!

Salivary glands
The salivary glands consist of parenchymal (functional) and stromal (support) components.

Each parenchymal unit is called a salivon, which consists of an acinus (from the Latin word for grape) and a duct (Fig. 2.10). The duct of the salivon modifies the secretions of the acinus. The striated segment of the duct is continuous with the excretory part of the duct.

Acini consist of serous or mucous cells. The parotid gland has only serous acini, the sublingual gland contains mostly mucous acini, and the submandibular gland contains predominantly serous acini. The minor salivary glands are mucous, except for von Ebner's glands and those in the tip of the tongue, which are serous.

The structure of the salivary glands is very similar to that of the pancreatic exocrine glands, which secrete a wide range of digestive enzyme precursors.

Lymphoid tissue
There are a number of aggregations of lymphoid tissue in the oral cavity and pharynx. The lingual tonsils (located in the posterior third of the tongue), the palatine tonsils (between the pillars of the fauces), the pharyngeal tonsils (adenoids) and other smaller aggregations form a protective ring around the oro- and nasopharynx, called Waldeyer's ring. The tissue is also described as mucosa-associated lymphoid tissue (MALT).

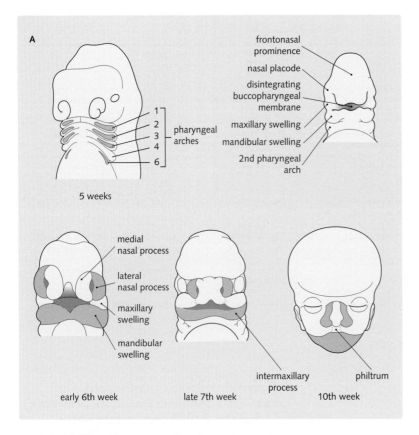

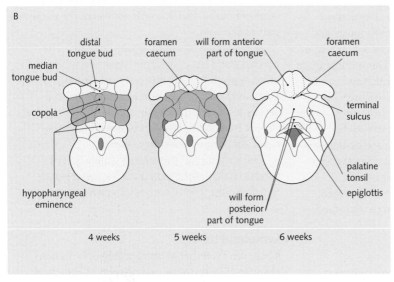

Fig. 2.9 Development of the mouth and pharynx (A) and the tongue (B).

Organization of the oesophagus

The oesophagus is a fibromuscular tube, approximately 25 cm in length, extending from the pharynx to the stomach. Its primary function is to convey food and fluids from the pharynx to the stomach during swallowing. It has cervical, thoracic, and abdominal parts.

Regional anatomy

The oesophagus begins in the neck, at the inferior border of the cricoid cartilage, where it is continuous

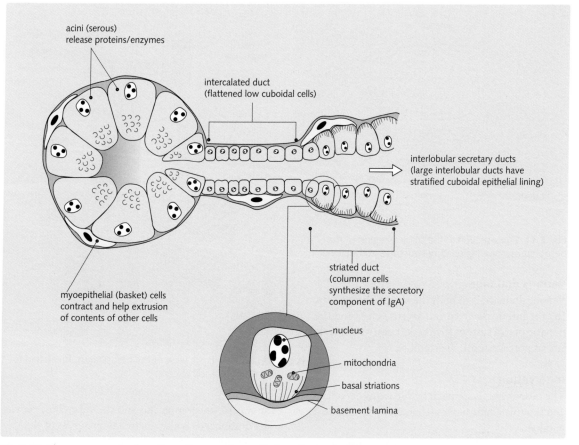

acini (serous)
release proteins/enzymes

intercalated duct
(flattened low cuboidal cells)

interlobular secretary ducts
(large interlobular ducts have
stratified cuboidal epithelial lining)

striated duct
(columnar cells
synthesize the secretory
component of IgA)

myoepithelial (basket) cells
contract and help extrusion
of contents of other cells

nucleus

mitochondria

basal striations

basement lamina

Fig. 2.10 The components of a salivon, the secreting unit of a salivary gland.

with the pharynx (Fig. 2.11). Initially it inclines to the left, but it is moved medially by the aortic arch (at the level of T4). Inferior to the arch, it inclines to the left and passes through the diaphragm just left of the median plane.

In the superior mediastinum, it lies anterior to the 1st four thoracic vertebrae and posterior to the trachea, left main bronchus, and the left recurrent laryngeal nerve. The azygos vein lies on the right of the oesophagus; the aortic arch and thoracic duct lie on the left.

At the level of T5 (the 5th thoracic vertebra), the oesophagus moves forward and to the left, accompanied by the right and left vagal nerves, to descend behind the fibrous pericardium and in front of the descending aorta. The oesophagus enters the abdomen through the muscular part of the diaphragm at the level of T10.

The abdominal part of the oesophagus is only about 2 cm long, and it is lined by columnar epithelium. It joins the stomach at the cardiac orifice, at the level of T11 (Fig. 2.12) and just

Impressions, or constrictions in the thoracic part of the oesophagus, are made by the arch of the aorta, the point where the left main bronchus crosses, and the diaphragm, as it passes through the oesophageal hiatus.

posterior to the 7th costal cartilage. This part is also covered by peritoneum and encircled by the oesophageal plexus of nerves.

Blood supply
Blood supply is from the inferior thyroid artery, branches of the thoracic aorta, and branches of the left gastric artery and left inferior phrenic artery (both ascend from the abdominal cavity).

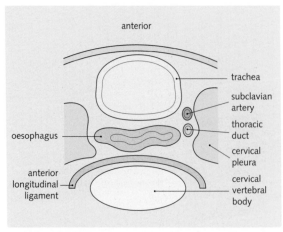

Fig. 2.11 Cross-section of the cervical region of the oesophagus, showing relating structures at that level.

Venous drainage

Venous drainage is to both the systemic circulation (by the inferior thyroid and azygos veins) and the hepatic portal system (by the left gastric vein). It is a site of portosystemic anastamosis.

Innervation

The oesophagus is supplied by the vagus nerve (X) and the splanchnic nerves (thoracic sympathetic trunks).

Striated muscle in the upper part is supplied by somatic motor neurons of the vagus from the nucleus ambiguus, without synaptic interruption.

The smooth muscle of the lower part is innervated by visceral motor neurons of the vagus that synapse with postganglionic neurons, whose cell bodies lie in

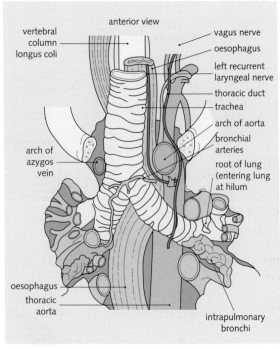

Fig. 2.12 Anterior view of the oesophagus, in relation to the other thoracic viscera.

the wall of the oesophagus and the splanchnic plexus. The oesophagus is also encircled by nerves of the oesophageal plexus.

Development

At about four weeks of gestation, the respiratory diverticulum (lung bud) begins to form at the ventral wall of the foregut. The diverticulum becomes

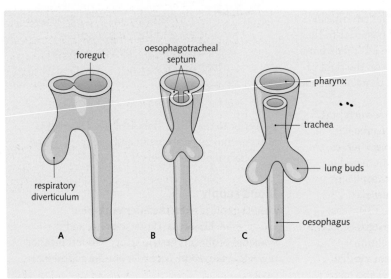

Fig. 2.13 The development of the pharynx and oesophagus. (A) Development by end of week 3 of gestation. (B and C) Development in the course of week 4. Abnormalities at this stage of development can lead to atresia and fistulae, which can result in death for the infant.

separated from the dorsal part of the foregut by the oesophagotracheal septum (Fig. 2.13).

The dorsal portion of the foregut becomes the oesophagus, which, although short initially, lengthens with the descent of the heart and lungs.

The ventral portion becomes the respiratory primordium, and the surrounding mesenchyme forms the oesophageal muscle layers. Congenital abnormalities are described later in the chapter.

Tissues

The layers of the oesophagus are essentially the same as in other parts of the gastrointestinal tract (Fig. 2.14).

The serosa covers the oesophagus inside the abdominal cavity, and the adventitia is a connective-tissue covering that blends with the surrounding connective tissue in the neck and thorax.

The muscularis externa consists of an outer longitudinal and an inner circular layer (the opposite arrangement from that in the urethra).

The upper third of the oesophagus is striated muscle (a continuation of the muscular layer of the pharynx—the lowest part of cricopharyngeus forms the upper oesophageal sphincter). The middle third is made up of striated and smooth muscle, and the lower third is smooth muscle. The lower oesophageal sphincter is described below.

The muscular layers of the upper 1/3 of the oesophagus are made up of striated muscle. The middle 1/3 has both striated (inner circular) and smooth (outer longitudinal) muscle and the lower 1/3 has only smooth muscle.

The submucosa contains numerous branched tubular glands, more abundant in the upper region, which produce mucus to lubricate the oesophagus.

The mucosa is lined by non-keratinized, stratified squamous epithelium, and it has a lamina propria similar to that in other parts of the body, but the muscularis mucosa is thicker than in the rest of the digestive tract.

Numerous mucous glands are usually present in the uppermost part and mucus-producing 'cardiac

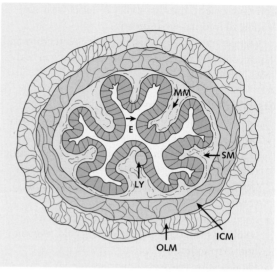

Fig. 2.14 Cross-sectional view of oesophageal tissue. (LY, lymphoid nodule; E, epithelium; MM, muscularis mucosae; SM, submucosa; ICM, inner circular muscle layer; OLM, outer longitudinal muscle layer.)

glands' (resembling the glands in the cardiac region of the stomach) are found in the lowermost part.

The lumen appears branched in cross-section, because the oesophagus is usually collapsed anteroposteriorly.

Oesophageal sphincters

The oesophagus has two sphincters:
- The upper oesophageal sphincter, which is a striated muscular sphincter and part of the cricopharyngeus. It is normally constricted to prevent air entering the oesophagus.
- The lower oesophageal sphincter, which is a physiological sphincter and made up of the lower 2–3 cm of oesophageal smooth muscle. This is the intra-abdominal segment of oesophagus. It acts as a flap valve and, with the muscosal rosette formed by folds of gastric mucosa, helps to occlude the lumen of the gastro-oesophageal junction. Normally there is tonic contraction of the circular muscles and the basal tone is regulated by vagal nerves.

Functions of the upper gastrointestinal tract

Food intake and its control

The control of food intake is complex and the hypothalamus plays an important role.

Young people burn off excess intake as heat and through physical activity. They maintain a relatively constant weight, but this ability reduces with age, leading to middle-aged spread.

Our genetics have a huge influence on feeding and can account for up to 70% of the difference in body mass index in later life.

Signals that affect appetite

There are a number of factors that regulate appetite.

- Blood glucose concentration activates glucoreceptors in the hypothalamus, either acting to upregulate hunger when blood glucose levels fall, or upregulate satiety when blood glucose concentrations rise.
- Amino acids in food raise body temperature, resulting in starving people feeling cold, even in hot surroundings.
- Fat ingestion releases cholecystokinin (CCK), which slows stomach emptying, making us feel full. Injection of CCK into the hypothalamus inhibits appetite, suggesting a central as well as peripheral role.
- Calcitonin, a peptide hormone secreted by the thyroid gland, acts to reduce appetite.
- Insulin acts to upregulate appetite, but glucagon downregulates it.
- Deposition of fat may lead to control of appetite by neuronal and hormonal signals. Leptin, a protein secreted by white fat cells, acts on the leptin receptors in the hypothalamus. This is thought to be part of the main satiety centre in the brain. Leptin produces a feedback mechanism between adipose tissue and the brain, acting as a 'lipostat', thus controlling fat stores. Leptin inhibits neuropeptide Y, the most potent peptide to stimulate feeding.
- Cold environments stimulate appetite, whereas hot environments inhibit it.
- Distension of a full stomach inhibits appetite, but contraction of an empty stomach stimulates it. However, denervation of the stomach and intestines seems to have no effect on food intake.

Central controls

As mentioned previously, the satiety centre is found in the ventromedial wall and the paraventricular nucleus of the hypothalamus. Stimulation of this inhibits food intake (aphagia), but lesions in this area may result in hyperphagia.

Glucostats in the brain measure the utilization of glucose. Diabetic patients feel hungry, despite high blood glucose concentrations, because they lack insulin and, therefore, the cellular ability to take up glucose.

A feeding centre (not specific for hunger) is found in the lateral hypothalamus. Stimulation of this area increases eating and lesions here result in aphagia.

Other important central nervous system controls include opioids, somatostatin, and growth hormone releasing hormone (GHRH), all of which increase appetite. 5-Hydroxytryptamine (5-HT, serotonin), dopamine and γ-aminobutyric acid (GABA) all decrease appetite.

Cortical and limbic centres

Habit and conditioning play a role in controlling appetite.

Diurnal variation

We principally metabolize carbohydrates during the day and fats at night. The hypothalamus is responsible for the switch between the two.

Mastication

Mastication breaks up large food particles, mixing them with salivary secretions, and aiding subsequent digestion. Molecules dissolve in salivary secretions and stimulate taste buds. Odours are released that activate the olfactory system, leading to the initiation of reflex salivation and gastric acid secretions.

The muscles of mastication cause movement of the mandible at the temporomandibular joint.

The digastric and mylohyoid muscles open the mouth, and the infrahyoid muscles stabilize the hyoid bone during mastication.

The teeth, gums, palate, and tongue also play an important role, manipulating food and immobilizing it between the crushing surfaces of the teeth. The tongue then propels the bolus of food along the palate towards the pharynx, initiating the swallowing reflex.

Salivation

The average rate of saliva secretion is 1–2 L per day. Saliva composition varies according to the rate and site of production, but the main components are water, proteins, and electrolytes. Primary secretion from the acini produces an isotonic fluid that is modified in the ducts (Fig. 2.15).

Control of secretion

Chemoreceptors in the mouth and oropharynx are activated by smell and taste: amyl nitrate and citric acid produce copious secretion. Saliva secretion is

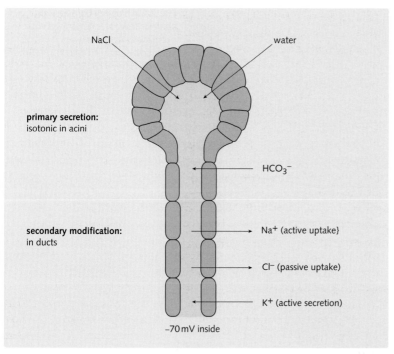

primary secretion:
isotonic in acini

secondary modification:
in ducts

NaCl

water

HCO_3^-

Na^+ (active uptake)

Cl^- (passive uptake)

K^+ (active secretion)

−70 mV inside

Fig. 2.15 Secretion of saliva. The primary secretion is released into the blind-ending acini and the fluid then flows through a series of converging ducts for secondary modification, before entering the oral cavity. The parotid glands produce the most serous secretions.

controlled from the medulla, and both parasympathetic and sympathetic pathways are involved. Parasympathetic innervation causes an upregulation in secretion and sympathetic innervation causes a downregulation. Parasympathetic cholinergic stimulation produces a watery secretion that is blocked by atropine. This is given before surgery to reduce the risk of aspiration of saliva.

Sympathetic adrenergic and noradrenergic stimulation produce thick mucoid secretions that add to the dry mouth sensation during the fright–fight–flight response.

Denervation causes dribbling. This is known as Canon's law of denervation hypersensitivity. Normally receptors are localized at neuroeffector junctions, but, if nerves are cut, receptors spread all over the gland and it becomes excessively sensitive to circulating acetylcholine, producing copious amounts of saliva.

Chewing produces saliva secretion by stimulating receptors in the masticatory muscles and joints. Paradontal mechanoreceptors around the teeth can also stimulate saliva.

There are four main sites at which the sympathetic and parasympathetic nerves can act to modify saliva secretion:
- The acini producing the primary secretion.
- The ducts, which modify the secretions.
- The blood vessels providing substances required for secretion and energy-containing nutrients, and removal of waste.
- The myoepithelial cells, surrounding the ducts and acini.

Salivary electrolytes

The major electrolytes found in saliva are Na^+, K^+, Cl^- and HCO_3^-. The concentrations vary according to the rate of flow (Fig. 2.16). Levels of Na^+ and Cl^- in saliva are hypotonic, but levels of HCO_3^- and K^+ are hypertonic at higher rates of flow. Saliva is hypotonic overall (about 200 mmol/L) and alkaline, although the exact pH varies with flow.

Salivary proteins

Salivary proteins include amylase, ribonuclease, R protein (which protects vitamin B_{12} as it passes through the duodenum, jejunum, and ileum), lipase (important in cystic fibrosis when pancreatic lipase is lost), lysozyme, secretory IgA (immunoglobulin A), IgG, and IgM.

Epidermal growth factor (EGF) is also secreted in saliva. This has a protective role at the gastroduodenal mucosa, by preventing the development of ulcers and promoting healing. Blood group antigens A, B, O (H), and Le[a] have also been identified in saliva.

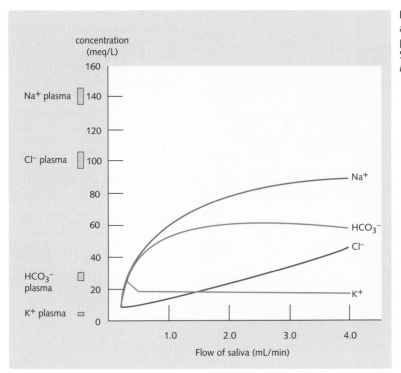

Fig. 2.16 Salivary composition against flow rate. (Redrawn with permission from Thaysen JH et al. Secretion control in salivation. *Am J Physiol* 1954; **178**: 155.)

Functions of saliva and the salivary glands

The functions of saliva and the salivary glands include:

- General cleansing and protection of the buccal cavity.
- Moistening of the buccal cavity for speech and breastfeeding (saliva forms a seal around the mother's nipple).
- Secretion of digestive enzymes, especially α-amylase, which attacks 1,4-linkages in starch.
- Dissolving many components and contributing to taste.
- Lubrication of the buccal cavity by mucus-secreting units of glands (under sympathetic and parasympathetic control).
- Secretion of the antibacterial enzyme, lysozyme, which protects teeth.
- Secretion of IgA by plasma cells in connective tissue, which act to protect the body from invasion of microorganisms. The secretory component of IgA is synthesized by striated duct cells.

Oral absorption

Most drugs are administered orally. Although this is the most convenient method for patients, it results in the most complicated pathway to the tissues and exposes drugs to first-pass metabolism in the liver.

Drugs given orally must dissolve in the gastrointestinal (GI) fluids and penetrate the epithelial cells lining the GI tract by passive diffusion or active transport. Some drugs are poorly absorbed orally or are unstable in the GI tract. Most drugs require an un-ionized state to move passively through the gut mucosa, which may be difficult to achieve because of the pH of the gastric acid.

Sublingual administration allows diffusion into the systemic circulation through the capillary network of the oral cavity, bypassing the liver and avoiding first-pass metabolism. Lower doses can, therefore, be given. Glyceryl trinitrate (GTN) used in angina treatment is commonly given this way.

Oral defences
Salivary defences

The alkaline pH of saliva neutralizes acid in food or in gastric contents following vomiting. Calcium and phosphate in saliva protect teeth by mineralizing newly erupted teeth and repairing pre-carious white spots in enamel.

Salivary proteins cover teeth with a protective coat called an 'acquired pedicle'. Antibodies and antibacterial agents retard bacterial growth and tooth decay. The MALT also plays an important role in protecting against microbial invasion at the mucosal membranes of the oral cavity.

Swallowing

We swallow about 600 times a day: 200 times while eating and drinking, 350 times while awake (but not eating or drinking), and 50 times while asleep.

Swallowing is the controlled transport of a food bolus from mouth to stomach, involving a sequential swallowing motor programme, which is generated in the medullary centres and consists of three phases: buccal, pharyngeal, and oesophageal (Fig. 2.17).

The buccal phase is voluntary and occurs when the mouth is closed. The bolus of food is pushed upwards and backwards against the hard palate, forcing it into the pharynx. This phase initiates the subsequent phases, which are involuntary.

The pharyngeal phase is initiated by the bolus stimulating mechanoreceptors in the pharynx and firing impulses in the trigeminal (V), glossopharyngeal (IX), and vagus (X) nerves. Efferent fibres pass to the tongue and the pharyngeal muscles through the trigeminal, facial, and hypoglossal nerves.

This results in:
- The nasopharynx being closed off by the soft palate.
- The epiglottis closing the larynx.

- The relaxation and opening of the upper oesophageal sphincter (UOS) for 0.5–1 s (once the bolus has passed through the upper oesophageal sphincter, it contracts tightly).

The oesophageal phase involves transport of the bolus along the oesophagus and takes between 6–10 s. Both primary and secondary peristaltic contractions are required.

The primary peristaltic wave is initiated by swallowing, and it sweeps down the entire length of the oesophagus. It involves sequential activation of the vagal efferents, which supply the striated muscle in the upper oesophagus directly. The smooth muscle is supplied by the enteric nerve plexus.

The bolus of food begins to move towards the stomach with the aid of gravity. The secondary peristaltic wave is triggered in response to local distension of the oesophagus, and it begins on the orad (mouth) side of the bolus and runs to the lower oesophageal sphincter (LOS). This occurs by an enteric reflex, and it helps clear food residues. Tertiary waves are common in the elderly, but they are not peristaltic or propulsive.

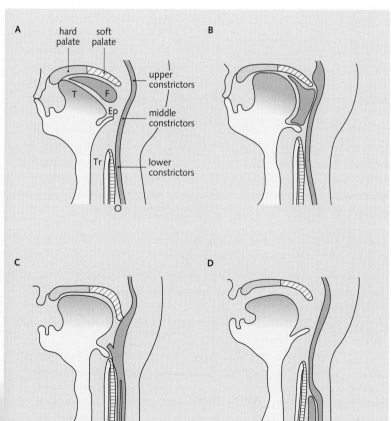

Fig. 2.17 The stages of swallowing. (A) The bolus of food (F) is pushed into the pharynx by the tongue (T). (B) The bolus is propelled further back and the soft palate shuts off the nasopharynx. (C) The epiglottis (Ep) closes the opening to the trachea (Tr) and the bolus moves through the upper oesophageal sphincter. (D) Peristalsis now propels the bolus towards the lower oesophageal sphincter and stomach. (O, oesophagus.)

The LOS relaxes when the peristaltic wave meets it. It opens for 5–10 s, allowing the bolus to pass into the stomach. Precision of tone is given by the vagal excitatory fibres (cholinergic) and the vagal inhibitory fibres (non-adrenergic non-cholinergic; NANC). These act reciprocally.

To tighten the LOS, an upregulation in vagal excitatory fibre stimulation is required (coupled with a downregulation in vagal inhibitory fibre stimulation). The opposite is true in relaxing, or opening the LOS.

Vomiting

Vomiting (emesis) is one of the most common symptoms of illness, especially in children (when it is associated with almost any physical or emotional illness), pregnancy, alcohol dependency, and some metabolic disorders (e.g. uraemia).

Vomiting centres (Fig. 2.18) in the lateral reticular formation of the medulla are stimulated by:

- Chemoreceptor zones in the area postrema, which are themselves stimulated by circulating chemicals, drugs, motion sickness (induced by prolonged stimulation of vestibular apparatus), and metabolic causes.
- Vagal and sympathetic afferent neurons from the gut, stimulated by mucosal irritation.
- The limbic system—less is known about these circuits, but sights, smells, and emotional circumstances can induce vomiting.

Lesions of the chemoreceptor zones abolish vomiting induced by some emetic drugs, uraemia, and radiation sickness, but not gastrointestinal irritation.

Vomiting involves a retrograde giant contraction from the intestines, which expels some intestinal contents (e.g. bile), as well as gastric contents.

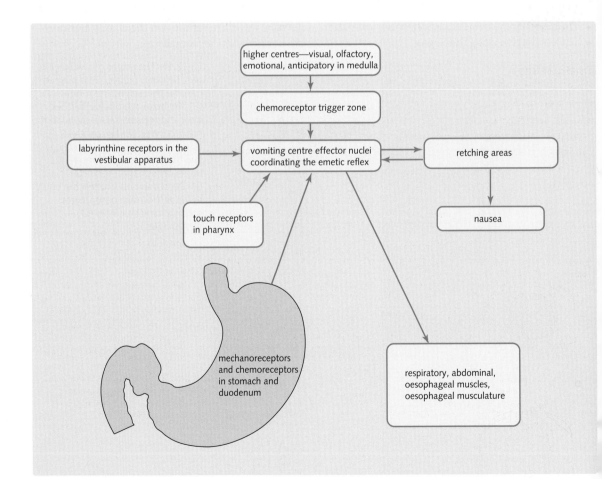

Fig. 2.18 Control of vomiting. This protective mechanism requires complex input from many centres in the brain.

Stages of vomiting

- A feeling of nausea is often accompanied by autonomic symptoms of sweating, pallor, and hypersalivation (which protects the mucosa of the mouth from the acid contents of the stomach).
- A deep breath is taken and the epiglottis closes, protecting the trachea and lungs.
- At the same time, the retrograde giant contraction moves the contents of the upper intestine into the stomach.
- The breath is held, fixing the chest. The muscles of the abdominal wall contract, increasing intra-abdominal pressure.
- The oesophageal sphincters relax allowing expulsion of gastric contents through the mouth by reverse peristalsis.

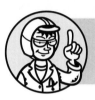

To quote a surgeon: 'It doesn't matter how many times you do it, vomiting only has one "t".'

Emetic drugs

Emesis is sometimes induced if the patient has swallowed poison and gastric lavage would be difficult (for example, small children are given paediatric ipecacuanha). More usually, vomiting is an unwanted side effect of drugs given for other reasons (e.g. cytotoxic drugs and opioids).

Antiemetic drugs

These should only be prescribed when the cause of vomiting is known, otherwise they may delay diagnosis. Metoclopramide and domperidone are prokinetic drugs, and they act to upregulate gut motility by acting as serotonin (5-HT) antagonists.

Disorders of the mouth and oropharynx

Congenital abnormalities

Cleft lip and cleft palate are common defects, which present with abnormal facial appearance and defective speech. Overall, cleft lip is more common than cleft palate (1/1000 births compared with 1/2500 births). Cleft lip is more common in male babies than female babies. A lateral cleft lip (hare lip) may result from incomplete fusion of the maxillary and medial nasal prominences, and a cleft palate from failure of fusion of the palatine shelves. Cleft lip and palate may occur together or one may be seen without the other (Fig. 2.19).

The palatine shelves in the female fetus fuse about 1 week later than they do in the male; cleft palate on its own is more common in female babies. Of every nine affected babies, two have a cleft lip, three a cleft palate, and four have both. About 20% of babies with cleft lip or palate also have other malformations.

Unlike babies with a cleft lip, those with a cleft palate cannot be breastfed (but they may be given expressed breast milk or formula milk by a bottle with a special teat).

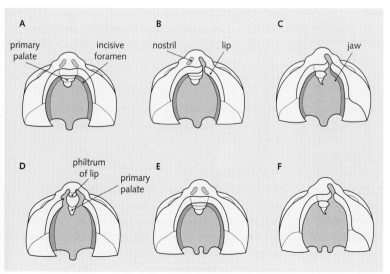

Fig. 2.19 Congenital abnormalities of the mouth and oropharynx. These result in variations of cleft palates and cleft lips. (A) Normal. (B) Unilateral cleft lip extending into the nose. (C) Unilateral cleft lip involving the lip and jaw and extending to the incisive foramen. (D) Bilateral cleft lip involving the lip and jaw. (E) Isolated cleft palate. (F) Cleft palate combined with unilateral anterior cleft. (Reproduced with permission from Sadler TW. *Langman's Medical Embryology*, 8th edn. Philadelphia: Lippincott, 2000.)

Median cleft lip is much more rare, and it is caused by incomplete fusion of the two medial nasal prominences in the midline. Infants with midline clefts often have brain abnormalities, including loss of midline structures. These defects occur early in neuralation (days 19–21). The infants are usually mentally retarded.

Failure of the maxillary prominence to merge with the lateral nasal swelling causes an oblique facial cleft, exposing the nasolacrimal duct.

Repair is surgical and it is normally carried out after 3 months in the case of cleft lip and about 1 year in cleft palate. Genetic and environmental factors have been identified. Trisomy 13 (Patau's syndrome) and a number of teratogens (most notably anticonvulsants such as phenytoin and phenobarbitone and also folic acid antagonists) are associated with both cleft lip and cleft palate.

Many parents are distressed by the birth of a child with a cleft lip but the results of surgery are usually excellent. It is often helpful to show such parents photographs of other children whose cleft lips have been repaired.

Infections and inflammation

The oral cavity and its mucosa are the target of many insults: infections, chemicals, and physical agents. The oral mucosa is, therefore, affected by a number of inflammatory disorders, either restricted to the mouth, or as part of a systemic disease.

Herpes simplex virus

Herpes simplex virus 1 (HSV-1) infection usually affects the body above the waist and herpes simplex virus 2 (HSV-2) below it. Changes in sexual practices, however, have led to an increase in herpes simplex virus 1 infections below the waist and 2 above it.

The primary infection may be asymptomatic or produce a severe inflammatory reaction. Presentation is usually with fever and painful ulcers in the mouth, which may be widespread and confluent.

The virus can remain latent in the trigeminal ganglia, but it may be reactivated by stress, trauma, fever, and UV radiation. This recurrent form of the disease presents as cold sores.

About 70% of the population are infected with HSV-1, and recurrent infections are found in 1/3 of those affected. Complications of HSV-1 include spread to the eye and acute encephalitis.

HSV infection in the immunocompromised, such as those undergoing cytotoxic chemotherapy for cancer, or those with human immunodeficiency virus (HIV) infection, is very dangerous. The infection can spread easily, leading to death in severe cases. Treatment for HSV involves topical or systemic administration of aciclovir, an antiviral drug.

HIV-1 and -2 are the viruses that lead to AIDS. AIDS can be said to have developed when an AIDS-defining illness has occurred, typically 10–15 years after infection with HIV-1 (slightly longer with HIV-2).

Oral candidiasis (thrush)

Candidiasis is caused by the yeast *Candida albicans*; it looks similar to leucoplakia (described below), but it can be scraped off with a spatula. Although it is the most common fungal infection in humans, all the species that are pathogenic to humans are normal oropharyngeal and gastrointestinal commensals! Usually candidiasis is found secondary to immunosuppression or a disturbance in the natural flora (e.g. after broad spectrum antibiotic therapy). Therefore, these commensals can act as opportunists.

Candidiasis causes lesions in neonates, the immunocompromised, and those whose natural flora has been disturbed by broad-spectrum antibiotics. It is common in acquired immune deficiency syndrome (AIDS) patients, in whom it may also cause lesions in the oesophagus.

Oral infections respond well to nystatin, oral amphotericin, or miconazole. Systemic infections require parenteral therapy with amphotericin or ketoconazole for up to 3 weeks.

Aphthous ulcers

Aphthous ulcers have a grey/white centre with a haemorrhagic rim, and they usually heal spontaneously within a few days. Ulcers can occur for a number of reasons. The most common are minor aphthous ulcers, which recur, but have an unknown aetiology.

Sometimes nutritional deficiencies are found, such as iron, folic acid, or vitamin B_{12} (with or without gastrointestinal disorders). Trauma to the oral mucosa, infections, and some drugs (antimalarial drugs and methyldopa) can also cause ulcers. Ulceration is also associated with inflammatory bowel diseases (Crohn's and ulcerative colitis) and coeliac disease.

Glossitis
Glossitis describes inflammation of the tongue, resulting from anaemia and certain other deficiency states, most notably vitamin B_{12} deficiency. It occurs after trauma to the mouth from badly fitting dentures, jagged teeth, burns, or the ingestion of corrosive substances.

The combination of glossitis, iron deficiency anaemia, and an oesophageal web causing dysphagia occurs in Plummer–Vinson syndrome (Paterson–Brown–Kelly syndrome), most commonly seen in women with iron deficiency.

Sialadenitis
Sialadenitis describes inflammation of the salivary glands. This uncommon condition may be caused by infection or obstruction of salivary ducts. Mumps (infectious parotitis) can also be the cause.

Saliva has antibacterial properties but individuals with reduced amounts of saliva (e.g. in Sjögren's syndrome) are at increased risk of sialadenitis.

Oral manifestations of systemic disease
Many infections, dermatological conditions, haematological diseases and other disorders can present with oral manifestations.

As previously mentioned, ulcers can be indicative of inflammatory bowel disease. Other systemic diseases presenting this way include systemic lupus erythematosus (SLE), Behçet's disease, cyclic neutropenia, and immunodeficiency disorders.

Neoplastic disease
Neoplasms are new and abnormal growths, which may arise from any tissue and be benign or malignant.

Premalignant and benign neoplasms
These include:
- Leucoplakia (hyperkeratosis and hyperplasia of squamous epithelium)—a premalignant condition that takes its name from the Greek for 'white patches' and is associated with excess alcohol,

poor dental hygiene, and in particular, smoking. It is regarded as a premalignant condition.
- Erythroplakia (dysplastic leucoplakia)—lesions which have a higher malignant potential than leucoplakia.
- Squamous papilloma (nipple-like growth) and condyloma acuminatum (raised wart-like growth)—these are both associated with human papilloma viruses 6 and 11 and they are largely benign.

Leucoplakia and erythroplakia are more common in men, particularly those aged between 40 and 70 years.

Malignant tumours
In the UK, malignant tumours of the mouth account for 1% of all malignant tumours. Squamous cell carcinoma is by far the most common malignant tumour (95%); however, adenocarcinoma, melanomas, and other malignant tumours may occur.

Alcohol and smoking (and, even more so, chewing tobacco) predispose to squamous cell carcinoma. The risk of a drinker who smokes developing squamous cell carcinoma is about 15 times that of the rest of the population.

Squamous cell carcinoma may arise in areas of leucoplakia and also on the lip, where it is associated with exposure to sunlight.

Treatment is by radiotherapy and/or surgery.

Neoplasms of the salivary glands
Neoplasms of the salivary gland account for 3% of all tumours, worldwide. The majority occur in the parotid gland and pleomorphic adenomas are the most common, accounting for 2/3 of all salivary tumours. An adenoma is a benign epithelial growth derived from glandular tissue. Only 15% of pleomorphic adenomas (mixed tumours) become malignant.

Warthin's tumour (an adenolymphoma) is a tumour of the parotid salivary gland. It contains both epithelial and lymphoid tissues, with cystic spaces. It accounts for 5–10% of all salivary gland neoplasms.

Disorders of the oesophagus

Congenital abnormalities
The oesophagus and trachea both develop from the embryonic foregut, at around 4 weeks of gestation.

Atresia and fistulae

Atresia is the congenital absence or narrowing of a body opening. A fistula is an abnormal connection between two epithelial lined surfaces (Fig. 2.20).

Atresia is a common condition, affecting 1/200 births and is caused by a failure of the oesophageal endoderm to grow quickly enough when the embryo elongates in week 5.

In 90% of cases, oesophageal atresia and fistula occur together, but either may occur without the other (10% of cases).

In the most common form of atresia, the upper part of the oesophagus has a blind ending but the lower end forms a fistulous opening into the trachea.

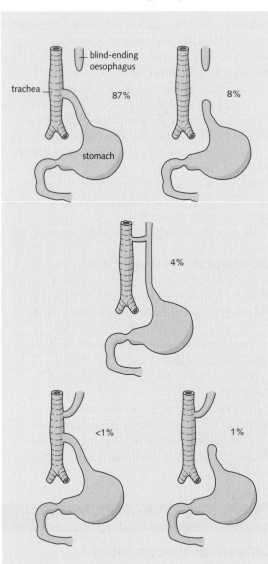

Fig. 2.20 Different forms of oesophageal atresia and fistulae and their occurrence as percentages.

This means that the infant cannot swallow milk or saliva and the diagnosis becomes apparent shortly after birth. The infant is at risk of aspiration pneumonia and of fluid and electrolyte imbalances.

Atresia should be suspected in a fetus where there is hydramnios (abnormally large amounts of amniotic fluid, i.e. over 2 L). Normally a fetus swallows amniotic fluid and some fluid is reabsorbed into the fetal circulation. Where there is atresia, the fetus cannot swallow, amniotic fluid is not reabsorbed, and excess fluid accumulates causing a distended uterus.

Hydramnios may also be caused by a failure of development of the fetal neurohypophysis (pituitary gland) that results in very little or no antidiuretic hormone (ADH) secretion and decreased reabsorption of water from the distal convoluted tubules in the fetal kidney. Treatment of atresia and fistulae is by surgery.

Agenesis

This is the complete absence of an oesophagus and it is much rarer than atresia or fistula.

Treatment is surgical.

Stenosis

Stenosis is the abnormal narrowing of a passage or opening.

Congenital stenosis may occur, but acquired stenosis is more common, and it is described below.

Inflammation of the oesophagus

Oesophagitis may be acute or chronic.

Acute oesophagitis is more common in immunocompromised individuals, for example, in HIV infection.

Oral and oesophageal candidiasis are common in AIDS patients, and they may cause dysphagia or retrosternal discomfort. They give rise to white plaques with haemorrhagic margins.

Herpes simplex and cytomegalovirus may also cause focal or diffuse ulceration of the gut. The herpes simplex ulceration is more common at the upper and lower ends of the gastrointestinal tract, cytomegalovirus lesions are more common in the bowel, but either may affect any part of the tract from the mouth to the anus.

Acute oesophagitis may also be caused by the deliberate or accidental swallowing of corrosive substances.

Chronic oesophagitis is most commonly caused by reflux of acidic gastric content through the lower oesophageal sphincter. This is called gastro-oesophageal reflux disease (GORD). In GORD, one or more of the following mechanisms implicate the pathogenesis:

- The resting LOS tone is low or absent.
- The LOS tone fails to increase when lying flat, or when the intra-abdominal pressure has increased (e.g. during pregnancy, or while wearing tight clothing).
- Poor oesophageal peristalsis leads to reduced clearance of acid in the oesophagus.
- A hiatus hernia can impair the function of the LOS and the diaphragm closure mechanism.
- Delayed gastric emptying increases the chance of reflux.

The squamous mucosa of the lower oesophagus is not designed to cope with acid.

Reflux causes injury to, and desquamation of, oesophageal cells. Normally the cells shed from the surface of the epithelium are replaced by basal cells, which mature and move up through the layers of squamous epithelium. Increased loss due to reflux is compensated for by a proliferation of basal cells (basal cell hyperplasia) (Fig. 2.21).

Basal cell hyperplasia in reflux oesophagitis causes an elongation of the connective tissue papillae.

A number of inflammatory cells are usually present, and these are a normal response to cell injury.

Ulcers form if basal cell formation cannot keep pace with cell loss, and these may haemorrhage, perforate, or heal by fibrosis (sometimes forming a stricture) and epithelial regeneration. The premalignant disorder, Barrett's oesophagus (a columnar cell lined oesophagus) may also result.

Factors associated with GORD are:

- Pregnancy or obesity.
- Fat, chocolate, coffee, or alcohol ingestion.

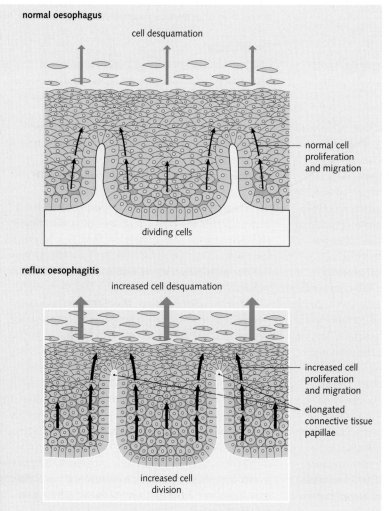

Fig. 2.21 Cell desquamation and proliferation in the normal oesophagus and in gastro-oesophageal reflux (GORD). Oesophagitis can be graded from I to IV; I being mild and IV being serious with danger of perforation. Often ulceration is seen with oesophagitis, and the premalignant disorder called Barrett's oesophagus may result.

- Large meals.
- Cigarette smoking.
- Anti-cholinergic drugs, Ca^{2+} channel antagonists and nitrate drugs.
- Hiatus hernia.
- Treatment for achalasia.

Treatment for GORD includes loss of weight, raising the head of the bed at night so that the patient does not lie flat, and taking antacids. A reduction in alcohol consumption and cessation of smoking is usually advised too.

The reduction of acid production can be achieved by using H_2 receptor antagonists and proton pump inhibitors.

Metoclopromide, a motility stimulant, may enhance peristalsis and help acid clearance in the oesophagus.

Lesions associated with motor dysfunction

Motor dysfunction may be caused by:
- A failure of innervation.
- A defect in the muscle wall of the oesophagus.
- A combination of the two above.

Achalasia

Achalasia is an uncommon condition that can present at any age, but it is rare in childhood. It involves the loss of coordinated peristalsis of the lower oesophagus and spasm of the lower oesophageal sphincter, thereby preventing the passage of food and liquids into the stomach. The aetiology is unknown.

It may be caused by damage to the innervation of the oesophagus, for example in Chagas' disease, where trypanosomes invade the wall of the oesophagus, damaging the intrinsic plexuses.

Degenerative lesions are found in the vagus with a loss of ganglionic cells of the myenteric nerve plexus in the oesophageal wall. Two thirds of patients with achalasia have autoantibodies to a dopamine-carrying protein on the surface of the cells in the myenteric plexus.

Diagnosis is by radiography. A barium swallow shows dilatation of the oesophagus, with a beak deformity at the lower end, caused by a failure of relaxation of the lower oesophageal sphincter. Manometry shows an absence of peristalsis and a high-resting lower oesophageal sphincter pressure.

The patient usually has a long history of sporadic dysphagia for both solids and liquids. Regurgitation of food is common, especially at night. Retrosternal chest pain is felt, due to the vigorous non-peristaltic contractions of the oesophagus.

Treatment consists of endoscopic balloon dilatation of the lower oesophageal sphincter or surgery (Heller's operation) to weaken the sphincter. Reflux is common after surgery unless a fundoplication is also performed.

Hiatus hernia

Hiatus hernia describes the herniation of part of the stomach through the diaphragm. Hernias can be sliding, where the gastro-oesophageal junction slides through the hiatus and lies above the diaphragm, or rolling (para-oesophageal), where a part of the fundus of the stomach rolls up through the hernia next to the oesophagus (Fig. 2.22).

Sliding hernias are more common, occurring in 30% of over 50 year olds. Symptoms are usually associated with reflux, but many are asymptomatic.

The rolling hernias usually require surgical correction to prevent strangulation.

Diverticula

Diverticula (out-pouchings) may form in the proximal or distal oesophagus, particularly where there is a disorder of motor function in the oesophagus.

A pharyngeal pouch (Killian's dehiscence or Zenker's diverticulum) may form in the area of weakness between the thyropharyngeus and cricopharyngeus (the two parts of the inferior pharyngeal constrictor) (Fig. 2.7). Killian's dehiscence is more common in elderly men. Food may collect in the pouch and later be regurgitated, and dysphagia is common. A swelling may be felt in the neck.

Diagnosis is by barium swallow and treatment is surgical.

A traction diverticulum may form in the lower oesophagus, particularly where fibrosis of the lower oesophagus has occurred.

Oesophageal varices

Oesophageal varices are dilated veins at the junction of the oesophagus and the stomach (the site of portal systemic anastomosis). They are found in patients with cirrhosis of the liver and portal hypertension.

The enlarged veins protrude into the lumen of the lower oesophagus (visible on endoscopy), and they may burst, resulting in haematemesis, which may rapidly be fatal.

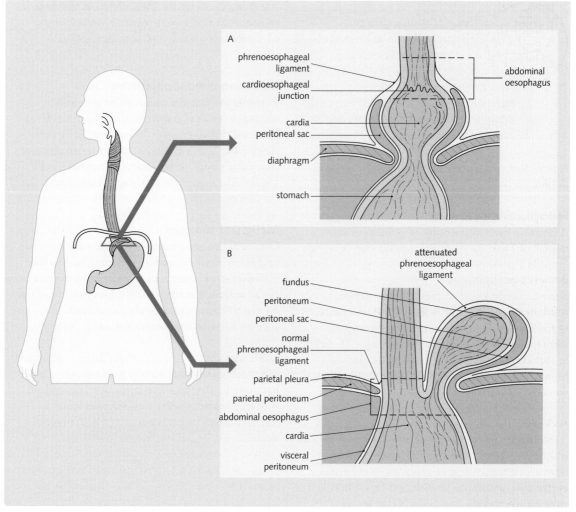

Fig. 2.22 The sliding (A) and rolling (B) hiatus hernias. The sliding hernia is more common, especially in people over 50 years old, and it can exacerbate reflux.

Prognosis following bleeding varices is poor, particularly when jaundice, ascites, encephalopathy, or hypoalbuminaemia may be present. Overall, mortality from a first bleed from oesophageal varices is 40%.

Cirrhosis carries a particularly bad prognosis as clotting factors made in the liver are reduced as a result of cirrhotic damage.

Cirrhosis is the cause of 90% of varices in the UK, but schistosomiasis (bilharzia) is the major worldwide cause.

The management of acute variceal bleeding requires resuscitation involving restoring blood volume and taking measures to stop the bleeding. Urgent endoscopy is required and vasoconstrictor drugs (e.g. vasopressin and octreotide, a somatostatin analogue) can be given.

Sclerotherapy and banding are widely used techniques to stem the loss of blood. Both are performed by endoscopy, and they can help prevent rebleeding. Sclerotherapy involves injecting the varices with a sclerosing agent to produce vessel thrombosis and arrest bleeding.

Banding involves placing a tight fitting band around the varix to stop it bleeding.

Mallory–Weiss syndrome

Mallory–Weiss syndrome is haematemesis from a tear at the gastro-oesophageal junction. It is caused by prolonged retching or coughing and a sudden increase

Never biopsy anything protruding into the lower oesophagus if there is any possibility it may be an oesophageal varix. Massive haemorrhage and haematemesis may occur, resulting in the patient's death.

in intra-abdominal pressure. It is most common in alcoholics.

Neoplastic disease

As in other parts of the body, neoplasms of the oesophagus may be classified as malignant or benign.

Barrett's oesophagus

Barrett's oesophagus is a premalignant condition resulting from prolonged reflux of the acid contents of the stomach into the oesophagus through an incompetent lower oesophageal sphincter. It occurs in approximately 20% of symptomatic cases of reflux, and it is most commonly seen in middle aged men.

Diagnosis requires biopsies to be taken during endoscopy for analysis of any histological changes.

Normally the epithelium of the lower oesophagus is squamous but in cases of prolonged injury the normal epithelium may be replaced by columnar epithelium (a metaplastic change). This is believed to occur when prolonged injury to the lower oesophagus causes ulceration. Pluripotent stem cells form a replacement epithelium. However, because acid contents are refluxing into the oesophagus, the pH in the area is lower than normal. This causes the stem cells to differentiate into the sort of epithelium seen in areas of low pH, such as gastric epithelium (found in the cardiac or fundic regions of the stomach) or intestinal epithelium.

Gastric and intestinal epithelium are more resistant to injury from the refluxing acid.

Adenocarcinoma is 30–40 times more likely to occur in a Barrett's oesophagus than in the normal oesophagus.

Benign tumours

These are much less common than malignant tumours, and they account for only about 5% of all neoplasms of the oesophagus.

Leiomyomas are the most common of benign tumours but fibromas, lipomas, haemangiomas, neurofibromas, and lymphangiomas may also arise.

Benign squamous papilloma

This is an epithelial tumour, and it may also occur as a result of human papilloma virus (HPV) infection. There are over 70 different HPVs and their role in the causation of cancer is becoming increasingly well understood. For example, HPV 16, 18, and 31 cause particularly aggressive carcinoma of the cervix.

Malignant tumours

Cancer of the oesophagus is the 8th most common cancer in the world, and it is mainly found in the 60–70-year-old age group. Cancers in the upper third of the oesophagus are very rare, but tumours of the middle third are squamous cell carcinoma and these account for 40% of oesophageal malignancy (Fig. 2.23).

Tumours in the lower third are adenocarcinomas, and these account for 45% of malignancies. These have usually developed from Barrett's oesophagus.

Kaposi's sarcoma is a complication found in AIDS patients, and it is associated with herpes virus 8.

Causes of squamous carcinoma of the oesophagus
Oesophageal disorders Chronic oesophagitis Achalasia Plummer–Vinson syndrome
Predisposing factors Coeliac disease Ectodermal dysplasia, epidermolysis bullosa Tylosis Genetic predisposition
Dietary Vitamin deficiency (A, C, riboflavin, thiamine, pyridoxine) Mineral deficiency (zinc, molybdenum) Fungal contamination of foodstuffs Nitrites/nitrosamines in foodstuffs
Lifestyle Alcohol Smoking

Fig. 2.23 Causes of squamous carcinoma of the oesophagus.

Clinical manifestations of oesophageal malignancies begin with persistent dysphagia and weight loss. Anorexia and lymphadenopathy are also common. Unfortunately, by the time symptoms are present, the carcinoma has usually spread and the 5-year survival is only about 5%.

Anorexia nervosa is a potentially fatal psychiatric disorder, primarily of adolescent girls, in which patients persistently perceive themselves as overweight and, although obsessed with food, voluntarily starve.

Bulimia nervosa is a psychiatric disorder characterized by binge eating and compensatory vomiting, purging, or both.

Disorders of food intake

In Fröhlich's syndrome, a hypothalamic tumour causes obesity through excessive intake.

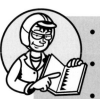

- Draw a labelled diagram of the open oral cavity to describe the regional anatomy.
- Describe the muscles and basic anatomy of the tongue. State the motor and sensory nerve supplies to each region of the tongue.
- Where are the taste buds located in the mouth? Draw a diagram depicting where each taste is 'sensed' by the receptors.
- Briefly discuss the development of the mouth and oropharynx from the pharyngeal arches.
- Draw a labelled diagram showing the functional components of a salivary gland. Where are the major salivary glands situated in the mouth and what kind of saliva do they secrete?
- Briefly describe the anatomy of the oesophagus in terms of the structures surrounding it and the different regions of the body through which it travels.
- How does the oesophagus develop in the embryo?
- Compare and contrast the upper and lower oesophageal sphincters.
- What are the mechanisms regulating hunger and satiety?
- Briefly describe the mechanisms involved in mastication. What are the muscles of mastication and how are they innervated?
- What components make up saliva?
- Describe the process of swallowing.
- What happens when someone vomits? Describe the physiological processes.
- What are the differences between a cleft lip and a cleft palate? What factors are associated with these congenital abnormalities?
- Describe the common infections and inflammatory conditions affecting the mouth.
- What are the common neoplasms found in the mouth?
- List the common congenital abnormalities that may occur in the oesophagus. How do they present?
- What causes oesophagitis, and what is the mechanism causing the inflammation?
- What lesions are caused by motor dysfunction in the oesophagus?
- What are varices? What causes them, and how are they treated?
- How does Barrett's oesophagus develop, and what is the outcome if untreated?
- What neoplasms may occur in the oesophagus?

3. The Stomach

Organization of the stomach

The stomach is a mobile, muscular organ that mixes food with digestive juices to form chyme. It receives food and fluid from the oesophagus, and it releases its contents into the duodenum. Gastric contents are broken down both by the churning action of the stomach and by being squirted through the narrow pylorus.

It acts as a reservoir for food, and it is very distendible, capable of holding up to 2–3 L of food.

The stomach wall is impermeable to most substances, but alcohol, water, salts, and some drugs may be absorbed through it. Most other substances are absorbed from more distal parts of the gastrointestinal tract.

Regional anatomy

The stomach lies between the oesophagus (proximally) and the duodenum (distally). It varies widely in size and shape depending on the person, the food content, and the posture of the body. It is J-shaped normally and the pyloric part lies horizontally or ascends to meet the proximal part of the duodenum.

Anatomically, the stomach is divided into 3 parts (Fig. 3.1):

- Fundus—the superior part of the stomach, this lies above the imaginary horizontal plane passing through the cardiac orifice.
- Body—this lies between the fundus and the antrum, and it is the largest part of the stomach.
- Antrum—this lies in the imaginary transpyloric plane and to the right of the angular notch (incisura angularis). It joins the pyloric canal on its right.

The physiological lower oesophageal sphincter (LOS) protects the oesophagus from reflux of the acidic gastric contents. The pyloric sphincter controls the flow of gastric contents into the duodenum.

The cardiac (gastro-oesophageal) orifice of the stomach lies behind the 7th left costal cartilage about 2–4 cm to the left of the median plane. The pylorus lies 1 cm to the right of the midline, in or below the transpyloric planes, and it is joined to the cardiac orifice by the lesser curvature. The position of the greater curvature varies greatly.

Fig. 3.1 Structure of the stomach.

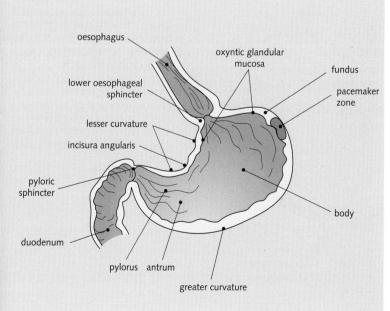

oesophagus

oxyntic glandular mucosa

fundus

pacemaker zone

lower oesophageal sphincter

lesser curvature

incisura angularis

pyloric sphincter

duodenum

pylorus   antrum

greater curvature

body

The anterior and posterior surfaces of the stomach are covered by peritoneum, and they meet at the greater and lesser curvatures. The peritoneum is reflected at the greater curvature to become the greater omentum, a double layer of fatty peritoneum suspended from the greater curvature. It is an apron-like structure hanging off the stomach, and it has a remarkable ability to stick to damaged or perforated parts of the gastrointestinal tract, sealing off leaks and giving some protection against peritonitis.

Excess fat may be stored on the greater omentum, especially in men (who have different distributions of fat from women). This is how the infamous beer belly came to be!

The lesser omentum is made up of peritoneum reflected at the lesser curvature to extend to the liver. The mucosa of the stomach is folded into large longitudinal rugae (wrinkles), which can be seen in a barium meal.

Relations

The anterior surface is in contact with:

- The diaphragm (in the fundal region).
- The anterior abdominal wall.
- The left lobe of the liver.

The spleen lies posterolateral to the fundus.

The diaphragm, left suprarenal gland, upper part of the left kidney, splenic artery, pancreas, transverse mesocolon, and, in some people, the transverse colon lie posteriorly forming the 'bed of the stomach'. They are separated from the stomach by the omental bursa (lesser sac of the peritoneum).

Blood supply

There is a rich blood supply to the stomach (Fig. 3.2), derived from three branches of the coeliac artery:

- The left gastric artery.
- The splenic artery.
- The common hepatic artery.

The left gastric artery supplies both anterior and posterior surfaces of the stomach, running along the lesser curvature. It anastomoses with the right gastric artery, and it also supplies the lower oesophagus.

The splenic artery follows a tortuous route across the posterior abdominal wall. It gives rise to the left gastroepiploic artery, which runs along the greater curvature and anastomoses with the right gastroepiploic artery.

The common hepatic artery gives rise to the right gastric artery and the gastroduodenal artery. The gastroduodenal artery passes behind D1 of the duodenum and gives rise to the right gastroepiploic

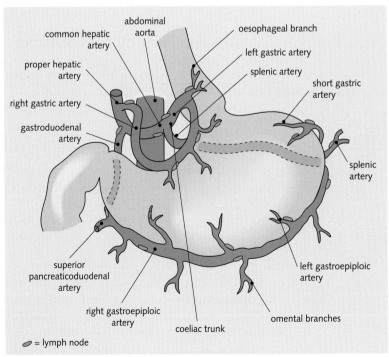

Fig. 3.2 The blood supply and lymphatic drainage of the stomach. The lymphatics follow the arteries. The lymphatics following the right gastric artery drain to the pyloric, hepatic and left gastric nodes. Those following the right gastroepiploic artery drain to the right gastroepiploic and pyloric nodes. Those following the left gastroepiploic and splenic arteries drain to the pancreaticosplenic nodes, and those following the left gastric artery drain to the left gastric nodes.

and the superior pancreaticoduodenal arteries (the latter supplies the pancreas and the duodenum!).

 Remember, there is a gastroduodenal artery that gives rise to the right gastroepiploic and superior pancreaticoduodenal arteries, but there is no gastroduodenal vein!

Venous drainage

The stomach drains, like most of the alimentary system, to the hepatic portal system. The gastric veins accompany the arteries.

Drainage of specific veins is as follows:

- The right and left gastric veins drain into the portal vein itself.
- The short gastric and left gastroepiploic veins drain into the splenic vein and its tributaries.
- The right gastroepiploic vein usually drains into the superior mesenteric vein.
- Oesophageal tributaries of the left gastric vein form an important portacaval anastomosis with tributaries of the azygos vein in the thorax.

Lymphatic drainage

The lymphatics follow the distribution of the arteries. There are four major groups of lymph nodes:

- The left gastric nodes.
- The pancreaticosplenic nodes.
- The right gastroepiploic nodes.
- The pyloric nodes.

Lymph drains from the anterior and posterior surfaces of the stomach towards its curvatures where many of the gastroepiploic nodes are situated.

These nodes all drain to the coeliac nodes and then to the cisterna chyli. From the cisterna chyli, lymph drains to the thoracic duct, which is the largest lymphatic vessel in the body and, unlike most of the lymphatic system, is visible to the naked eye. Knowledge of this is essential when gastric cancer occurs. The lymphatic drainage can spread metastases to the liver, pelvis, and the rest of the body, via the thoracic duct.

Throughout the alimentary system, the lymphatic system takes up finely emulsified fat absorbed from the diet.

Nerve supply

The stomach is supplied by both sympathetic and parasympathetic systems.

Sympathetic supply

The sympathetic supply is from the autonomic coeliac plexus through the periarterial plexus, which runs along the arteries of the stomach. Presynaptic sympathetic fibres come from the splanchnic nerves (from T6 to T9 of the spinal cord).

It causes vasoconstriction of the gastric blood vessels, relaxation of the gastric muscles, and decreased activity of gastric glands. These also carry pain fibres from the stomach.

Parasympathetic supply

The parasympathetic supply is from the vagus (X). Anterior and posterior vagal trunks from the oesophageal plexus pass through the diaphragm with the oesophagus and divide into anterior and posterior gastric branches on the anterior and posterior surfaces of the stomach. Posterior branches contribute to the coeliac plexus.

Gastric branches form Auerbach's and Meissner's plexuses, described below. Upregulation of parasympathetic innervation causes an increase in gastric motility and secretion.

Development

The stomach develops from a fusiform dilation of the foregut, which appears at about week 4 of gestation (Fig. 3.3). Its appearance and position change greatly during development as it rotates around both a longitudinal and an anteroposterior axis.

The posterior wall grows faster than the anterior wall, and it forms the greater and lesser curvatures.

Tissues

All parts of the stomach have the same basic structural layers (Fig. 3.4):

- Mucosa.
- Submucosa.
- Muscularis externa.
- Serosa.

Mucosa

The mucosa and submucosa are folded into longitudinal rugae, when the stomach is empty. The mucosal surface is lined with simple columnar epithelium (which has a lifespan of about 1 week) and forms numerous gastric pits that are openings for the gastric glands. The mucous cells lining the gastric

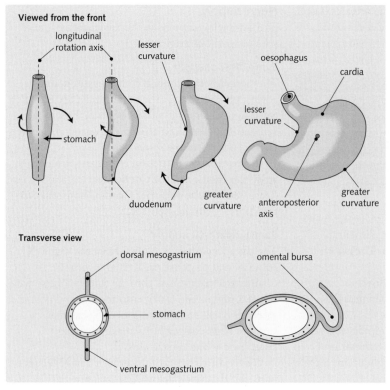

Viewed from the front

longitudinal rotation axis

lesser curvature

oesophagus

cardia

stomach

lesser curvature

duodenum

greater curvature

anteroposterior axis

greater curvature

Transverse view

dorsal mesogastrium

omental bursa

stomach

ventral mesogastrium

Fig. 3.3 Formation of the stomach. The stomach rotates 90° around its longitudinal axis, causing the left vagus to innervate the left, now anterior surface and the right vagus to innervate the right, now posterior surface. The longitudinal rotation also causes the formation of the space behind and to the left of the stomach, called the omental bursa (lesser sac), which is continuous with the coelomic cavity behind the stomach. (Redrawn with permission from Sadler TW. *Langman's Medical Embryology*, 6th edn. London: Williams & Wilkins, 1990.)

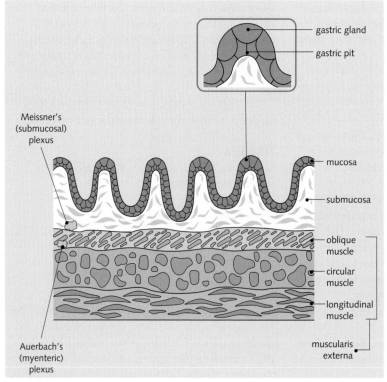

gastric gland

gastric pit

Meissner's (submucosal) plexus

mucosa

submucosa

oblique muscle

circular muscle

longitudinal muscle

Auerbach's (myenteric) plexus

muscularis externa

Fig. 3.4 Cross-section of the stomach wall.

lumen secrete mucus as well as bicarbonate ions (HCO_3^-).

The depth of the gastric mucosa is divided into three histological zones (Fig. 3.5):

- A superficial zone.
- A neck zone.
- A deep zone.

The superficial zone is composed of surface mucous cells with openings to the gastric pits. The neck zone, between the superficial and deep zones, is composed of mostly immature stem cells, but it has some neck mucous cells. The immature stem cells eventually proliferate and move upwards to replace mucous cells in the superficial zone.

 Stem cells are very important in the cell regeneration and healing of a gastric ulcer.

In the deep zone, glands are found. These vary in structure, according to where they are situated. Each of the three main areas of the stomach—the cardiac, gastric (or body) and the pyloric regions—have their own arrangement of gland (Fig. 3.5).

The lamina propria contains numerous cells of the immune system, migrant cells from the blood, and resident connective tissue cells. The muscularis mucosa consists of two thin layers of muscle.

Submucosa

This is made up of collagen, fibroblasts, and acellular matrix with blood vessels, nerves and lymphatics. It also contains autonomic ganglion cells and lymphoid aggregates, which make up the gut-associated lymphoid tissue (GALT). This structure is consistent throughout the digestive tract.

Muscularis externa

This consists of three layers of smooth muscle:

- An outer longitudinal muscle layer (absent from much of the anterior and posterior surfaces of the stomach).
- A middle circular muscle layer (poorly developed in the paraoesophageal region).
- An inner oblique muscle layer.

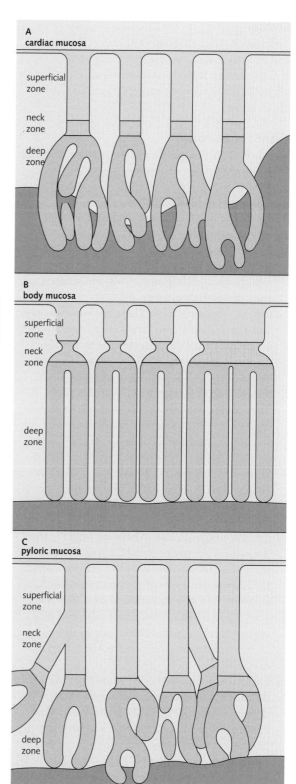

Fig. 3.5 The different types of gland found in the stomach. (A) Cardiac mucosa. (B) Body mucosa. (C) Pyloric mucosa. (Redrawn with permission from Stevens and Lowe, 1997.)

Serosa

This consists of an inner layer of connective tissue and an outer layer of simple squamous epithelium. It is also known as the visceral peritoneum, and it allows for frictionless movement of organs within their cavities.

Glands of mucosa

The three main groups of glands are named after the region in which they are found.

Gastric (body or fundic) glands

These are the most numerous, and they contain several types of cells:

- Mucous neck cells—These are found just below gastric pits, and they contain mucinogen granules, well-developed Golgi apparatus, and rough endoplasmic reticulum (RER).
- Parietal (oxyntic) cells—These are found deeper than mucous neck cells. They are pyramidal cells, which look triangular in section, with the apex pointing towards the gland lumen, and they have a spherical nucleus. They secrete HCl and intrinsic factor (for vitamin B_{12} absorption). They contain numerous mitochondria to provide energy for HCl production. Parietal cells are absent in achlorhydria ('absence of acid'); thus, no intrinsic factor is produced in this condition. Histamine, gastrin, and acetylcholine all stimulate HCl production (Fig. 3.6). Their internal appearance changes when food has been eaten (Fig. 3.7).
- Chief (zymogen) cells—These are found in the deepest part of gastric glands, and they are typical protein-secreting cells. They secrete pepsinogen, the inactive precursor of pepsin (a proteolytic enzyme), which is converted to pepsin by acid. They are rich in mitochondria, Golgi, and RER, required for the production of pepsinogen. The enzyme precursor is delivered to the lumen by exocytosis.
- Enteroendocrine cells—These are also called APUD cells (amine precursor uptake and decarboxylation cells). They are found on the epithelial basement membrane, and they secrete peptide hormonal substances, such as vasoactive intestinal polypeptide (VIP) and somatostatin. In the gastric region, the most common type of endocrine cell is the enterochromaffin-like (ECL) cell. These are 20 times smaller than parietal cells, and they secrete histamine into the lamina propria of the mucosa.

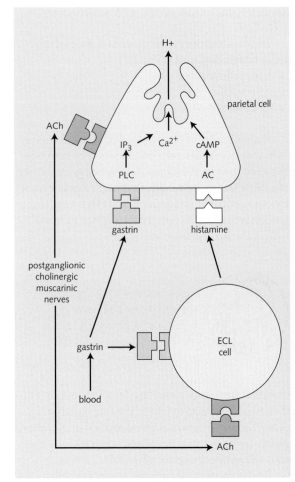

Fig. 3.6 Stimulation of secretion of HCl by parietal cells. (ACh, acetylcholine; AC, adenylate cyclase; ECL, enterochromaffin-like; IP$_3$, inositol triphosphate; PLC, phospholipase C.) (Redrawn with permission from Johnson, 2000.)

- Undifferentiated stem cells—Stem cells are precursors of all the mucosal epithelial cells. When undifferentiated, they show no cytoplasmic specialization, and they are capable of becoming any of the cell types present in the gastric mucosal glands. They are usually located in the neck zone.

Cardiac glands

As the name suggests, the cardiac glands are found in the cardiac region. They are mostly mucus secreting, coiled tubular glands (but may be branched). Some undifferentiated stem cells are present in the neck region and enteroendocrine (APUD) cells are scattered throughout. Some parietal cells may also be seen.

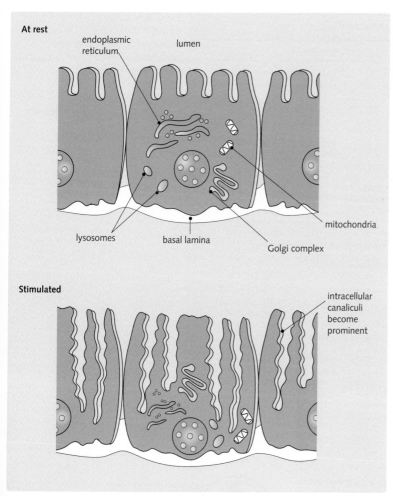

Fig. 3.7 Morphological changes in parietal cells. At rest, the parietal cells have numerous tubulovesicles derived from smooth endoplasmic reticulum (SER). These contain H$^+$ pumps, and they do not connect with the apical surface membrane. After stimulation of acid secretion, the tubulovesicles merge and become deep trough-like invaginations of the apical surface, called secretory canaliculi. These communicate with the lumen of the gland. The surface area is also increased by numerous microvilli.

Pyloric glands

The pyloric glands are coiled (but less so than cardiac ones) and often branched. They contain mainly mucous cells, but they have parietal, enteroendocrine and stem cells scattered throughout. In particular, the enteroendocrine cells secrete gastrin in this area. These cells are called G cells, because they secrete gastrin. D cells, another type of enteroendocrine cell, secrete somatostatin in paracrine fashion. The cell types found in each region of the stomach are summarized in Fig. 3.8.

Nerve fibres

There are two major networks of nerve fibres:
- Auerbach's (myenteric) plexus, between the inner oblique and the middle circular muscle layer.
- Meissner's (submucous) plexus, between the inner oblique muscle layer and the mucosa.

Both plexuses are interconnected, and they contain nerve cells with processes that originate in the wall of the gut or mucosa.

The mucosa has mechanoreceptors and chemoreceptors, which are sensitive to stretch of the gut wall and composition of the stomach contents, respectively.

Nerve cells innervate hormone-secreting cells (see gastric functions) and all the muscle layers in the mucosa.

The plexuses are sometimes described as a third division of the autonomic system—the enteric nervous system.

Gastric function

Storage of food

The stomach acts as a reservoir for food, releasing the gastric contents into the duodenum at a steady rate. Relaxation of the LOS and arrival of food in the stomach is followed by a receptive relaxation of the fundus and body of the stomach.

Cell types of the stomach			
Cell type	**Area of stomach**		**Function**
Mucous cells	Cardiac	Many	Secrete mucus to protect the epithelium from acid secretions
	Gastric	Fewer	
	Pyloric	Many	
Parietal cells (oxyntic cells)	Cardiac	Few	Secretion of HCl and intrinsic factor (for vitamin B_{12} absorption)
	Gastric	Many	
	Pyloric	More near the pyloric sphincter	
Chief cells (zymogen)	Cardiac	Many	Secretion of pepsinogen, the precursor of pepsin, a proteolytic enzyme
	Gastric	Few	
	Pyloric		
Enteroendocrine (APUD)	Cardiac	Few	Secretion of protein hormones such as VIP and somatostatin. (Gastrin is secreted in the pyloric region)
	Gastric	Many	
	Pyloric	Few	
Stem cells	Cardiac	Present	These give rise to new cells to replace the old mucosal and glandular epithelial cells
	Gastric	Present	
	Pyloric	Present	

Fig. 3.8 Summary of the cell types found in the stomach. (APUD cells, amine precursor uptake and decarboxylation cells; VIP, vasoactive intestinal polypeptide.)

This is mediated by a vagal reflex, which inhibits the smooth muscle tone in this area (via the vagal inhibitory fibres with release of VIP and nitric oxide). The vagal inhibitory fibres cause relaxation by inducing hyperpolarization.

The muscle wall is thinner in the fundus and body, resulting in generally weaker muscle contractions than in the antral area. These factors allow the fundus and body of the stomach to store food and accommodate up to 1.5 L without a marked increase in intragastric pressure.

The muscles in the antral region contract vigorously, mixing the food with gastric secretions to continue digestion. Salivary digestion is still occurring, particularly at the centre of the mass. The smooth muscle in the antral area has a higher resistance to stretch than that of the fundus and body.

Food may remain in the stomach, unmixed, for up to 1 hour. Fats form an oily layer on top of other gastric contents. A fatty meal delays gastric emptying but liquids generally empty more quickly.

 Rennin is an enzyme produced in neonatal stomachs, which converts caseinogen (milk protein) to insoluble casein. This ensures the milk stays in the stomach for as long as possible, to be digested by other enzymes.

Gastric secretions and their control
Secretions of the stomach
The average adult produces 2–3 L of gastric juice every 24 hours. Gastric juice contains mucus, digestive enzymes (pepsinogen and lipase), HCl, and intrinsic factor.

Resting juice
Resting juice is an isotonic juice secreted by the surface cells. It is similar to plasma, but it has an alkaline pH of 7.7 and a higher concentration of HCO_3^-.

Mucus

Mucus is secreted by goblet cells of the surface epithelium and mucus neck cells, especially in the pyloric antrum.

The alkaline mucus of the stomach is a thick, sticky mucopolysaccharide. It is secreted with HCO_3^- ions, which are exchanged for Cl^- ions by the epithelial cells. It plays an important role in the protection of the stomach against its acid contents.

Mucus forms a water-insoluble gel that adheres to the surface of the stomach lumen. It reduces the flow of H^+ ions and acts as a barrier to pepsin. Although pepsin can degrade mucus, the HCO_3^- secretions increase the pH and make the enzyme less active.

Pepsin

Pepsin is secreted from the chief cells in the gastric pits in the form of its precursor, pepsinogen. HCl activates pepsinogen (42 kDa) by cleaving off nine amino acid residues to form pepsin (37.5 kDa).

Pepsin is a proteolytic enzyme that acts on proteins and polypeptides, by hydrolysing internal peptide bonds.

Lipase

Gastric lipase is an enzyme that acts on triglycerides to produce fatty acids and glycerol. It is useful in facilitating subsequent hydrolysis by pancreatic lipases, but it is of little physiological importance except in pancreatic insufficiency.

Hydrochloric acid

HCl is produced by the parietal (oxyntic) cells.
The concentration of HCl depends on:
- The rate of HCl secretion.
- The amount of buffering provided by the resting juice, ingested food and drink, and the alkaline secretion of the pyloric glands, duodenum, pancreas, and bile.
- Gastric motility.
- The rate of gastric emptying.
- The amount of diffusion back into the mucosa.

The pH of the contents of the stomach after feeding is normally about 2–3.

Gastric HCl is not essential for life, but it has a number of important functions. It provides a defence mechanism that is non-specific in killing ingested microorganisms. It also aids protein digestion (by enabling the activation of pepsin from pepsinogen), and it stimulates the flow of bile and pancreatic juice.

The secretion of HCl by parietal cells is stimulated by histamine, acetylcholine, and gastrin (Fig. 3.6). It is also stimulated by caffeine (through the activation of cyclic AMP).

Secretion is inhibited by vagotomy (which removes acetylcholine stimulation), by blocking the histamine receptor on the parietal cells by drugs (e.g. ranitidine), or, more effectively, by blocking the proton pump with a drug (e.g. omeprazole).

Intrinsic factor

Intrinsic factor is made in the parietal cells of the stomach; it is a glycoprotein vital for the absorption of vitamin B_{12} in the terminal ileum. Without intrinsic factor, vitamin B_{12} is digested in the intestine and not absorbed.

R protein in the saliva protects vitamin B_{12} until it reaches the stomach.

Most diets contain excess vitamin B_{12} and stores are built up in the liver. These stores last for 2–3 years; thus, it takes considerable time for a dietary deficiency to produce symptoms. However, once body stores have been used up, pernicious anaemia develops.

Control of gastric secretion

The control of gastric secretion is brought about by a combination of nervous, hormonal, and paracrine messages. There are three phases of stimulation (Fig. 3.9):
- The cephalic phase.
- The gastric phase.
- The intestinal phase.

The cephalic phase

The cephalic phase is the smallest phase, and it is initiated by the sight, smell, and taste of food. It usually begins before the meal and lasts up to 30 minutes into the meal. This allows the stomach to prepare itself for the imminent arrival of food.

It is mediated entirely by the vagus nerve (vagotomy of the stomach leads to cessation of the cephalic phase).

Acid secretion is upregulated by acetylcholine (ACh) released from neurons of the intramural plexus acting:
- Directly, by stimulation of the parietal cells.
- Indirectly, by causing release of gastrin from antral G cells, which stimulates the parietal cells too. The mediator at the G cell is gastrin-releasing peptide (GRP).

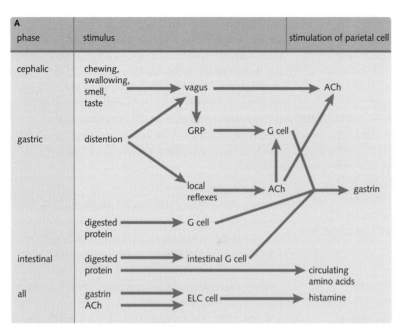

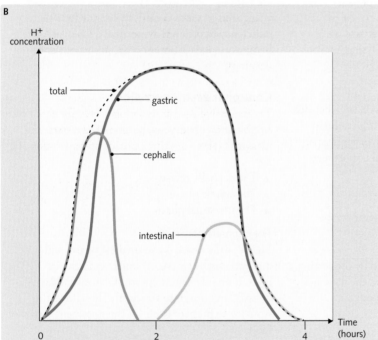

Fig. 3.9 The three phases of gastric secretion. (A) The control mechanisms for each phase of gastric secretion. ACh, acetylcholine; GRP, gastrin releasing peptide; ELC, enterochromaffin-like cells. (Redrawn with permission from Johnson, 2000.) (B) A graphical presentation of the three stages.

• Indirectly, by causing the release of histamine from ECL cells, which also upregulates acid production.

The gastric phase

This is the largest phase, lasting for up to 2½ hours after the start of the meal. It is triggered by the presence of food in the stomach in response to distension of the stomach, and the presence of amino acids and peptides (products of pepsin degradation). Most acid secretion in response to a meal takes place during the gastric phase.

Distension of the body or antrum of the stomach stimulates mechanoreceptors that cause local (enteric) and central vago-vagal cholinergic reflexes.

Amino acids and peptides activate vagal chemoreceptors and also antral G cells, which are sensitive to peptides. These secrete gastrin in response.

The gastrin and acetylcholine activate ECL cells to produce histamine, which further increases acid secretion from the parietal cells.

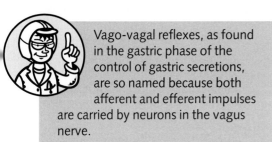
Vago-vagal reflexes, as found in the gastric phase of the control of gastric secretions, are so named because both afferent and efferent impulses are carried by neurons in the vagus nerve.

The intestinal phase

The intestinal phase is brought about by the presence of chyme in the duodenum. The amino acids and peptides in the chyme stimulate gastrin release and the levels of gastrin in the duodenum contribute to serum gastrin level during a meal.

However, the intestinal phase can have an inhibitory effect on gastric acid secretion. The presence of acid in the duodenum (with a pH less than 2) has the following results:

- Somatostatin is released from D cells. This acts directly on the parietal cells to inhibit acid secretion.

- Acid mediates the release of secretin into the bloodstream. This inhibits the release of gastrin by G cells and reduces the response of parietal cells to gastrin.
- Fatty acids (from triglyceride digestion) in the duodenum and proximal jejunum cause the release of gastric inhibitory polypeptide (GIP) and cholecystokinin (CCK), which both act to inhibit secretion of acid by parietal cells. GIP also suppresses gastrin release.

Secretin, GIP, and CCK are collectively called enterogastrones, because they have an inhibitory effect on gastric secretion. Hypertonic solutions in the duodenum also suppress gastric secretion. This is mediated by an unidentified enterogastrone. The inhibition of gastric secretions is also controlled by an enteric reflex, which is integrated with higher controls from the medulla oblongata.

The loss of volume in the stomach and the distension of the duodenum (as chyme passes from one to the other), both activate the local enteric reflex, via mechanoreceptors. Chemoreceptors in the duodenum can also activate the reflex ion response to irritants, reduced pH, and hypertonic solutions. The mechanisms for inhibiting acid secretion are summarized in Fig. 3.10.

Mechanisms for inhibiting gastric acid secretion		
Stimulus	Mediator	Action
Acid (pH <2)	Somatostatin	Directly inhibits parietal cells
	Secretin	Inhibits gastrin release. Decreases response of parietal cells to gastrin
	Enteric reflex	Directly inhibits parietal cells
Fatty acids	Gastric inhibitory peptide (GIP)	Directly inhibits parietal cells Inhibits gastrin secretion from G cells
	Cholecystokinin (CCK)	Adds to the inhibition of parietal cells
Hypertonic solutions	Unidentified enterogesterone	Inhibits acid secretion
	Enteric reflex	Inhibits acid secretion
Distention of duodenum	Mechanoreceptor initiated enteric reflex	Decreases acid secretion
Emptying of stomach	Enteric reflex	Decreases acid secretion

Fig. 3.10 Summary of the mechanisms for inhibiting gastric acid secretion.

Gastric motility and emptying

Gastric motility and emptying are carefully regulated to ensure that chyme is delivered to the duodenum at a rate at which it can be absorbed.

Gastric motility

Motility in the stomach is initially brought about by the reflex receptive relaxation, which allows food to enter from the oesophagus. This process is mediated by vagal inhibitory fibres.

Mixing of the food with gastric secretions follows and takes place in the distal body and antrum of the stomach (the caudal region). The muscularis externa is thicker in this area of the stomach. The contractions involved in mixing and emptying the stomach contents are brought about by the three smooth muscle layers, which are coordinated by intrinsic and extrinsic nerves.

The most prominent plexus is Auerbach's plexus, situated in a three-dimensional matrix between the layers of smooth muscle in the stomach wall. It receives innervation from both sympathetic and parasympathetic systems. Axons from the plexus innervate both muscle fibres and glandular cells.

Interneurons connect intrinsic afferent sensory fibres with efferent neurons of smooth muscle and secretory cells, to ensure that gastric activity is fully coordinated, even in the absence of external innervation. Cholinergic stimulation from the vagus increases gastric motility and secretion, but adrenergic stimulation in the coeliac plexus has the opposite effect.

When the stomach is full of food, it undergoes a 'lag' phase. During this time, the stomach is not contracting, but intense secretions are digesting the food down to basic components to form chyme. Once the lag phase is over, there is a reversal of vagal discharge. There is an upregulation in vagal excitatory fibre activation and a decrease in vagal inhibitory fibre activation.

Large peristaltic contractions originate in the pacemaker zone of the distal body, on the greater curvature. They sweep down towards the antrum where the amplitude of contraction is greatest. The contractions occur at a rate of 3 per minute, lasting between 2 and 20 seconds (Fig. 3.11).

Between contractions, the pressure in the caudad region of the stomach nearly equals intra-abdominal pressure.

The contractions break off small boluses of food, carrying them towards the pylorus. Large pieces of food are refluxed back towards the gastric body for further degradation. This process is termed retropulsion, and it allows for the thorough mixing and mechanical breakdown of solid food material (Fig. 3.12).

The force and frequency of contractions depends on:

- The neural activity of intrinsic and extrinsic nerves.
- The myogenic properties of smooth muscle.
- The properties of paracrine and endocrine agents (gastrin and motilin upregulate the force of gastric contraction, but secretin inhibits it).

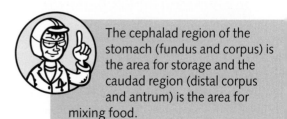

The cephalad region of the stomach (fundus and corpus) is the area for storage and the caudad region (distal corpus and antrum) is the area for mixing food.

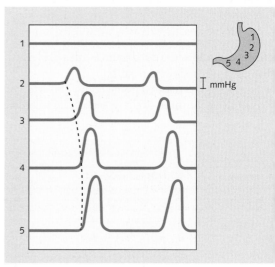

Fig. 3.11 Intraluminal pressures recorded from five areas in the stomach. (Redrawn with permission from Johnson, 2000.)

Gastric emptying

Emptying of gastric contents into the duodenum is a continuum of gastric mixing. As retropulsion occurs, the pyloric sphincter opens by a coordination of antral and duodenal contractions. Small digested particles are squirted through the sphincter into the duodenum. The rate at which the stomach empties depends on:

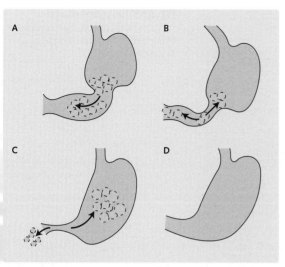

When the stomach is empty, it is small and relaxed. Peristaltic contractions are weak, but as hunger sets in, the muscle contractions increase in size and frequency. The tetanic contractions last for 2–3 min. Hunger pangs usually begin 12 hours after the previous meal. Low blood sugar increases the contractions.

Fig. 3.12 Effects of gastric peristaltic contractions on intraluminal contents. (Redrawn with permission from Johnson, 2000.)

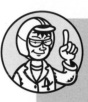

Liquids empty from the stomach at a faster rate than solids, unless they have a high lipid content. Solids and semi-solids undergo a lag phase of intense secretion before the stomach begins to empty.

- The type of food eaten. Carbohydrates are emptied most quickly, proteins more slowly, and fatty foods even more slowly to ensure that food is released into the duodenum at a rate at which it can be absorbed. Fatty acids or monoglycerides in the duodenum decrease the rate of gastric emptying by increasing the contractility of the pyloric sphincter. The presence of acidic contents with a pH of less than about 3.5 in the duodenum also slows gastric emptying, as may amino acids and peptides.
- The osmotic pressure of the contents of the duodenum. Duodenal osmoreceptors initiate a decrease in gastric emptying in response to hyperosmolar chyme.
- Vagal innervation. Antral and duodenal overdistension activates mechanoreceptors that stimulate a vago-vagal reflex. This acts to inhibit gastric contractile activity by vagal inhibitory fibres. Vagotomy results in a marked decrease in the rate of gastric emptying.
- The release of somatostatin, secretin, CCK, and GIP by the duodenum, in response to the presence of chyme. These all inhibit gastric emptying.

Protection of the gastric mucosa

The gastric mucosa is frequently subjected to the corrosive secretions of HCl and pepsin. Several mechanisms exist to prevent tissue damage by the gastric juices:

- Mucus, secreted by neck and surface mucous cells in the body and fundus and similar cells elsewhere in the stomach, forms a water-insoluble gel that coats the mucosa (Fig. 3.13). Prostaglandins stimulate mucus production.
- The surface cells secrete HCO_3^- which, together with the mucus, forms an adherent layer. This raises the pH around the mucus layer, thus making pepsin less active and preventing the enzymes degrading the mucus.
- The surface membranes of the mucosal cells, the tight junctions between them, and the ability to form a fibrin coat protect the cells.
- Prostaglandins may inhibit acid secretion.

Several factors cause a breakdown of the mucosal protection or an increase in acid production and predispose to gastric irritation and peptic ulceration:

- Acid secretion (from the parietal cells) is stimulated by histamine, acetylcholine, and gastrin (Fig. 3.6).
- Non-steroidal anti-inflammatory drugs (NSAIDs) and aspirin reduce mucus secretion and decrease bicarbonate secretion by inhibiting prostaglandin production.
- In Zollinger–Ellison syndrome, gastrin-secreting adenomas result in marked hyperacidity. The adenomas are usually found in the pancreas and

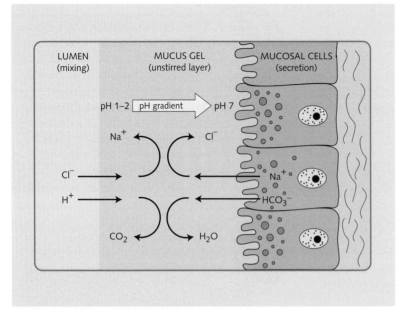

Fig. 3.13 Protection of gastric mucosa from low pH by mucus layer. (Redrawn with permission from Underwood, 1992.)

present as gastric or duodenal ulcers. The syndrome is rare.

- *Helicobacter pylori*, a Gram-negative bacterium that may infect individuals and live on the surface epithelium beneath the mucus layer in the stomach (but not further down the alimentary tract), has been isolated from about 80% of gastric ulcers and about 95% of duodenal ulcers. It attacks the surface cells causing a break in the mucosal barrier and an acute inflammatory reaction.
- Hyperparathyroidism predisposes to ulcer formation because increased levels of calcium stimulate acid production.
- Chronic exposure to nicotine from smoking causes an increase in acid secretion.
- Stress may also result in ulcer formation (this is rare).

Gastric and duodenal ulceration are common and a number of drugs have been developed to reduce acid secretion or increase mucosal protection. These are discussed later in the chapter.

Gastric defences against infection

The stomach has a number of defence strategies. Gastric acid and pepsin secretions act to kill aerobic microorganisms (they require oxygen) and other ingested bacteria, preventing infection of the gastric mucosa.

The intestines are colonized with millions of commensal anaerobic microorganisms. These prevent other organisms colonizing and causing damage or inflammation (however, rupture of the stomach or intestines may lead to peritonitis).

Other factors preventing infection include:

- Mucus production.
- Peristalsis and fluid movement.
- Seamless epithelium with tight junctions.
- A fast cell turnover.
- IgA secretions at mucosal surfaces.

Disorders of the stomach

Congenital abnormalities
Diaphragmatic hernia
The diaphragm develops from:

- The septum transversum.
- The pleuroperitoneal membranes.
- The dorsal mesentery of the oesophagus.
- Muscular components of the body wall.

The pleuroperitoneal folds appear at the beginning of week 5, and they fuse with the septum transversum and the oesophageal mesentery in week 7, separating the abdominal and thoracic cavities. This primitive diaphragm then fuses with a ring of muscle that develops from the body wall.

If there is incomplete fusion, the contents of the abdomen may push up into the pleural cavity, forming a diaphragmatic hernia (usually on the left side), pushing the heart forwards and compressing the lungs. The incidence is about 1 in 2000 births, and treatment is surgical.

Pyloric stenosis

Pyloric stenosis (narrowing) occurs in about 1 in 150 male infants and 1 in 750 female infants. There is a genetic factor involved.

Stenosis is caused by hypertrophy of the circular muscles of the pylorus, obstructing the flow of contents from the stomach into the duodenum. Typically, it presents 4–6 weeks after birth with projectile vomiting within half an hour of a feed. There is no bile in the vomit because the obstruction is above the ampulla of Vater.

Peristaltic waves are visible in the child, a sausage-shaped mass (the enlarged pylorus) can be felt in the right upper quadrant, and the hypertrophied pyloric muscle can be observed using ultrasonography. Treatment is by surgery.

Stenosis may also be acquired in adult life, usually caused by scarring from peptic ulceration or because of malignancy obstructing the outflow. It is diagnosed by barium meal and gastroscopy.

When treating a patient who is vomiting, always test the vomit for the presence of bile. Bile joins the intestinal contents at the ampulla of Vater. Vomit will only contain bile if the lesion is below the ampulla.

Inflammation of the stomach

Inflammation of the stomach (gastritis) may be acute or chronic.

Acute gastritis

This involves an acute inflammatory reaction at the superficial mucosa, with the infiltration of neutrophils. Acute gastritis is almost always caused by drugs (especially NSAIDs such as aspirin) or by alcohol causing chemical exfoliation of the surface epithelial cells and decreasing the secretion of protective mucus.

The drugs or chemicals often inhibit prostaglandins, which protect the gastric mucosa by stimulating mucus and HCO_3^- production and inhibiting acid secretion (despite their role in inflammation).

The degree of damage depends on the amount of toxic substance and the time it has been there. It also varies from erosions (a partial loss of mucosa) to ulcers (involving the full thickness of the mucosa).

H. pylori has been implicated in both acute and chronic gastritis. *H. pylori* was first isolated from the human stomach in 1983, and it is also involved in gastric and duodenal ulcers, and non-ulcer dyspepsia. It is found beneath the mucus barrier and helps protect itself by catalysing urea to ammonia with urease. Urease and ammonia are both proinflammatory agents. *H. pylori* may be eradicated by triple therapy (two antibiotics and a proton pump inhibitor).

NSAIDS, such as aspirin, inhibit the enzyme cyclooxygenase (COX), which is necessary for prostaglandin production. Concurrent therapy with a proton pump inhibitor can prevent gastritis and ulcer formation.

Chronic gastritis

Chronic inflammatory changes in the mucosa cause atrophy and epithelial metaplasia (which may develop into carcinoma). Chronic gastritis is classified as:
- Type A (autoimmune).
- Type B (bacterial infection).
- Type C (reflux).

Other, less common forms exist, most notably lymphocytic, eosinophilic, and granulomatous gastritis.

Type A gastritis

Inflammation is caused by antibodies against gastric parietal cells and intrinsic factor binding sites. Intrinsic factor is needed to absorb vitamin B_{12}. In its absence, macrocytic anaemia develops once liver stores of vitamin B_{12} have been used up.

Pernicious anaemia occurs where autoimmune gastritis and macrocytic anaemia exist together. It is associated with other autoimmune diseases such as thyroid disease, vitiligo, Addison's disease, and myxoedema. Pernicious anaemia predisposes to carcinoma of the stomach.

The body of the stomach is always affected and often this type of gastritis involves the entire stomach.

Vitamin B_{12} is needed for the synthesis of DNA. Normally, the nucleus is extruded from red blood cells before they are released into the peripheral blood from the bone marrow. In vitamin B_{12} deficiency, however, maturation of the nucleus is delayed relative to the cytoplasm and macrocytic blood cells are seen in the peripheral blood.

Type B gastritis

H. pylori infection is present in about 90% of cases of active chronic Type B gastritis. It provokes an acute inflammatory response and the release of proteases, which destroy gastric glands, leading to atrophy.

Type B gastritis usually begins in the antrum, but it may cause atrophy, fibrosis, and metaplasia of the entire stomach.

Type C gastritis

This reflux gastritis is caused by regurgitation of duodenal contents into the stomach through the pylorus, and it is more common where pyloric or duodenal motility has been compromised. This type of gastritis is caused by irritants such as NSAIDs, alcohol, and biliary reflux.

It may present with dyspepsia and bilious vomiting.

Less common forms of gastritis

Lymphocytic gastritis is so named because of numerous mature lymphocytes in the gastric epithelium.

In eosinophilic gastritis large numbers of eosinophils are found, possibly as a result of an allergic reaction to an antigen in the diet.

Granulomatous gastritis may be seen in granulomatous disease, such as Crohn's and sarcoidosis. Gastric granulomas may also be found in the absence of systemic granulomatous disease, however. Complications include haemorrhage and perforation, which may lead to peritonitis.

Ulceration

Ulcers arise when damaging factors overwhelm the natural protection of the mucosal lining of the gastrointestinal tract. They can result from a decrease in protective factors, an increase in damaging factors, or both.

Peptic ulcers are chronic lesions occurring in the upper gastrointestinal tract where gastric acid and pepsin are present, and they are caused by hyperacidity, *H. pylori* infection, reflux of duodenal contents, NSAIDs, and smoking. Genetic factors play a role, as peptic ulceration is more common in patients with blood group O and first-degree relatives of people with duodenal ulcers are three times more likely to develop them themselves.

Peptic ulcers are most common in:
- The duodenal cap.
- The stomach (especially at the junction of the antrum and body).
- The distal oesophagus, particularly in a Barrett's oesophagus.
- A Meckel's diverticulum (particularly where ectopic gastric mucosa is present).
- Where a gastroenterostomy has been performed.

Like ulcers elsewhere, they may haemorrhage (leading to blood loss and anaemia), perforate, or heal by fibrosis, thus causing a stricture.

Duodenal ulcers (DU) are 2–3 times more common than gastric ulcers (GU), occurring in about 15% of the population. There is an increase in incidence of peptic ulcer above the age of 45 years. Both duodenal and gastric ulcers are common in the elderly.

About 95% of DU and 80% of GU are associated with *H. pylori*, and NSAID treatment is associated with the rest.

Gastric ulcers may also occur in response to acute gastritis or extreme hyperacidity, as in Zollinger–Ellison syndrome.

Severe stress and trauma, such as after burns (Curling's ulcer), and ischaemia of the gastric mucosa can also cause ulceration.

Zollinger–Ellison syndrome is a rare condition due to gastrin-secreting pancreatic adenomas causing excess acid production. It can lead to acute ulcers in the antrum, duodenum, and, in severe cases the jejunum.

Acid secretion reducers

H_2 histamine receptor antagonists (e.g. cimetidine and ranitidine) reduce acid secretion, relieve the pain, and increase the rate of ulcer healing.

M_1 muscarinic receptor antagonists (e.g. pirenzepine) selectively block M_1 receptors, reducing acid secretion with fewer muscarinic side effects than non-selective blockers, such as dry mouth, blurred vision, and urinary retention. Pirenzipine is not in use anymore. Proton-pump (H^+/K^+ ATPase) inhibitors (e.g. omeprazole and lansoprazole) irreversibly inhibit the proton pump, reducing the transport of H^+ ions out of parietal cells. Proton pump inhibitors are the most powerful acid inhibiting and ulcer healing drugs available.

The acid inhibiting drugs and their sites of action are shown in Fig. 3.14.

Mucosal strengtheners

Mucosal strengtheners act as a buffering agent to neutralize acid and to protect the mucosa.

Sucralfate forms a polymerized, sticky gel in acid conditions of less than pH 4 that adheres to the base of ulcers. It has very few side effects.

Bismuth chelate has a similar mechanism of action to sucralfate and it may eradicate *H. pylori*.

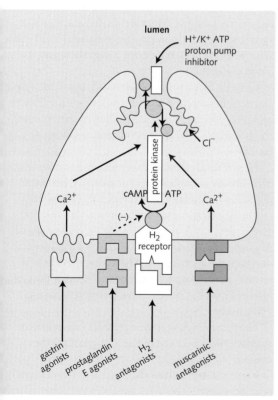

Fig. 3.14 Strategies for inhibiting oxyntic/parietal cell acid secretion.

Prostaglandin analogues

Misoprostol is a synthetic prostaglandin analogue, which can prevent NSAID-associated ulcers. It is contraindicated in pregnancy (prostaglandins induce the onset of labour) and breastfeeding.

Helicobacter pylori eradication

Triple therapy regimes provide higher eradication rates than dual ones and result in long-term ulcer remission. Current regimes include the following:

- Amoxycillin, metronidazole, and omeprazole.
- Clarithromycin, tinidazole, and omeprazole.

Metronidazole should be avoided during the first trimester of pregnancy.

Gastric varices

Gastric varicese are uncommon, but they may occur in submucosal veins below the gastro-oesophageal junction, as a result of portal hypertension.

Like oesophageal varices, they should never be biopsied or they will haemorrhage with potentially fatal consequences.

Treatment includes injecting with a sclerosing agent to arrest bleeding by thrombosis or banding to cut off the blood flow to the damaged vessel. Bleeding ulcers can be injected with adrenaline (epinephrine) or a sclerosing agent.

Hypertrophic gastropathy

Hyperplasia of mucosal epithelial cells causes enlargement of the rugae (which may be mistaken for a neoplasm on radiographs) and an increase in acid secretion. It may occur secondary to excess gastrin release in Zollinger–Ellison syndrome.

Hypertrophy also occurs in Ménétrièr's disease, where loss of parietal and chief cells is found with mucosal cell hyperplasia and glandular proliferation. Hyperplasia of the parietal and chief cells is known as hypertrophic hypersecretory gastropathy.

Delayed gastric emptying

Gastric emptying can be delayed by mechanical or non-mechanical obstructions.

Mechanical obstructions include tumours, duodenal, gastric, or pyloric stenosis, and a bezoar (a mass of swallowed foreign material, which has collected and is obstructing emptying).

Non-mechanical delayed gastric emptying is known as gastroparesis. This is an uncommon complication of diabetes, but it can also occur due to gastric arrhythmias, myotonic dystrophy, collagen-vascular diseases, neuropathies, and after vagotomy.

Mechanical delayed gastric emptying must be excluded before non-mechanical aetiologies can be explored. Quite often, the cause is unknown and the problem is typed idiopathic gastroparesis, but is probably due to gastric arrhythmias. Diabetic gastroparesis is associated with peripheral neuropathy.

Patients can be asymptomatic, or they may have a combination of symptoms, including bloating, abdominal pain, persistent belching, nausea (with or without vomiting), anorexia, early satiety, and weight loss.

Treatment includes:
- Nutritional supplement.
- Prokinetic drugs (e.g. metoclopramide or cisapride).
- Surgery.

Drugs to improve motility

Motility stimulants (e.g. metoclopramide and cisapride) act on the gut to mimic the natural pattern of activity. These drugs are used to treat delayed gastric emptying, and they can increase oesophageal peristalsis and LOS tone. They also stimulate colonic propulsion.

Metoclopramide is a dopamine antagonist and cisapride is an agonist at the 5-HT$_4$ receptor (5-hydroxytryptamine (serotonin) type 4 receptor) in the neurons of the myenteric plexus.

Metoclopramide is also an effective antiemetic. Cisapride has recently been removed from the national formulary, due to cardiac side effects.

Neoplastic disease

Neoplasms may be malignant or benign. They are described according to their tissue of origin.

Benign neoplasms

These include:
- Hyperplastic polyps (regenerative polyps)—elongated gastric pits separated by fibrous tissue, usually found in association with *H. pylori* infection in the antrum.
- Simple fundic polyps (glandular cystic dilatation in the body of the stomach).
- Hamartomas (overgrowth of mature tissue, displaying disordered arrangement and proportion) are most commonly seen in Peutz–Jeghers syndrome, a hereditary disorder.
- Ectopic (heterotopic) pancreatic tissue.

- Leiomyomas, arising from smooth muscle, which may bleed from ulceration. These are the most common benign gastric tumours.
- Adenomas (benign tumours of glandular origin) make up 5–10% of polypoid lesions in the stomach, and they may contain proliferative dysplastic epithelium with the potential for malignant transformation. They are much more common in the colon but, if present in the stomach, are usually in the antrum. They may be pedunculated (with a stalk) or sessile (without a stalk), and they are more common in males. The incidence of adenomas increases with age.

Malignant neoplasms

Adenocarcinoma is the most common gastric neoplasm and accounts for 90% of all malignant neoplasms in the stomach. Malignant lymphomas account for 5% of gastric malignant neoplasms and other malignancies, such as carcinoid and malignant spindle cell tumours occur rarely.

In the UK, 15 in 100 000 men are affected each year and the incidence increases with age, affecting men more than women.

A number of conditions are premalignant, such as atrophic gastritis, some chronic gastric ulcers, pernicious anaemia, Ménétrièr's disease, and post-gastrectomy (carcinomas often develop 15–20 years after surgery). The incidence is slightly higher in blood group A.

Genetic factors may be involved, but a decrease in gastric acid secretion and corresponding increase in bacteria (which are normally killed by gastric acid), particularly *H. pylori*, are common aetiological factors.

H. pylori infections cause chronic gastritis, which occasionally becomes atrophic gastritis, leading to metaplasia, dysplasia, and ultimately carcinoma.

Dietary factors may act to initiate or promote carcinogenesis. A diet high in salt increases the risk. Also, dietary nitrates are converted to carcinogenic nitrosamines by bacteria. Therefore, diets high in nitrates predispose to carcinoma. The incidence is high in Japan but much lower amongst Japanese living in the USA.

Diets high in fruit and vegetables can help protect against cancer because of the anti-oxidants they contain.

Presentation is often late, with a correspondingly poor prognosis.

Four different appearances may be recognized:
- Malignant ulcers with raised, everted edges.

- Polypoid tumours.
- Colloid tumours (which appear gelatinous).
- Linitis plastica (leather bottle stomach, so named because the stomach becomes small, thick, and contracted).

Carcinomas may spread through:
- The lymphatic system.
- The bloodstream.
- Direct spread locally.
- Transfusion through a body cavity (transcoelomically).

Metastases can occur in the liver, bone, brain, and lung. Through peritoneal seeding, metastases can also be found in the ovary (Krukenberg's tumour).

Signs and symptoms include:
- Epigastric pain.
- Nausea and vomiting (especially if the tumour is at the pylorus, causing obstruction).
- Anorexia.
- Anaemia from occult bleeding.
- Haematemesis.
- Weight loss.
- Palpable epigastric mass (in 50% of patients).
- Abdominal tenderness.

A patient with gastric carcinoma may develop acanthosis nigricans—abnormal pigmentation of the skin of the axilla—a condition also associated with breast carcinoma.

Generally, the 5-year survival is less than 10%, but it is much better for diagnosis of early carcinoma, confined to the mucosa and submucosa. Treatment includes radiotherapy and surgery to excise the tumour and any affected lymph nodes.

Partial or total gastrectomy may be necessary in some cases. Screening is important for patients who have had a previous gastrectomy for peptic ulceration.

Never ignore it if one of the supraclavicular lymph nodes on the left side of the body is enlarged. Lymph from the cardiac region of the stomach drains to these nodes and they may become enlarged due to metastatic spread (Virchow's node or Troisier's sign) from gastric carcinoma.

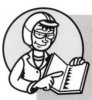

- Draw an annotated diagram depicting the stomach and its major regions.
- Briefly describe the stomach in relation to its neighbouring anatomical structures.
- Describe the arterial supply, and venous and lymphatic drainage of the stomach.
- How does the stomach develop from the foregut?
- List the layers and cell types of the stomach. What functions do the cell types have?
- How does the stomach 'store' food?
- What components make up the gastric secretions?
- Describe the control of gastric secretion.
- Briefly describe the physiology of gastric motility.
- What factors determine the rate of gastric emptying?
- How is the gastric mucosa protected against damage by acid and pepsin?
- List factors that stop mucosal protection and predispose to gastric mucosal damage?
- How does the stomach protect against infection?
- What are the congenital abnormalities associated with the stomach?
- Compare and contrast the different types of acute and chronic gastritis.
- Where is peptic ulceration found? What causes it, and what might it lead to?
- What treatments are available for gastritis and peptic ulcers?
- What is hypertrophic gastropathy?
- What causes delayed gastric emptying? What symptoms are seen with gastroparesis?
- What drugs are given to stimulate gut motility? How do they work?
- List the benign neoplasms associated with the stomach.
- Briefly describe the main malignancies found in the stomach, the factors involved in their aetiology, and the treatments available for gastric carcinoma.
- What are the different appearances of gastric carcinoma?
- How do gastric carcinomas spread, and which sites in the body are metastases from these found?

4. The Liver and Biliary Tract

Organization of the liver and biliary tract

The liver is the largest abdominal organ and also the largest gland in the body. It is vital for life, and it has many metabolic, endocrine, and detoxifying functions.

The biliary system removes waste products from the liver and carries bile salts to the intestine where they aid digestion.

Regional anatomy

The liver is a soft reddish-brown organ, weighing about 1.5 kg and situated under the diaphragm. It is surrounded by a capsule of strong connective tissue (Glisson's capsule).

It lies in the right upper quadrant and occupies most of the right hypochondriac region, extending into the left hypochondriac and epigastric regions (see Fig. 1.1).

It is protected by the rib cage and moves during respiration, owing to its attachment to the diaphragm by the falciform, coronary, and triangular ligaments (Fig. 4.1).

The lesser omentum connects the stomach to the liver, and it is continuous with the left triangular ligament. The liver has diaphragmatic and visceral surfaces. The sharp inferior border separates the two surfaces.

The visceral surface is related to:

- The abdominal oesophagus.
- The fundus and body of the stomach.
- The lesser omentum.
- The gall bladder.

In life, the liver is soft and jelly-like in substance. In death, the capsule of connective tissue (Glisson's capsule) gives it a definite shape, as seen in the cadaver.

- The superior part of the duodenum.
- The transverse colon (including the hepatic flexure).
- Many associated vessels and nerves.

Peritoneum covers the visceral surface (except the gall bladder and porta hepatis) and the superior part of the liver, except the posterior part known as the bare area. This area is in direct contact with the diaphragm and is situated between the reflections of the coronary ligament. The inferior vena cava and the right adrenal gland also lie next to the bare area (Fig. 4.2).

The liver is divided into two functional lobes, the left and right, by the plane passing through the gall bladder and inferior vena cava. Each lobe receives its own blood supply (Fig. 4.3). There are also two minor lobes (used for descriptive purposes) called the caudate and quadrate lobes. The left lobe includes the caudate lobe and most of the quadrate lobe.

Blood supply

The liver has a very rich blood supply from two main sources:

Fig. 4.1 Summary table of ligaments attaching the liver to the diaphragm.

Ligaments attaching liver to diaphragm	
Ligament	**Attachments**
Falciform ligament (remnant of the ventral mesentery of the abdominal foregut)	Attaches the anterior and superior surfaces of the liver to the anterior abdominal wall and the diaphragm
Coronary ligament	Attaches the posterior surface of the right lobe to the diaphragm
Right triangular ligament	An extension of the coronary ligament
Left triangular ligament	Attaches the posterior surface of the left lobe to the diaphragm

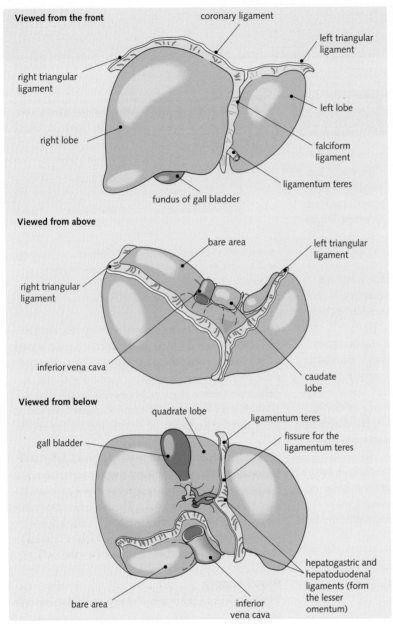

Fig. 4.2 Three different views of the liver, showing the anterior, superior, and inferior sides. The bare area on the posterior part of the liver is not covered with peritoneum.

Viewed from the front

- coronary ligament
- left triangular ligament
- right triangular ligament
- left lobe
- right lobe
- falciform ligament
- ligamentum teres
- fundus of gall bladder

Viewed from above

- bare area
- left triangular ligament
- right triangular ligament
- inferior vena cava
- caudate lobe

Viewed from below

- quadrate lobe
- ligamentum teres
- gall bladder
- fissure for the ligamentum teres
- hepatogastric and hepatoduodenal ligaments (form the lesser omentum)
- bare area
- inferior vena cava

- The hepatic artery (a branch of the coeliac trunk), which divides into left and right branches to supply the left and right lobes.
- The portal vein, which carries venous blood from the GI tract, full of digestion products. It divides into left and right branches to supply the two functional lobes. An accessory left hepatic artery, often arising from the left gastric artery, may be found. Variations in the hepatic arterial supply are common. The arterial blood connects to the central vein of each liver lobule.

The hepatic veins drain from the central veins of each lobule into the inferior vena cava.

Lymphatic drainage
The lymphatics of the liver drain to deep and superficial vessels.

The deep vessels come together at the porta hepatis and end in the hepatic lymph nodes scattered along the hepatic vessels (e.g. the cystic lymph node near the neck of the gall bladder). These then drain to the coeliac lymph nodes to enter the thoracic duct.

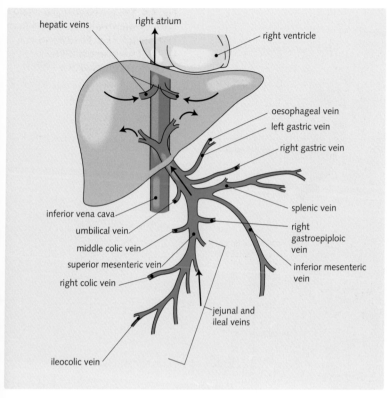

Fig. 4.3 The hepatic portal venous system. (Redrawn with permission from Hall-Craggs ECB. *Anatomy as a Basis for Clinical Medicine.* London: Waverly Europe, 1995.)

Some deep lymph vessels follow the hepatic veins through the diaphragm to end in the phrenic lymph nodes.

The superficial lymph vessels follow the same drainage as the deep vessels, but they can also drain to the mediastinal lymph nodes.

Nerve supply

The liver receives both sympathetic and parasympathetic innervation. The nerve fibres reach the liver via the hepatic plexus, which is derived from the coeliac plexus. It also receives parasympathetic innervation from the right phrenic nerve and left and right vagi.

The hepatic nerves follow the blood supply of the liver and enter at the porta hepatis.

The porta hepatis is a deep fissure on the visceral surface of the liver, and it contains the hepatic artery (proper), portal vein, hepatic nerve plexus, hepatic ducts, and lymphatic vessels.

The gall bladder

The gall bladder is a pear-shaped sac that concentrates and stores bile secreted from the liver. It can hold between 30 and 60 mL of bile and, when stimulated, it releases its contents into the duodenum, through the cystic and biliary ducts.

It lies on the right edge of the quadrate lobe in the gall bladder fossa on the visceral surface, partly covered by peritoneum on its posterior and inferior surfaces.

It has a fundus, body, and neck (Fig. 4.4), which tapers and makes an S-shaped bend to join with the cystic duct. The cystic duct is 2–4 cm long, and it joins the common hepatic duct to form the bile duct.

This opens into the second part of the duodenum through the sphincter of Oddi (hepatopancreatic sphincter) at the ampulla of Vater (duodenal papilla).

The cystic duct has a spiral folding of its mucus membrane, forming a spiral valve. This keeps the cystic duct open constantly for two purposes:

- To allow bile to pass into the gall bladder from the liver when the bile duct is closed (by the sphincter of Oddi and the choledochal sphincter).
- To allow bile to be secreted into the duodenum when the gall bladder contracts.

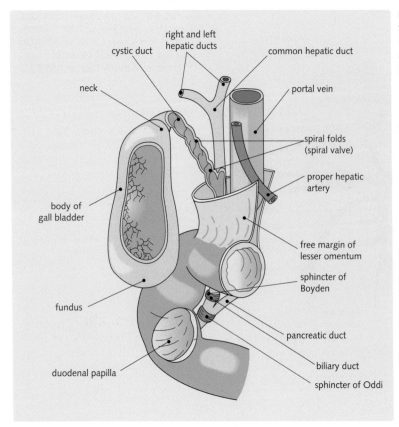

Fig. 4.4 The gall bladder and biliary tract. (Redrawn with permission from Hall-Craggs, ECB. *Anatomy as a Basis for Clinical Medicine.* London: Waverly Europe, 1995.)

Labels: right and left hepatic ducts; cystic duct; common hepatic duct; neck; portal vein; spiral folds (spiral valve); proper hepatic artery; body of gall bladder; free margin of lesser omentum; sphincter of Boyden; fundus; pancreatic duct; duodenal papilla; biliary duct; sphincter of Oddi

Blood supply

The blood supply to the gall bladder is from the cystic artery (a branch of the right hepatic artery). Variations in the cystic artery are common.

Venous drainage occurs in three ways:

- Directly to the liver.
- Joining the portal vein.
- Joining the gastric, duodenal, and pancreatic veins (which then join the portal vein).

Lymphatic drainage

Lymph from the gall bladder passes to the hepatic nodes via the cystic nodes, near the neck of the gall bladder. These drain to the coeliac lymph nodes.

Nerve supply

The innervation to the gall bladder is from the coeliac plexus (sympathetic), the vagus nerve (parasympathetic), the right phrenic nerve (sensory), and the hepatic plexus. The nerves follow the cystic artery.

The biliary tract

The biliary tract conveys bile from the liver to the duodenum. The left and right hepatic ducts join to form the common hepatic duct, which descends in the free edge of the lesser omentum and joins the cystic duct to form the bile duct.

The bile duct is approximately 8 cm in length. The duct descends in the free edge of the lesser omentum with the hepatic artery and portal vein. It continues its descent behind the superior part of the duodenum and head of the pancreas.

There are two sphincters involved in the movement of bile:

- The choledochal sphincter (sphincter of Boyden)—at the distal end of the bile duct. Contraction of this prevents bile entering the ampulla and duodenum.
- The sphincter of Oddi—around the ampulla of Vater, which controls the secretion of both bile and pancreatic juice into the duodenum.

The sphincter of Oddi at the ampulla of Vater is 10 cm beyond the pylorus. The main pancreatic duct opens into the duodenum at the same point.

Development

The liver develops from the liver bud (hepatic diverticulum) that appears as an outgrowth of the endodermal epithelium at the distal end of the primitive foregut in the middle of the 3rd week (Fig. 4.5).

The liver bud is composed of rapidly proliferating cells, which penetrate the mesodermal septum transversum. The connection between the liver bud and the foregut (duodenum) narrows and forms the bile duct.

A small ventral outgrowth from the bile duct gives rise to the gall bladder and cystic duct. The structure of the liver is formed by epithelial liver cords that mix with the vitelline and umbilical veins to give rise to hepatic sinusoids.

The liver cords differentiate into the hepatocytes (parenchyma), the bile canaliculi, and the hepatic ducts. The mesoderm of the septum transversum gives rise to:

- Haematopoietic cells.
- Kupffer cells.
- Connective tissue cells.

The liver is the major haematopoietic organ in the embryo, and, by the 4th week, haematopoiesis has already begun.

The lesser omentum and the falciform ligament are both derived from the mesoderm of the septum transversum, located between the foregut and liver, and the ventral abdominal wall and the liver, respectively.

The rotation of the stomach, liver and spleen occurs between the 6th week and 11th week of embryonic development (Fig. 4.6).

At about the 12th week, the hepatocytes begin to form bile. This is able to enter the duodenum, as the biliary tract and gall bladder are all fully formed.

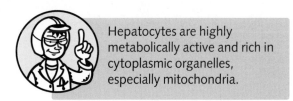

Hepatocytes are highly metabolically active and rich in cytoplasmic organelles, especially mitochondria.

Tissues of the liver and biliary tract

Traditionally, there are three ways of describing the arrangement of the liver (Fig. 4.7):

- Classic lobule.
- Portal lobule.
- Acinus.

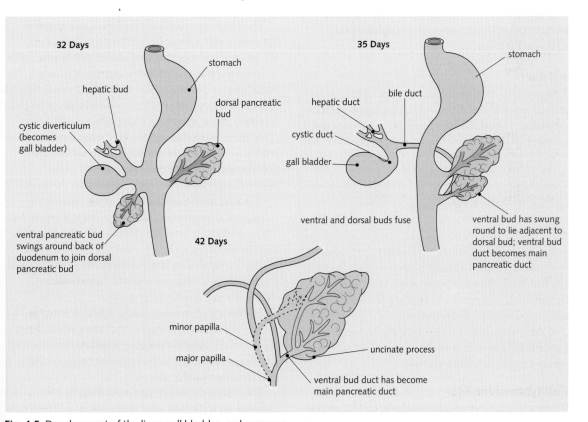

Fig. 4.5 Development of the liver, gall bladder, and pancreas.

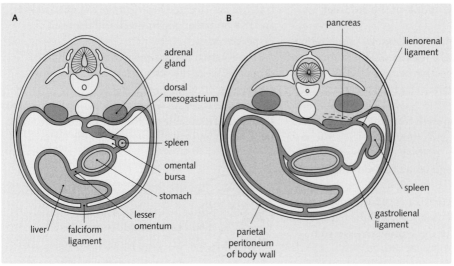

Fig. 4.6 Rotation of the stomach and the liver during the 6th week of embryonic development, shown in transverse section. (Reproduced with permission from Sadler TW. *Langman's Medical Embryology*, 8th edn. Philadelphia: Lippincott, 2000.)

Classic lobule

Each lobule may be thought of as a hexagon with a central vein at its centre and a portal triad at its outer corners. A portal triad consists of a branch of the hepatic artery, a branch of the portal vein, and a bile duct.

Portal lobule

This views the liver as being made up of a series of triangles with a central vein at each corner and a portal triad at the centre, and it emphasizes the exocrine function.

Acinus

This is an elliptical arrangement with a portal triad at the centre and a central vein at each pole, and it emphasizes the endocrine function. It reflects the gradient of metabolic activity found in the liver, and it is divided into three zones for descriptive purposes:

- The periportal zone (zone 1).
- The mid zone (zone 2).
- The centrilobular zone (zone 3).

Most oxygenated blood is found in the centre of the acinus around the portal triad (zone 1); this zone is most susceptible to damage from toxins carried to the liver in the hepatic portal vein. Most of the metabolic activity of the liver takes place here. This zone makes up the limiting plate.

Conversely, zone 3, being furthest from the portal triad and closest to the central vein, is most susceptible to ischaemic damage.

Cell types of the liver

There are a number of different cells making up the architecture of the liver. These are the hepatocytes,

Kupffer cells, haematopoietic cells, and perisinusoidal cells.

The functions of these cells are summarized in Fig. 4.8.

Sinusoids, spaces of Disse, and bile canaliculi

The hepatocytes are arranged in 'cords', which radiate out in a spoke-like fashion from the central vein (Fig. 4.9).

They have a network of capillaries, or sinusoids, between them, which are lined with discontinuous fenestrated endothelium and phagocytic Kupffer cells.

In between the hepatocytes and the sinusoidal endothelial cells is the space of Disse (the perisinusoidal space). This contains perisinusoidal cells (Ito cells) that secrete collagen, providing a supportive mesh.

At their sinusoidal surface, the hepatocytes have numerous short microvilli, which extend into the perisinusoidal space. Between the bases of the microvilli, lie coated pits that are used for endocytosis.

The microvilli increase the surface area for the transfer of digestive products, nutrients, oxygen, and other substances between the blood in the sinusoids and the hepatocytes.

Two surfaces of each hepatocyte communicate with a space of Disse and two surfaces communicate with a bile canaliculus (Fig. 4.10).

Bile canaliculi are formed by a groove between surfaces of adjacent hepatocytes. The canaliculi are about 0.5–2.5 μm in diameter and they are sealed by zonulae occludentes, which prevent leakage of bile into the intercellular spaces.

The canaliculi form rings around the hepatocytes and approach the bile ductules in the portal tracts by opening into canals of Hering.

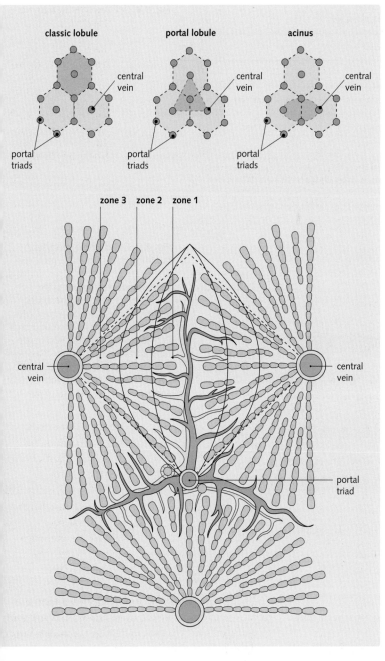

Fig. 4.7 The arrangement of the liver.

These are short corridors lined with cuboidal cells that drain bile into the ductules of the portal tracts.

In the fetal liver, islands of haematopoietic cells are found within the spaces of Disse for the production of blood cells.

Portal canal and limiting plate

The portal canal consists of the portal triad (hepatic portal vein, hepatic artery, and bile duct) surrounded by connective tissue.

A small space (the space of Mall) exists between the connective tissue covering and the surrounding hepatocytes. Lymph is thought to originate in the space of Mall.

The limiting plate (the hepatocytes of the periportal zone) that surrounds the portal tract, makes up a protective layer of cells, which are first to be exposed to toxins in the systemic or portal blood. Breaching the plate can lead to liver damage, in particular cirrhosis.

Cell types of the liver	
Cell type	**Function**
Kupffer cells	Phagocytosis, found in sinusoids
Hepatocytes	Perform most of the functions of the liver (Fig. 4.11)
Ito cells (perisinusoidal cells)	Replace damaged hepatocytes and secrete collagen
Endothelial cells	Scavenger cells for denatured collagen, harmful enzymes, and pathogens: they line the sinusoids
Haemopoietic cells	Haemopoiesis in the fetus, and in adults with chronic anaemia

Fig. 4.8 Cell types of the liver.

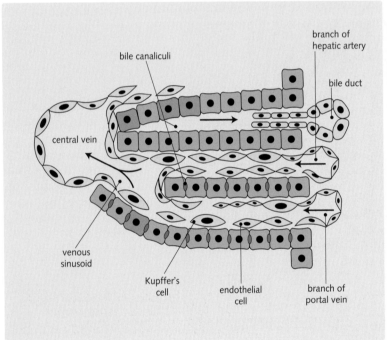

Fig. 4.9 Cords of hepatocytes radiating out from the central vein. The space of Disse (the perisinusoidal space) is located between the hepatocytes and the fenestrated endothelial cells, interspersed with Kupffer cells, that line the sinusoids. Perisinusoidal cell (Ito cells) reside here and secrete collagen. (Redrawn with permission from Marshall W. *Clinical Chemistry*, 3rd edn. London: Mosby.)

Nerves

The liver is innervated by both the sympathetic and parasympathetic systems.

Nerves enter the liver at the porta hepatis and travel in the portal canals with the vessels of the portal triad.

Sympathetic fibres innervate blood vessels.

Cell bodies of parasympathetic neurons may be found near the porta hepatis. Parasympathetic fibres innervate large ducts with smooth muscle in their walls, and they may innervate blood vessels.

Blood vessels

The liver receives blood from the hepatic artery and the hepatic portal vein, both of which extend into the portal triad.

The hepatic artery has a smaller lumen than the hepatic vein and a thicker, muscular wall. It supplies oxygenated blood to the connective tissue, the larger portal canals, and the sinusoids.

Blood flows from the smaller vessels in the portal triad into the sinusoids and drains to the central vein. From there, it flows into the sublobular vein and the systemic system and is returned to the heart.

Apart from the sinusoids, all the hepatic blood vessels are lined with the usual vascular endothelial cells, and they have the basic structure of intima (connective tissue), media (smooth muscle), and adventitia (elastic and fibrocollagenous connective tissue).

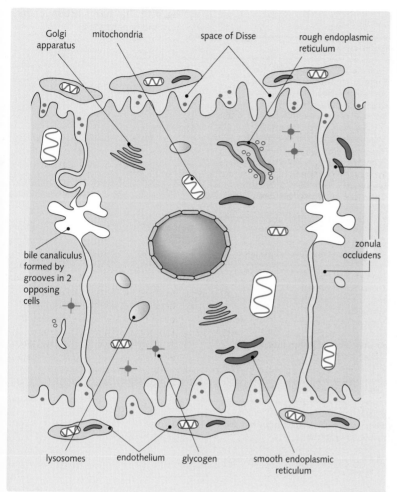

Fig. 4.10 Two sides of each hepatocyte communicate with a sinusoid (via the space of Disse), and bile canaliculi are formed by a groove between adjacent hepatocytes.

Labels in figure:
Golgi apparatus — mitochondria — space of Disse — rough endoplasmic reticulum — zonula occludens — bile canaliculus formed by grooves in 2 opposing cells — lysosomes — endothelium — glycogen — smooth endoplasmic reticulum

Tissues of the biliary tract

The intrahepatic bile ducts are lined by cuboidal or low columnar epithelial cells. Increasing amounts of fibroelastic connective tissue surround the epithelium as the ducts become larger near the porta hepatis. The largest ducts have smooth muscle in their walls. The wall of the gall bladder consists of a mucous membrane, muscular layer, adventitia, and a serous membrane.

The mucous membrane is made up of simple columnar epithelium and a lamina propria of loose connective tissue. The columnar epithelial cells have a brush border of many microvilli on their apical surfaces, and they are absorptive cells. The mucosa is thrown into folds, particularly when the gall bladder is empty.

The muscularis consists of layers of smooth muscle with collagenous elastic fibres between the layers.

The adventitia is made up of collagen and elastic fibres, and it contains a rich lymphatic network.

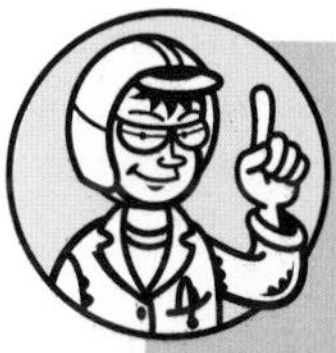

The gall bladder epithelial cells are highly specialized for absorption. They have a brush border of microvilli; they are rich in mitochondria; and they have numerous Na^+/K^+ ATPase transporters at their lateral surfaces.

Metabolic functions of the liver

Overview of liver metabolism

The liver performs many functions vital for life, and it has a substantial capacity to regenerate after injury. The main functions of the liver are protein, fat, and carbohydrate metabolism; bile production; storage of vitamins, minerals, and glycogen; biotransformation; and detoxification and protection (by filtration of portal blood). These are summarized in Fig. 4.11.

Functions of the liver	
Function	Processes involved
Protein metabolism	Synthesis and secretion of albumin Synthesis of plasma proteins Formation of urea from ammonia Deamination of amino acids Synthesis of coagulation factors, e.g. factors V, VII, IX, X and prothrombin Metabolism of polypeptide hormone
Fat metabolism	Formation of lipoproteins and fatty acids Synthesis of cholesterol Conversion of cholesterol to bile salts Conversion of carbohydrates and protein to fat Ketogenesis Metabolism and excretion of steroid hormones
Carbohydrate metabolism	Gluconeogenesis Synthesis and breakdown of glycogen
Bile secretion	Production of bile salts Elimination of bilirubin
Storage	Glycogen Vitamins (A and B_{12})
Biotransformation and detoxification	Of drugs and exogenous substances Gonadal hormones Aldosterone Glucocorticoids Nitrogenous gut toxins
Protection	Filtration of portal blood Removal of bacteria/antigens by Kupffer cells (phagocyctosis)
Haematopoiesis	The fetal liver is the major source of blood cell production

Fig. 4.11 The main functions of the liver and hepatocytes.

To maintain these functions, the liver must receive 25% of the cardiac output through the portal vein and hepatic artery. Nutrients and other substances are absorbed from the sinusoids into the hepatocytes.

Functional heterogeneity of hepatocytes

As mentioned previously, the acinar architecture can be divided into three zones: the periportal (zone 1), the mid (zone 2), and the centrilobular (perivenous zone 3) zones. The cells in each zone differ in ultrastructure, function, and distance from the blood supply. Zone 1 of the acinus (the periportal area) is adjacent to the portal canal (Fig. 4.7), and it receives more oxygenated blood from the hepatic artery and blood from the hepatic portal vein. It is, therefore, particularly susceptible to damage from toxins absorbed from the alimentary tract and carried to the liver in the portal system, for example, in paracetamol poisoning.

Zone 3 (the centrilobular zone) is furthest from the arterial supply and particularly vulnerable to ischaemic damage, for example, in cardiac failure. These zones are contiguous and liver cell necrosis affecting this zone is often confluent.

Functional differences include:

- The periportal hepatocytes take up bile under normal circumstances, but during bile overload, this function is also adopted by the centrilobular (perivenous) hepatocytes too.
- The centrilobular hepatocytes contain enzymes required in esterification, but the periportal hepatocytes are rich in oxidative enzymes.

Carbohydrate metabolism

In the normal individual, blood glucose levels are carefully regulated. The liver plays an important role in glucose homeostasis.

Blood glucose levels rise transiently after a meal but the liver takes up the glucose and converts it to glycogen.

In the fasting state, glycogen is converted to glucose (glycogenolysis) (Fig. 4.12) and released into the bloodstream to keep levels within the range 3.5–5.5 mmol/L.

The liver contains approximately 80 g of glycogen. This is enough to keep blood glucose levels within the normal range for approximately 24 hours at rest, but for less time during heavy exercise.

The peptide hormones insulin and glucagon, both produced by the pancreas, control the levels of plasma glucose. Insulin promotes synthesis of

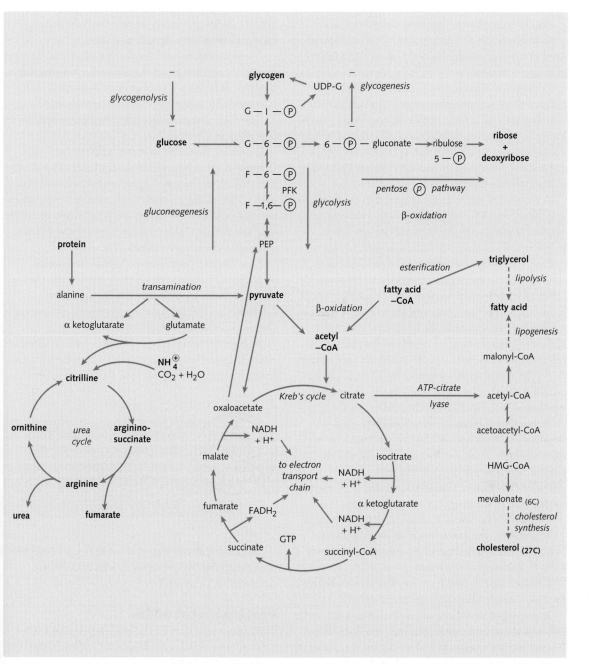

Fig. 4.12 Overview of metabolism. ℗, phosphate; G—1—℗, glucose-1-phosphate; F—6—℗, fructose-6-phosphate; PEP, phosphoenol pyruvate; GTP, guanosine triphosphate; ATP, adenosine triphosphate; NADH, reduced nicotinamide adenine dinucleotide; HMG-CoA, 3-hydroxy-3-methylglutaryl CoA; FADH$_2$, reduced flavin adenine dinucleotide; (6C), six carbon atoms; (27C), 27 carbon atoms.)

glycogen, protein, and fat, while inhibiting gluconeogenesis and lipolysis.

Glucagon acts on the liver primarily, and it has no effect on muscle. It upregulates gluconeogenesis and ketogenesis.

During hypoglycaemia, glucagon is stimulated and this upregulates production and release of glucose, free fatty acids, and ketone bodies into the blood (via glycogenolysis, gluconeogenesis, and ketogenesis).

Carbohydrates and amino acids (but not fats) are used to make glycogen. Its synthesis is catalysed by glycogen synthetase.

Glycogen is also present in muscle, but its sole purpose there is to provide energy for muscle contraction. It makes no direct contribution to blood glucose levels. Glycogen is a highly branched polysaccharide and it is made exclusively from α-D-glucose with α-1,4 and α-1,6 linkages. Branched chains are added to existing glycogen remnants in cells (primers).

A number of enzymes are involved in the synthesis and breakdown of glycogen, and defects in one or more of them lead to glycogen storage disorders (e.g. Pompe's disease, McArdle's syndrome, Hers' disease, Cori's disease, and von Gierke's disease).

Glycogen phosphorylase cleaves the α-1,4-glycosidic bond, glucosyltransferase transfers residues to other branches, and further enzymes act to release glucose.

The liver also contains the hydrolytic enzyme glucose-6-phosphatase, which allows for glucose release. This enzyme is absent in the brain and muscle.

As the synthesis and degradation of glycogen has an effect on blood glucose levels, both are carefully controlled, principally by cyclic AMP.

Adrenaline inhibits synthesis and activates breakdown of glycogen in the liver and muscle. In fight-or-flight situations we need normal blood glucose levels and do not want to make it into glycogen for storage. Therefore, it has a similar effect to glucagon in the liver (but not in muscles).

Conversely, insulin increases synthesis of glycogen.

In diabetes, the utilization of carbohydrates is impaired and ketone bodies are formed in the liver from β-oxidation of fatty acids.

Ketones are released from hepatocytes and carried to other tissues where they are metabolized.

In prolonged starvation, ketone bodies and fatty acids are used as alternative sources of fuel, and body tissues (except the brain) adapt to a lower glucose requirement.

Lipid metabolism

Most of the fat in the diet is in the form of triglycerides (esters of fatty acid and glycerol).

The essential fatty acids are linoleic, linolenic and arachidonic acids. These must be included in the diet, as they cannot be synthesized by the body, and they are required for synthesis of prostaglandins and cell membrane components. Non-essential fatty acids can be made by the body, and there is no requirement for them in the diet.

In developed countries, the fat component of an average diet is excessive, leading to an increased incidence of atherosclerosis and obesity.

Cholesterol is needed for the manufacture of steroid hormones and bile acids, and it can be synthesized in the liver. It is also a component of most diets, and it is found in all animal products, especially eggs.

The digestion and absorption of dietary lipids is described in Chapter 7.

Lipids are insoluble in water, and they are assembled into lipoproteins (complexes of lipid and protein) in the liver, for transport in the blood (Fig. 4.13). Depending on their composition, lipoproteins are classified into chylomicrons (the lowest density), very low density, intermediate density, low-density, and high-density lipoproteins (Fig. 4.14).

Low-density lipoproteins (LDLs) have been implicated in atheroma and their level in the plasma should be kept low. Conversely, high-density lipoproteins (HDLs) have a protective function and their levels should be higher.

The apoprotein element of the polar coat is made in the liver and intestine, and defects in its synthesis have important effects on lipid metabolism.

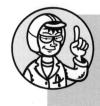
It is easy to remember the ideal levels of circulating lipoproteins. Low-density ones should be LOW and high-density ones should be HIGH!

Hyperlipidaemia may also result from a defect in lipid receptors. Alcoholic fatty liver changes are described in Chapter 5.

Protein metabolism

The liver synthesizes all the plasma proteins except γ-globulins. Amino acids from the intestines and muscles enter the liver and by controlling their metabolism (especially via transamination and gluconeogenesis) the plasma protein concentrations can be regulated.

Urea metabolism

Amino acids are transaminated and deaminated (via oxidative pathways) in the liver to form ammonia, which is converted to urea via the urea (ornithine) cycle. This occurs mainly in the periportal cells (hepatocytes adjacent to the portal canals).

The cycle occurs partly in the mitochondria and partly in the cytoplasm, so the enzymes are situated in one or the other, according to their function in the cycle.

In liver failure, there is decreased synthesis of urea and increased levels of ammonia—a toxic product. Ammonia can depress cerebral blood flow and cerebral oxygen consumption. Ammonia toxicity is usually due to cirrhosis, but it is also seen in inherited deficiencies of urea cycle enzymes.

Transamination of amino acids is the interconversion of amine groups (NH_2) from amino acids to α-ketoacids, to produce different amino acids. This is catalysed by transaminase in the liver.

Vitamins

The liver is the main store of the fat soluble vitamins (A, D, E, and K). Vitamin deficiency may occur when there is malabsorption of fat, due to a variety of hepatic and extrahepatic causes.

Vitamin B_{12} is absorbed from the diet in the terminal ileum, provided intrinsic factor is made by the parietal cells of the stomach, and enough is stored in the liver to last 2 or 3 years. Deficiency eventually leads to megaloblastic anaemia (pernicious anaemia).

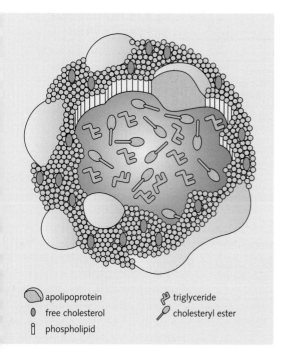

apolipoprotein
free cholesterol
phospholipid
triglyceride
cholesteryl ester

Fig. 4.13 Structure of a lipoprotein particle. Lipoproteins are complexes of lipids and proteins. They have a triglyceride and cholesterol ester middle and a polar coat, made up of phospholipids, apoproteins, and unesterified cholesterol. (Reproduced with permission from Gaw et al, 1999.)

The protein concentration of plasma is 60–80 g/L and is made up of mainly albumin, globulin, and fibrinogen. The plasma proteins synthesized by the liver are summarized in Fig. 4.15.

Fig. 4.14 The density classes of plasma lipoproteins.

Density classes of plasma lipoproteins			
Class	Abbreviation	Sources	Mean diameter (nm)
Chylomicrons	CHYLO	Intestine	500
Very low density lipoproteins	VLDL	Liver	43
Intermediate density lipoproteins	IDL	Catabolism of very low density lipoproteins and chylomicrons	27
Low-density lipoproteins	LDL	Catabolism of very low density lipoproteins	22
High-density lipoproteins	HDL	Catabolism of chylomicrons and very low density lipoproteins; liver and intestine	8

Plasma proteins synthesized by the liver	
Protein	Function
Albumin	Maintain colloid osmotic pressure Transport of hydrophobic substances e.g. bilirubin, hormones, fatty acids, drugs
Lipoprotein	Transport of lipids in the blood
Transferrin	Carrier molecule for iron
Caeruloplasmin	Carrier molecule for copper
Globulins (not γ-globulins)	Antibody functions Transport of lipids, Fe, or Cu in the blood
α_1-antitrypsin	Protein inhibitor of the enzyme trypsin
α_1-fetoprotein	Secreted by yolk sac and embryonic liver epithelial cells In adults is produced by proliferating liver cells and can be used as an indicator of liver cancer
Fibrinogen	Blood clotting factors
Prothrombin	
Factors V, VII, IX, X, XII (not VIII)	
Complement cascade proteins	Immune function upregulators and coordinators Inflammatory functions

Fig. 4.15 Plasma proteins synthesized by the liver.

The liver stores folate and converts it to its active form, tetrahydrofolate. Folate is needed as a coenzyme for the transfer of 1-carbon groups and its deficiency also leads to megaloblastic anaemia, but more quickly than vitamin B_{12} deficiency because body stores of folate are only sufficient for a few months. Folate deficiency in early pregnancy may also lead to neural-tube defects in the fetus. Dietary deficiency of folate is much more common than vitamin B_{12} deficiency, and it is seen in alcoholics and others on a poor diet or suffering from a severe illness where folate utilization is increased (e.g. in cancer).

In general, a deficiency of any substance may result from:
- Increased utilization.
- Increased excretion.
- Decreased manufacture.
- Decreased absorption.

Drug and hormone metabolism

The liver metabolizes drugs and hormones via biotransformation in three stages:
- Phase I (oxidation).
- Phase II (conjugation).
- Phase III (elimination).

Phase I reactions often produce more active metabolites of the drug (it can change the pro-drug into the active drug). Phase II reactions make the drug more water soluble, to facilitate phase III. Phase III occurs via ATPase pumps.

Phase I reactions
The mixed function oxygenase system of the smooth endoplasmic reticulum catalyses oxidation reactions. Several enzymes are involved, most notably cytochrome P_{450}. A large family of cytochrome P_{450} exists to cope with the diversity of toxins.

Oxidation may also be carried out by other enzymes such as xanthine oxidase and monoamine oxidase, present in other tissues as well as the liver.

Reductive reactions also involve microsomal enzymes, but they are less common than oxidative ones.

A number of drugs induce microsomal enzymes, affecting the metabolism of other drugs taken at the same time, and this should be borne in mind when deciding what dose to prescribe.

Notable examples of enzyme-inducing drugs include phenobarbitone, ethanol, and phenylbutazone.

Phase II reactions

A number of groups are conjugated with drugs or their metabolites in the liver, including glucuronyl, acetyl, methyl, glycyl, sulphate, and glutamyl groups, of which glucuronyl is the most common.

Conjugation is important in the metabolism of paracetamol. It is inactivated by conjugation to form a glucuronide or sulphate, but the liver has a limited capacity. If the normal conjugation pathway is saturated, mixed-function oxidases form a toxic metabolite instead. The toxic metabolite is itself inactivated by conjugation with glutathione, but stores of glutathione are limited.

In paracetamol overdose, the saturation of liver enzymes and depletion of glutathione lead to liver necrosis and damage to kidney tubules by toxic metabolites. Treatment is with acetylcysteine, which increases the formation of glutathione, or with methionine.

Phase III reactions

The elimination of conjugated substances is via the blood, which then results in excretion through the kidneys, or via bile through the intestines.

ATPase pumps are required to actively transport the substance out of the hepatocyte. Some pumps are specific for the conjugating molecule (e.g. glutathione).

Some drugs are rapidly inactivated by the liver (e.g. propranolol). The amount of active drug reaching the circulation is reduced and the drug is said to undergo significant first-pass metabolism. Drug metabolism in the liver is summarized in Fig. 4.16.

Paracetamol has a narrow therapeutic index (the difference between a beneficial and a toxic dose is small), and accidental or deliberate paracetamol overdose is common.
Damage to the liver is not immediate and patients often wake up a few hours after large overdoses thinking they are fine, and do not seek help. Symptoms of liver necrosis develop later (often too late for treatment to be effective) and death may follow.

Protection

The portal blood supply to the liver allows for toxins and microorganisms to be filtered out before the blood returns to the systemic circulation. This protects the rest of the body from any harmful substances that may have breached the gut defence

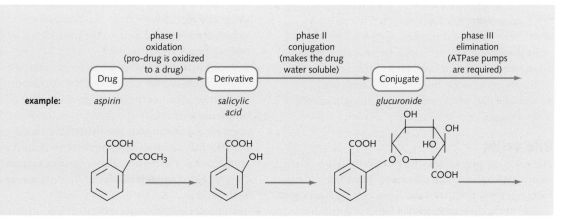

Fig. 4.16 Summary of drug metabolism in the liver. (Adapted from Rang et al, 1999.)

mechanisms. Kupffer cells in the sinusoids facilitate this, via phagocytosis.

Haematopoiesis

In embryonic life, the liver is the main site of haematopoiesis. This occurs from the 2nd month to the 7th month, but ceases before birth.

By five months of gestation, the bone marrow is supplementing the liver in this function.

Between conception and the 2nd month, haematopoiesis takes place in the yolk sac. The liver and spleen can resume their haematopoietic role (extramedullary haematopoiesis) if necessary.

Bile production and function

Bile is a greenish-yellow liquid produced by the liver to:

- Eliminate endogenous and exogenous substances from the liver.
- Emulsify fats in the small intestine and facilitate their digestion and absorption.

Bile consists of bile acids, cholesterol, phospholipids, bile pigments (bilirubin and biliverdin), electrolytes (Na^+, K^+, Ca^{2+}, Cl^-, HCO_3^-) and water.

Waste products found in bile include cholesterol and the bile pigments, bilirubin and biliverdin, which give bile its colour.

Bile passes out of the liver through the bile ducts, and it is concentrated and stored in the gall bladder. During and after a meal, it is excreted from the gall bladder by contraction and passes into the duodenum through the common bile duct.

Most of the bile acids are reabsorbed from the terminal ileum and recycled by the liver (Fig. 4.13). Bile pigments are normally excreted in the faeces, which they colour dark brown.

Reabsorption through enterohepatic recirculation means we only need a small pool of bile acids. Normally about 250–500 mg of bile acids are produced a day, which replaces the amount excreted in the faeces.

Bile acids

Bile acids are detergents which emulsify lipids. They have a hydrophobic and a hydrophilic end, and they form micelles in aqueous solutions.

Bile acids are synthesized in hepatocytes from cholesterol and excreted into bile. They account for approximately 50% of the dry weight of bile.

The rate-limiting step in the production of bile acids is catalysed by cholesterol-7α-hydroxylase.

The principal primary bile acids are cholic acid and chenodeoxycholic acid. They are made more soluble by conjugation with taurine or glycine.

Intestinal bacteria convert them into the secondary bile acids: deoxycholic acid (from cholic acid) and lithocholic acid (from chenodeoxycholic acid) by 7α-decarboxylation.

Of the bile acids excreted into the intestine, 95% are reabsorbed (mostly in the terminal ileum) and recycled by the liver. The total pool of bile acids is recirculated six to eight times a day.

Bile acids are taken up into hepatocytes from the blood by:

- An Na^+-dependent facilitated transport for conjugated bile acids.
- Anion exchange of unconjugated bile acids for OH^- or HCO_3^- ions.
- Simple diffusion of unconjugated bile acids.

Functions of bile acids

The main functions of bile acids are:

- Triglyceride assimilation—bile acids emulsify lipids with the aid of lecithin (found in high concentrations in bile) and break them down to 1 μm diameter droplets. This provides a large surface area for digestive enzymes to act on.
- Lipid transport—bile acids form mixed micelles with the products of lipid digestion and facilitate transport to the brush border, where they are absorbed.
- Bile flow induction—bile acids stimulate the flow of bile by osmotically attracting water and electrolytes as they are secreted. It is also thought that some bile acids are secreted in an unconjugated form. They are absorbed without water and electrolytes from the bile ducts to be quickly carried back to the liver for resecretion.
- Regulation of bile acid synthesis—normal reabsorption of bile acids from the intestines inhibits hepatic synthesis of bile acids. Not all bile acids are equally effective: chenodeoxycholic acid and lithocholic acid significantly reduce cholic acid formation. It is thought that the feedback mechanism acts on the rate limiting step involving cholesterol 7α-hydroxylase.
- Water and electrolyte secretion—if bile acids are present in the colon, they stimulate water and electrolyte secretion. This can result in diarrhoea.

A deficiency of bile acids results in malabsorption of fat.

Bile pigments

The principal pigment in bile is bilirubin, which is yellow and gives bile its colour.

Most bilirubin is formed by the breakdown of haemoglobin from worn-out red cells (Fig. 4.17), but about 15% results from the breakdown of other haem-containing proteins such as myoglobin, cytochromes, and catalases.

Bilirubin is insoluble, and it is transported to the liver in the plasma, bound to albumin. There, most of it dissociates from albumin, and it is extracted from the blood in the sinusoids by the hepatocytes. It binds to cytoplasmic proteins in the hepatocytes, and it is conjugated with glucuronic acid to form bilirubin diglucuronide (a reaction catalysed by glucuronyl transferase, found mainly in smooth endoplasmic reticulum).

Bilirubin diglucuronide is water soluble, unlike bilirubin, and it is actively transported against its

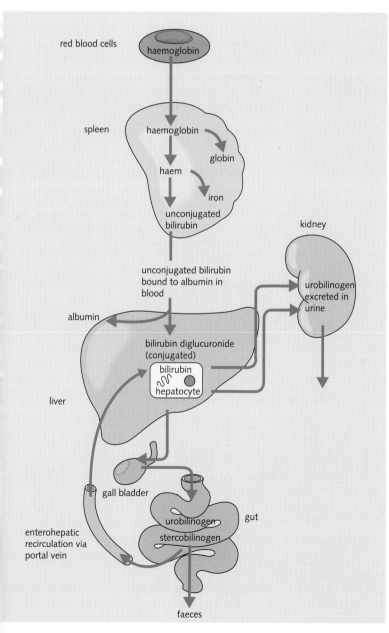

Fig. 4.17 Production and fate of bilirubin. The daily output of bile is between 700 and 1200 mL and bile acids are the major organic component. These, however, are recycled after use. During the breakdown of haemoglobin (which produces iron, bilirubin, and globin), the iron and globin are recycled too.

concentration gradient into the bile canaliculi. A small amount escapes into the blood, where it is transported bound to albumin, and it is then excreted in the urine.

The intestinal mucosa is permeable to unconjugated bilirubin and to urobilinogen (a colourless derivative of bilirubin produced by intestinal flora); some of the bile pigments and urobilinogens are reabsorbed from the gut into the portal circulation. The intestinal mucosa is relatively impermeable to conjugated bilirubin.

Some of the reabsorbed substances are excreted again by the liver but small amounts of urobilinogens enter the general circulation, and they are excreted in the urine.

Figs 4.17 and 4.18 summarize the production and excretion of bilirubin.

Control of bile production
Hepatocytes
There are three different mechanisms of control of bile production (Fig. 4.19):

- Bile acid dependent.
- Bile acid independent.
- Intrahepatic bile duct dependent.

The bile acid-dependent mechanism describes how water and electrolytes passively follow the movement of bile acids, which have been actively transported into the bile canaliculi and ducts. Movement of water and electrolytes is achieved by tight junctions between hepatocytes.

The tight junctions can become more permeable in response to bile acids, vasopressin, adrenaline, and angiotensin II.

It is thought that bile acids are secreted across the canalicular membrane into bile by protein-mediated facilitated transport, driven partly by the electrochemical difference across the membrane.

The bile acid-independent mechanism involves active transport of water and electrolytes across the

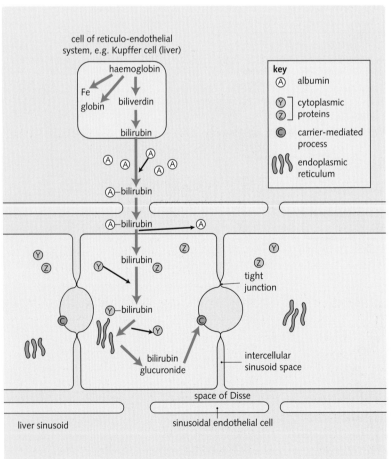

Fig. 4.18 The fate of bilirubin after processing in the hepatocyte. (From Sanford PA. *Digestive System Physiology*, 2nd edn. London: Edward Arnold, 1992. Reproduced by permission of Hodder/Arnold Publishers.)

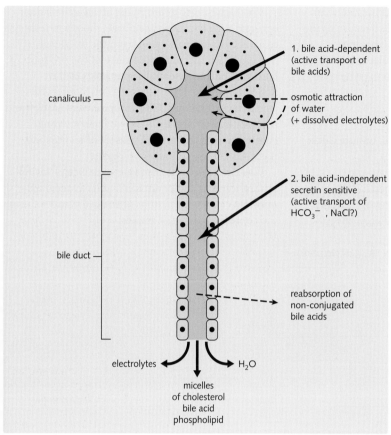

canaliculus

1. bile acid-dependent (active transport of bile acids)

osmotic attraction of water (+ dissolved electrolytes)

2. bile acid-independent secretin sensitive (active transport of HCO_3^-, NaCl?)

bile duct

reabsorption of non-conjugated bile acids

electrolytes ← → H_2O

micelles of cholesterol bile acid phospholipid

Fig. 4.19 The control of bile acid synthesis and secretion. This involves bile acid-dependent, bile acid-independent and intrahepatic bile duct-dependent control. (From Sanford, PA. *Digestive System Physiology*, 2nd edn. London: Edward Arnold, 1992. Reproduced by permission of Hodder/Arnold Publishers.)

hepatocyte membrane. This system occurs in animals, but not in humans.

The intrahepatic bile duct mechanism describes the aqueous secretion that makes up 50% of the total volume of bile.

The solution is secreted by epithelial cells lining the bile ducts, and it is isotonic, with sodium and potassium concentrations similar to those of plasma. It has a higher concentration of bicarbonate and a lower concentration of chloride.

Control of bile acid synthesis and secretion

Cholecystokinin increases the rate of bile acid secretion during the intestinal phase of digestion.

High concentrations of bile acids in the portal blood stimulate bile acid secretion and inhibit its synthesis during the intestinal phase.

Conversely, low levels of bile acids in the portal blood during the interdigestive phase stimulate the synthesis and inhibit the secretion of bile acids.

Secretin stimulates secretion by the bile duct epithelium and this effect is strongly potentiated by

cholecystokinin. Secretin alone has no effect on the concentration of bile acids in bile.

Role of the gall bladder
Functions of the gall bladder

The primary functions of the gall bladder are the concentration and storage of bile.

In the fasting state, the sphincter of Oddi (Fig. 4.4) is contracted, but it relaxes, and the gall bladder contracts releasing its contents, in response to stimulation during and after meals to aid digestion (Fig. 4.20). However, it is not essential for life.

Cholecystectomy is a common operation, following which bile is discharged into the duodenum at a constant, slow rate, and this allows the digestion of moderate amounts of fat in the diet.

Concentration of bile

The gall bladder stores bile secreted by the liver and has a capacity of about 35 mL (range 15–60 mL).

Stored bile is 5–20 times more concentrated than that secreted by the liver, principally because of the active transport of Na^+ from the gall bladder epithelium into the lateral intracellular spaces (Fig. 4.21). Water passively follows the active transport of Na^+ ions.

Gall bladder contraction

Gall bladder emptying begins several minutes after the start of a meal.

During the cephalic phase, the taste and smell of food and the presence of food in the mouth and pharynx cause impulses in branches of the vagus nerve that increase emptying of the gall bladder.

Distension of the stomach during the gastric phase also cause impulses in the vagus.

The highest rate of emptying of the gall bladder occurs during the intestinal phase, mostly in response to cholecystokinin released from the duodenal mucosa as a result of the presence of the products of fat digestion and essential amino acids in the duodenum.

Cholecystokinin (CCK) enters the circulation and reaches the gall bladder, where it causes strong contractions of the smooth muscle of its wall and relaxation of the sphincter of Oddi.

Gastrin, which has the same sequence of amino acid residues as cholecystokinin at its C-terminal, may also cause contractions of the gall bladder during the cephalic and gastric phases.

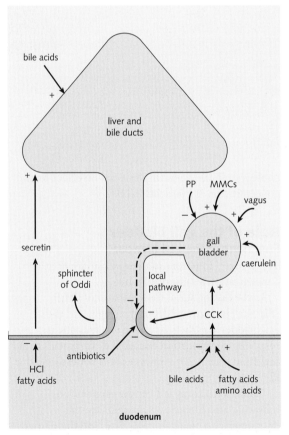

Fig. 4.20 Mechanisms controlling the secretion of bile into the duodenum. PP, pancreatic polypeptide; MMCs, migrating motor complexes; CCK, cholecystokinin. (From Sanford PA. *Digestive System Physiology*, 2nd edn. London: Edward Arnold, 1992. Reproduced by permission of Hodder/Arnold Publishers.)

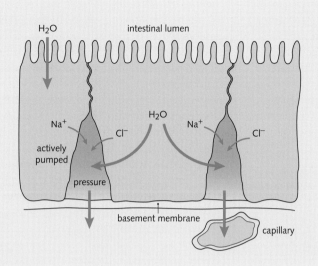

Fig. 4.21 The mechanism by which bile is concentrated in the gall bladder. The epithelial cells in the gall bladder mucosa have large lateral intercellular spaces near the basement membrane and tight junctions at the apices. Na^+ ions are coupled with Cl^- ions and actively transported into the intercellular spaces. Water passively diffuses into the spaces as it follows the osmotic gradient set up by the active transport of ions.

- Briefly describe the anatomy of the liver and biliary tract.
- How does the liver and biliary tract develop in the embryo?
- How can the arrangement of the liver be described?
- What are the 'zones' of the liver, and how do they differ?
- List each cell type found in the liver and what its function is.
- Describe the route of a digestion product if it were to move from the blood in the hepatic portal vein, into a hepatocyte. (Name all the cells it would come across and where they would be found.)
- Describe the tissues in the biliary tract and gall bladder.
- What features of the gall bladder epithelia make it so specialized for absorption?
- What are the functions of the liver?
- Compare and contrast the periportal and centrilobular zones in terms of their role in metabolism.
- How are lipids metabolized?
- How are carbohydrates metabolized?
- How are proteins metabolized?
- What are the plasma proteins synthesized by the liver, and what are their functions?
- Which vitamins are stored in the liver? What happens with a deficiency in vitamin B_{12} or folate?
- Briefly describe the phases of drug metabolism.
- Briefly describe what happens if someone takes a paracetamol overdose.
- What are the sites of haematopoiesis in embryonic life?
- What are the constituents of bile, and what are its functions?
- Describe the synthesis of bile acids. How are secondary bile acids made, and what are the functions of bile acids?
- How are bile pigments produced, and how are they ultimately excreted from the body?
- Describe the control of bile production.
- What are the functions of the gall bladder and how does it achieve them?
- What controls gall bladder contraction?

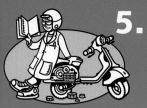

5. Disorders of the Liver and Biliary Tract

General aspects of hepatic damage

Patterns of hepatic injury

The liver is essential to life, and it has a remarkable capacity to regenerate. Damage from whatever cause (apart from trauma) results in similar pathology, usually an inflammatory reaction, some attempt at regeneration, and, if unsuccessful, cell death.

Damage may be acute or chronic, and the same agents may result in either.

The major causes of acute liver failure are:

- Viral infections.
- Injury from drugs.
- Injury from toxins.
- Injury from metabolic disturbances.
- Hypoxia.
- Tumours (usually metastases).

These can all produce diffuse liver injury. The pattern of injury may help identify the cause.

Necrosis

Hepatic necrosis can be described in a number of ways (Fig. 5.1):

- Apoptotic necrosis (Councilman's bodies) describes necrosis of individual hepatocytes. It is caused by acute viral hepatitis. Complete recovery with no long-term sequelae is the norm.
- Hydropic necrosis occurs when hepatocytes swell up and rupture.
- Focal necrosis describes small groups of necrotic hepatocytes. Macrophages and lymphocytes tend to accumulate around them in an effort to localize damage or infection. This type of necrosis is seen in acute viral or drug-induced hepatitis.
- Zonal necrosis describes hepatocytes within a particular zone, that are affected. Haemodynamic necrosis is a type of zonal necrosis because concentric bands of necrotic hepatocytes are seen around the central vein. This occurs in cardiac failure, stasis of hepatic venous blood, and paracetamol poisoning (centrilobular). Zone three is most affected by necrosis, and necrosis of zone two is rare, but seen in yellow fever. Coagulative or ischaemic necrosis involves a large number of hepatocytes in a band of necrosis, because zone three is most likely to be affected.

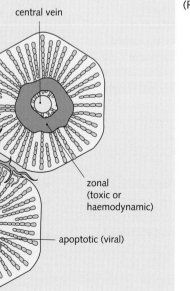

Fig. 5.1 Patterns of hepatic necrosis. (Redrawn from Underwood, 1996.)

79

- Confluent bridging necrosis involves a large number of hepatocytes in a 'band' of necrosis stretching between hepatic venules (central to central) or between hepatic venules and portal tracts (central to portal). This pattern of necrosis is caused by severe drug or viral induced hepatitis.
- Piecemeal necrosis occurs in chronic liver disease. It describes the necrosis of hepatocytes at the interface between the parenchyma and fibrous tissue. Lymphocytes, particularly plasma cells, infiltrate the area.
- Submassive or panacinar necrosis affects the entire acinus. Massive necrosis affects the entire liver. Both are caused by viral or drug induced injury. Massive necrosis can result in fulminant hepatic failure.

Degeneration

Degeneration is less serious than necrosis, and it is characterized by swollen, oedematous hepatocytes (ballooning degeneration) with irregularly clumped cytoplasm and large clear spaces. Diffuse, foamy, swollen hepatocytes suggest cholestasis.

Inflammation

In inflammation of the liver (hepatitis), an influx of acute or chronic inflammatory cells may occur secondary to hepatocellular necrosis.

Regeneration

Regeneration is the norm following injury. Hyperplasia and hypertrophy are common after injury. Hepatocyte proliferation results in a thickening of the cords radiating out from the central vein. The architecture may be disturbed unless the connective tissue framework remained intact.

The normal liver can restore its original weight, even if up to two thirds of the liver is removed. This allows for recovery from numerous injuries and even extensive surgical removal of tumours.

Fibrosis

Fibrosis from inflammation or a direct toxic insult may occur around the portal tracts, the central vein or within the spaces of Disse, disrupting the normal architecture and interfering with liver function. In severe cases, cirrhosis results.

Cirrhosis

Cirrhosis is a diffuse and irreversible condition that results from necrosis of hepatocytes followed by the formation of regeneration nodules separated by fibrosis.

The process causes architectural disturbances and interferes with normal liver blood flow and function. Portal hypertension, liver failure, and hepatocyte carcinoma are all possible sequelae.

Cirrhosis may be:
- Micronodular (nodules less than 3 mm in diameter).
- Macronodular (diameters greater than 3 mm).
- Mixed (both forms coexisting).

The causes of cirrhosis are summarized in Fig. 5.2. The consequences of cirrhosis are summarized in Fig. 5.3.

Treatment of cirrhosis

After performing a number of investigations, including liver function tests, liver biopsy, ultrasound, and computed tomography (CT) imaging, the severity and type of cirrhosis can be determined.

Treatment depends on the diagnosis and any complications that accompany the cirrhosis. Certain drugs are contraindicated in liver disease, and these should be avoided.

Patients require 6-monthly checks; involving ultrasound and serum α-fetoprotein measurements.

Causes of cirrhosis
Unknown (10% of cases)
Alcohol (50% of cases)
Hepatitis B (±D) and C
Iron overload (haemochromatosis)
Gall stones
Autoimmune liver disease
Wilson's disease (leading to deposition of copper in the liver)
α_1-antitrypsin deficiency
Type IV glycogenosis
Galactosaemia
Tyrosinaemia
Biliary cholestasis
Budd–Chiari syndrome
Drugs (e.g. methotrexate)
Biliary cirrhosis
Hepatic venous congestion
Cystic fibrosis
Glycogen storage disease

Fig. 5.2 Causes of cirrhosis.

Consequences of liver failure	
Feature	**Explanation**
Oedema	Decreased synthesis of albumin causing a reduced oncotic pressure gradient across the capillary wall and increased passage of fluid
Portal hypertension	Disturbed blood flow through the liver
Haematemesis	Ruptured oesophageal varices
Coma	Brain oedema and reduced elimination of false neurotransmitters
Ascites	Hypoalbuminaemia, portal hypertension and secondary hyperaldosteronism
Spider naevi and gynaecomastia	Reduced metabolism and excretion of oestrogen
Purpura and bleeding	Reduced synthesis of clotting factors
Increased infections	Reduced phagocytosis by Kupffer cells in the liver
Hepatic carcinoma	Hyperplasia caused by cirrhosis especially macromodular type

Fig. 5.3 Consequences of liver failure.

These will enable early detection of hepatocellular carcinoma development.

Portal hypertension

The normal pressure in the hepatic portal vein is about 7 mmHg, but this increases in portal hypertension.

The causes of portal hypertension may be classified as:

- Prehepatic—a blockage of the portal vein before the liver.
- Hepatic—a disruption or change of the liver architecture.
- Posthepatic—a blockage in the venous system after the liver.

Prehepatic causes include:

- Portal vein thrombosis.
- Arteriovenous fistula.
- Increased splenic bloodflow, secondary to splenomegaly or arteriovenous fistulae.

Hepatic causes include:

- Cirrhosis.
- Schistosomiasis.
- Sarcoidosis.
- Miliary tuberculosis (granulomata).
- Massive fatty change.
- Nodular regenerative hyperplasia.
- Alcoholic hepatitis.

Posthepatic causes include:

- Budd–Chiari syndrome (a rare condition caused by hepatic vein obstruction, sometimes associated with the oral contraceptive).
- Veno-occlusive disease.
- Severe right-sided heart failure (very rare with modern cardiac treatment).
- Constrictive pericarditis (very rare with modern cardiac treatment).

Cirrhosis results in disruption of the normal liver architecture, which increases hepatic vascular resistance and causes intrahepatic arteriovenous shunting. It is the most common cause of portal hypertension in the UK. Worldwide, cirrhosis due to viral hepatitis, is the main cause of portal hypertension.

Complications of portal hypertension

Many patients with portal hypertension are assymptomatic, and they only present with splenomegaly. Clinical features usually present once complications have begun. These include haematemesis or melaena (from ruptured gastro-oesophageal varices), ascites, and encephalopathy.

If the portal pressure rises above 12 mmHg, then dilatation of the venous system causes collateral vessels to form. They are found mainly at the gastro-oesophageal junction, rectum, diaphragm, left renal vein, the retroperitoneum, and the umbilical region of the anterior abdominal wall (via the umbilical vein).

Oesophageal varices can rupture, causing haematemesis and sometimes fatal consequences (oesophageal varices are described in Chapter 2). Enlargement of veins at other sites of portosystemic anastomoses may also occur forming caput medusae around the umbilicus, and haemorrhoids in the rectum.

A caput medusae at the umbilicus is so called because it looks like the serpents on the head of Medusa!

Ascites is the abnormal collection of fluid in the peritoneal cavity, and it is a common complication of cirrhosis.

It may form as a result of:

- Portal hypertension, which brings about a local hydrostatic pressure increase, resulting in an increased production of lymph in the hepatic and splanchnic regions. Transudation of the fluid into the peritoneal cavity causes ascites.
- Low serum albumin levels (hypoalbuminaemia), due to decreased liver synthesis, causing a low plasma oncotic pressure.
- Na^+ and water retention, due to peripheral arterial vasodilatation. This reduces effective blood volume and activates the renin–angiotensin system and sympathetic nervous system (both upregulate water and salt retention).

All three mechanisms can occur simultaneously. Clinically, ascites may be detected by abdominal swelling, some abdominal pain, a shifting dullness, and a fluid thrill. Many patients also have peripheral oedema, due to hypoalbuminaemia.

It should be managed by reducing sodium intake and increasing renal sodium excretion with diuretics (spironolactone and amiloride). Fluid may be removed by paracentesis (via a needle through the abdominal wall). However, there is a risk that fluid will accumulate again in the peritoneal cavity at the expense of the systemic circulation. This leads to shock, so intravenous albumin should also be given.

A peritoneovenous shunt (a catheter from the peritoneal cavity into the internal jugular vein) may be used to return the fluid to the systemic circulation. This is used in rare cases when diuretic therapy fails.

Portosystemic anastomoses

These occur at four sites in the body (Fig. 5.4):

(a) The lower end of the oesophagus, between the left gastric vein (portal) and the azygos vein (systemic).

(b) The lower part of the anal canal, between the superior (portal), middle, and inferior (systemic) rectal veins.

(c) The umbilical region of the anterior abdominal wall, between the epigastric veins and the paraumbilical veins in the falciform ligament of the liver.

(d) The bare areas of the gastrointestinal tract and its related organs, e.g. veins between the bare area of the liver and the diaphragm.

These anastomoses may enlarge if the portal vein is obstructed by a thrombus or the venous flow through the liver is impeded by cirrhosis.

Enlargement may result in oesophageal varices, haemorrhoids, and caput medusae (at the umbilicus).

Haemorrhoids are the most common cause of rectal bleeding, and they may also cause pruritus ani. If mild, they need no treatment. Diagnosis is by proctoscopy. Oesophageal varices are diagnosed by endoscopy. Haemorrhoids, like oesophageal varices, can be banded to prevent bleeding. Oesophageal varices are clinically the most important cause of bleeding in portal hypertension.

Splenomegaly

Splenomegaly is the term used to describe an enlarged spleen. It can be massive (extending into the right iliac fossa), and it has a large number of causes.

Normally the spleen weighs about 7 oz (200 g); it is oval in shape and found between the 9th and 11th ribs. It plays an important role in immune defence and the removal of expired or abnormal blood cells. The spleen normally has a rapid blood transit time of about 2 min.

Portal hypertension may cause moderate congestive splenomegaly, as may thrombosis of the extrahepatic portion of the portal vein or of the splenic vein.

A raised pressure in the inferior vena cava may be transmitted to the spleen through the portal vein, and is a cause of posthepatic splenomegaly. Ascites and hepatomegaly are also usually present.

More common causes of posthepatic splenomegaly include decompensated right-sided heart failure and pulmonary or tricuspid valve disease.

Splenomegaly may cause abdominal discomfort, and an enlarged spleen may occasionally rupture following minor trauma. Splenomegaly is easily detected on examination of the abdomen, as it is dull to percussion.

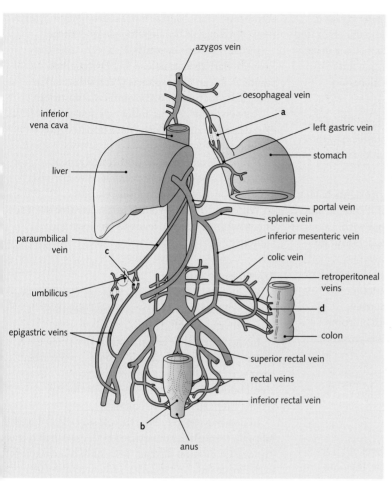

Fig. 5.4 Diagram showing the sites of portosystemic anastomoses, indicated by a–d.

azygos vein
oesophageal vein
inferior vena cava
a
left gastric vein
stomach
liver
portal vein
splenic vein
paraumbilical vein
inferior mesenteric vein
colic vein
c
retroperitoneal veins
umbilicus
d
epigastric veins
colon
superior rectal vein
rectal veins
inferior rectal vein
b
anus

Do not forget that other non-hepatic causes of splenomegaly include infections and inflammatory and haematological diseases, such as TB, infectious mononucleosis, septic shock, malaria, rheumatoid arthritis, and haemolytic anaemia.

Jaundice and cholestasis

Jaundice (icterus) is a clinical sign resulting from plasma levels of bilirubin exceeding 45 μmol/L, and it presents as a yellow pigmentation of skin, sclera, and mucosa. The colour of the sclera is the best indicator, but it must be examined in good white light!

Jaundice may be classified as:

- Prehepatic (haemolytic).
- Hepatic (congenital and hepatocellular).
- Posthepatic (obstructive or cholestatic).

Prehepatic jaundice

Bilirubin is formed from the breakdown of haemoglobin and, normally, it is conjugated with glucuronic acid by hepatocytes when it reaches the liver. This makes it more soluble. Unconjugated bilirubin only remains in the circulation when the liver is unable to conjugate all the bilirubin t hat is delivered to it. Unconjugated bilirubin is not soluble, and it cannot be excreted in the urine.

However, increased haemolysis may cause an excess of bilirubin, and this can overcome the liver's capacity to conjugate it.

Therefore, haemolytic jaundice results in raised levels of unconjugated bilirubin. Because unconjugated bilirubin is not soluble, it does not pass into the urine, so this type of jaundice is often called 'acholuric jaundice'. The urinary urobilinogen is increased.

Hepatic jaundice

This type of jaundice includes the congenital hyper-bilirubinaemias and hepatocellular jaundice, as the problems leading to jaundice all occur at the hepatocyte.

Gilbert's syndrome

This congenital disorder is caused by patients having a reduced amount of the enzyme, UDP-glucuronosyl transferase, which conjugates bilirubin with glucuronic acid. Other abnormalities in bilirubin handling have also been found.

This affects between 2% and 7% of the population, and it is not a serious disease. The reticulocyte (immature red blood cell) count is normal, there is only a slight increase in serum bilirubin (unconjugated), and the syndrome is asymptomatic. Treatment is not usually required.

Crigler–Najjar syndrome

This is an extremely rare disease that has two types:
- Type I (autosomal recessive)
- Type II (autosomal recessive).

Type II patients have a decreased level of UDP-glucuronosyl transferase and, therefore, they can survive into adulthood. This form is thought to be very similar to Gilbert's syndrome. Type I patients lack the enzyme altogether, and they do not survive, unless they undergo liver transplantation. Both types of patient have high serum levels of unconjugated bilirubin.

Dubin–Johnson syndrome

This is an autosomal recessive disorder where the liver fails to excrete conjugated bilirubin (caused by a mutation in the *c*analicular *m*ultispecific *o*rganic *a*nion *t*ransporter; 'CMOAT').

This results in jaundice, and the liver appears black because of deposits of a melanin-like pigment.

Rotor syndrome

This is very similar to Dubin–Johnson syndrome, with a defect in intracellular binding proteins for bilirubin. There is no pigment deposit.

Hepatocellular jaundice

Damage to the hepatocytes and the intrahepatic biliary tree leads to an increase in both unconjugated and conjugated serum levels of bilirubin. There is an increase in clotting time, serum alanine aminotransferase, and serum aspartate aminotransferase, because of the hepatocellular damage.

Viruses, such as hepatitis A, B, C, E, and the Epstein–Barr virus, can lead to hepatocellular jaundice, as can leptospirosis (Weil's disease), a bacterial infection spread by infected rat urine!

Autoimmune or drug-induced damage, as well as cirrhosis and tumours, can cause hepatocellular jaundice.

Haemochromatosis, an autosomal recessive disorder of iron metabolism can lead to cirrhosis, jaundice, and liver failure if untreated.

Wilson's disease, an autosomal recessive disorder of copper metabolism, leads to cirrhosis and jaundice.

Posthepatic jaundice

Normally, conjugated bilirubin passes from the liver to the gall bladder where it is stored and then released into the duodenum.

In the terminal ileum, intestinal flora convert it first to urobilinogen (some of which is reabsorbed and excreted in the urine) and then to stercobilinogen, which is excreted in the faeces (giving them their brown colour).

In posthepatic jaundice, the passage of conjugated bilirubin through the biliary tree is blocked, and it leaks into the circulation instead. It is soluble and excreted in the urine (making it dark). However, the faeces are deprived of their stercobilinogen and are pale.

There is no problem with the synthesis of any of the bile products in posthepatic obstructive (cholestatic) jaundice; only its release into the duodenum. Therefore, bile salts, along with conjugated bilirubin, escape into the circulation, and this causes itching (pruritus).

Causes of obstructive, cholestatic jaundice include gall stones, biliary stricture, congenital biliary atresia (complete blockage from birth), carcinoma of the pancreas or bile ducts, and pancreatitis.

The symptoms and causes of jaundice are summarized in Fig. 5.5.

Further investigations

Investigations other than liver function tests, a full blood count, serum bilirubin levels, virology screening, and urinanalysis that can be performed are:
- Ultrasound.
- Endoscopic retrograde cholangio-pancreatography (ERCP).
- Liver biopsy.

Causes and signs of jaundice		
Type of jaundice	Cause	Signs
Prehepatic	Haemolysis Ineffective erythropoiesis	Increased concentrations of unconjugated bilirubin (no bilirubin in the urine because it is insoluble)
Hepatic (congenital and hepatocellular)	• Gilbert's syndrome • Crigler–Najjar syndrome • Rotor syndrome • Dubin–Johnson syndrome • Viral infection, (e.g. Hep. A,B,C,E, and EBV) • Cirrhosis • Drugs • Autoimmune disease • Weil's disease • Wilson's disease	• Increased clotting time • Increased ALT and AST • Hepatocellular damage
Posthepatic (obstructive or cholestatic)	• Pancreatitis • Primary biliary cirrhosis • Gall stones • Drugs • Carcinoma (of head of pancreas or bile duct) • Lymphoma (with enlarged lymph nodes in the porta hepatis) • Biliary stricture • Congenital biliary atresia	• Dark urine (with bilirubin, not urobilinogen) • γ-GT and AP increase (canalicular enzymes raised due to damage to the biliary tree) • Pale stools • Itching

Fig. 5.5 The classification of the different types of jaundice, showing the causes and symptoms or clinical signs. (AST, serum aspartate aminotransferase; ALT, serum alanine aminotransferase; EBV, Epstein–Barr virus; γ-GT, γ-glutamyl transferase; AP, alkaline phosphatase.)

• Magnetic resonance cholangio-pancreatography (MRCP).

Lack of bile salts and, therefore, a lack of fat absorption causes the slow clotting time associated with jaundice. Vitamin K (a clotting factor) is a fat-soluble vitamin, which requires fat for absorption from the gut. In jaundice: decreased fat absorption = low vitamin K concentrations = slow clotting.

Hepatic failure

Despite its large capacity to regenerate after injury, the liver can sometimes fail due to severe acute liver injury (e.g. in viral hepatitis or drug toxicity), or chronic liver disease (e.g. cirrhosis).

The liver has a large number of vital functions, and its failure to perform these can lead to systemic consequences, from neurological problems to decreased coagulation or renal failure.

Hepatic encephalopathy

This is a neurological disorder caused by metabolic failure of the hepatocytes and the shunting of blood around the liver (due to cirrhosis or after portacaval anastomosis).

It may occur in both chronic and acute liver failure. It results in the exposure of the brain to abnormal metabolites, causing oedema and astrocyte changes.

Normally the liver eliminates the toxic nitrogenous products of gut bacteria. In liver failure, their elimination is reduced and some of them act as false transmitters (mimicking the normal neurotransmitters of the central nervous system). This results in central nervous system disturbances.

Other factors may play a part in the pathology, including ammonia and electrolyte disturbances, hypotension, changes in vascular permeability, and increased cerebral sensitivity due to the metabolic disturbances.

Symptoms include:
- Disturbances in consciousness (ranging from confusion to coma and death).
- Asterixis (a flapping tremor of outstretched hands).
- Fluctuating neurological signs (muscular rigidity and hyperreflexia).

There is no specific treatment, except to restrict protein intake, treat any infection, empty the bowels of nitrogen containing material, and correct the metabolic and coagulation disturbances. Flumazenil, a benzodiazepine receptor antagonist, can improve the encephalopathy in the short term.

Hepatorenal syndrome

This is the combination of renal failure in a previously normal kidney and severe liver disease. However, kidney function improves dramatically if the liver failure is reversed.

Renal failure is caused by a drop in renal blood flow and glomerular filtration rate, causing a fall in urine output and increased retention of sodium by the kidney. These mechanisms are brought about by upregulation of the renin–angiotensin–aldosterone system, noradrenaline and vasopressin. It may be fatal.

Liver transplantation

Liver transplantation is increasingly used in the treatment of:
- Acute and chronic liver disease.
- Alcoholic liver disease (provided the patient has given up drinking and is well motivated).
- Primary biliary cirrhosis, when serum bilirubin rises above 100 μmol/L.
- Chronic hepatitis B and C.
- Primary metabolic disease (e.g. Wilson's disease and α_1-antitrypsin deficiency).
- Other conditions including sclerosing cholangitis.

Absolute contraindications are human immunodeficiency virus (HIV) infection, active sepsis outside the hepatobiliary tree, and metastatic malignancy. If the patient lacks psychological commitment (as might occur in alcoholic liver disease), then transplantation is not an option. Patients aged over 65 years are not normally considered for surgery.

Most organs are taken from cadavers, but a relative may donate a single lobe to an infant.

The liver is less aggressively rejected than other organs but early (reversible), or late (irreversible) rejection may occur. Acute (cellular), or early rejection occurs within 5–10 days after the transplant. The patient develops pyrexia, general malaise, and abdominal tenderness due to hepatomegaly. This is caused by an inflammatory reaction.

Immunosuppressive therapy works very well in this situation.

Chronic (ductopenic) rejection occurs 6 weeks to 9 months after the transplant. This type of rejection cannot be reversed with immunosuppressive drugs and retransplantation is the only treatment. Graft-versus-host disease is very rare.

Ciclosporin has proved useful, but some patients require immunosuppression for life and they are, therefore, susceptible to opportunistic infection. However, 5 years after the transplant, 20–30% of patients no longer receive immunosuppressants.

Disorders of metabolism

Haemochromatosis (bronze diabetes)

Primary haemochromatosis is an inherited recessive disorder characterized by the absorption of too much iron, which then accumulates in the liver, pancreas, heart, and (to a lesser extent) in other organs, especially those of the endocrine system.

A gene defect on chromosome 6 (the HLA-A3 gene) causes excess absorption of iron from the small intestine even when the iron-binding protein, transferrin, is fully saturated. Iron stores may be many times greater than normal levels, rising from about 1 g to as much as 20 g.

Heterozygotes only have modest increases in absorption and generally they have normal iron stores compared to homozygotes. Symptoms are rare in women of child-bearing age as menstrual losses and pregnancy compensate for the excess iron absorption.

The presenting complaint in men is often loss of libido and hypogonadism, secondary to dysfunction of the pituitary gland. Diabetes occurs in two thirds of all cases.

The clinical features include:
- Liver enlargement.
- Fibrosis and cirrhosis.
- Bronze discolouration of the skin.
- Diabetes mellitus resulting from insufficient production of insulin by the pancreas.

- Cardiac arrythmias and other heart disorders.
- Presentation occurs most often after 40 years of age.

Untreated, the condition may lead to liver failure and primary hepatocellular carcinoma. Early in the disease, iron is deposited in periportal hepatocytes (as haemosiderin) and then in Kupffer cells, bile duct epithelium, and portal tract connective tissue.

Diagnosis is by blood tests (which characteristically show raised ferritin) and liver biopsy showing heavy deposits of iron (as haemosiderin) in hepatocytes.

Treatment is by phlebotomy (venesection), once or twice a week until iron levels return to normal, and then three or four times a year.

Chelation therapy (a drug that complexes with a metal ion for its removal) is very successful in patients who cannot have venesection, due to cardiac disease or anaemia. Desferrioxamine can be given continuously, or as and when required.

Secondary haemochromatosis may result from iron overload (e.g. in thalassaemia patients after repeated blood transfusions) or from excess iron absorption (e.g. in congenital haemolytic anaemias).

Wilson's disease

Wilson's disease (hepatolenticular degeneration) is a rare, autosomal recessive disorder (associated genes on chromosome 13) in which copper accumulates in the liver and the basal ganglia of the brain.

Normally copper is secreted into bile, but in Wilson's disease, biliary copper excretion is low, as is the copper-binding glycoprotein caeruloplasmin. Copper may be secreted into the blood, where it causes episodes of haemolysis.

Signs and symptoms may appear in patients at any age from about 5 years to 50 years, and they include hepatic and neurological abnormalities.

Faint, brown (Kayser–Fleischer) rings may appear in the eye at the junction of the cornea and sclera in Descemet's membrane. They are almost diagnostic.

Diagnosis is by measurement of the copper-containing protein caeruloplasmin in the blood (it is low in Wilson's disease) and by liver biopsy showing an excess of copper. Urinary copper concentrations are normally raised in Wilson's disease.

Treatment is with penicillamine, a chelating agent that binds to copper and enables it to be excreted.

Prognosis depends on the stage at which treatment is begun. If started early, before significant amounts of copper have been deposited, prognosis is good.

Neurological damage may be irreversible, and in hepatic failure or cirrhosis, the only treatment is transplantation.

Alpha$_1$-antitrypsin deficiency

Alpha$_1$-antitrypsin is a serum protein that is produced in the liver and has anti-protease effects. It is part of the *ser*ine *p*rotease *in*hibitors (SERPIN) superfamily. One in ten northern Europeans carry a deficiency gene, which is autosomal dominant in inheritance.

The gene controlling its production is located on chromosome 14 and a number of variants exist, including M, S, and Z alleles. The normal variant is M allele.

Homozygous deficiency occurs in about 1 in 5000 births.

Symptoms include emphysema in about 75% of homozygotes and liver cirrhosis in approximately 10%.

Emphysema is a lung disease characterized by enlargement of alveolar walls and destruction of elastin in the walls. Normally, α_1-antitrypsin inhibits neutrophil elastase in the lungs and prevents the elastase destroying the connective tissue of alveolar walls; in α_1-antitrypsin deficiency this protection is lost.

Liver disease only occurs with mutations, such as the Z allele, where α_1-antitrypsin accumulates by polymerization in hepatocytes, shown by PAS (Periodic Acid–Schiff) positive intracellular globules on liver biopsy. How cirrhosis develops is unknown.

Diagnosis is by measurement of serum α_1-antitrypsin (it is low in deficiency) and by liver biopsy.

Treatment is symptomatic. Patients should be advised to stop smoking.

Reye's syndrome

Reye's syndrome is a rare disorder affecting children up to 15 years of age. It is characterized by acute encephalopathy and infiltration of fatty microvesicles in the liver (steatosis). Symptoms begin as the child is recovering from a mild upper respiratory tract infection, influenza, or varicella. They include vomiting, lethargy, memory loss, disorientation, or delirium.

Seizures, deepening coma, disturbed cardiac rhythm, and cessation of breathing may occur because of swelling of the brain; jaundice and hypoglycaemia may result from liver damage.

The encephalopathy and hepatic microvesicular steatosis are caused by inhibition of β-oxidation and the uncoupling of oxidative phosphorylation in mitochondria. Aspirin has been implicated as a precipitating factor.

There is rapid progression to hepatic failure with neurological deterioration and eventual coma.

Histologically, the liver shows a foamy accumulation of triglycerides and alterations in the mitochondria; this is also seen in the brain.

Treatment is supportive, with corticosteroids and mannitol (to reduce brain swelling) and dialysis or transfusion to correct chemical imbalances resulting from liver damage.

Prognosis is worse in those whose symptoms include seizures, coma, or cessation of breathing. Brain damage or death may occur as a result of brain herniation or hypoxia. Overall mortality is about 50%, mainly due to cerebral oedema.

Neonatal hepatitis

Neonatal hepatitis is the end-result of a range of injurious processes including:

- Congenital infection with rubella.
- Cytomegalovirus and toxoplasmosis.
- α_1-antitrypsin deficiency.
- Tyrosinaemia.
- Cystic fibrosis.
- Storage disorders.
- Galactosaemia.
- Hepatitis A and B viruses.

The histological picture may include multinucleate giant cells and cholestasis or hepatocellular necrosis and inflammatory infiltrates in the portal tracts and lobules. Hyperbilirubinaemia is present.

The condition is often familial, inheritance being autosomal recessive.

It is very difficult to find the precise aetiology behind neonatal hepatitis.

Hyperlipidaemias

Hyperlipidaemias are a group of metabolic disorders characterized by high levels of lipids (chiefly cholesterol, triglycerides, and lipoproteins) in the blood. Several types of hyperlipidaemia have been described, depending on which lipid's levels are raised.

The disorder resulting in hyperlipidaemia can stem from:

- Abnormal expression of genes encoding apoproteins.
- Lipoprotein lipase deficiency.
- Low density lipoprotein (LDL)-receptor defects.

Hyperlipidaemia is closely associated with atheroma and cardiovascular disease, particularly in the West, where our diets contain too much fat.

Treatment for hyperlipidaemia includes the use of bile acid binding resins (such as cholestyramine and colestipol). These prevent the reuptake of bile acids from the terminal ileum and result in a greater de novo synthesis by the liver, using up cholesterol and lowering its circulating levels.

HMG-CoA reductase inhibitors, or 'statins' (e.g. pravastatin and simvastatin) inhibit the rate limiting step in cholesterol synthesis and can reduce LDL cholesterol by up to 40%.

Other treatments include fibric acid derivatives (e.g. gemfibrozil and ciprofibrate), nicotinic acid, and omega-3 marine triglycerides, which limit hepatic triglyceride synthesis, reduces free fatty acid concentrations, and reduces hepatic very low density lipoproteins (VLDL) secretion respectively.

Glycogen storage diseases

There are many different types of glycogen storage diseases, each caused by a different enzyme defect. All of these diseases are autosomal recessive, except type IX B, which is X-linked.

Hepatocytes are involved in types I, II, III, IV, VI, and VIII, with a different site for glycogen storage in each. Most patients present in childhood with hepatomegaly.

Type I can develop hepatocellular adenoma. Type IV can develop cirrhosis and usually results in death by the age of 5 years. The heart and skeletal muscle can be involved, resulting in myopathies and possible cardiac failure.

Convulsions may occur during severe metabolic disturbances, such as lactic acidosis and hypoglycaemia.

Treatment varies according to the type of glycogen storage disease. Extreme exercise must be avoided and oral glucose and fructose maintain blood glucose concentrations. Liver transplantation is a very successful treatment for glycogen storage diseases.

Lysosomal storage diseases

There are a number of lysosomal storage diseases, all of which have a specific enzyme defect. This results in the abnormal accumulation of the enzyme substrate in lysosomes.

Gaucher's disease is the most common type of lysosomal storage disease, and it has a deficiency of glucocerebrosidase. This leads to the abnormal storage of glucocerebroside (glycosylceramide) in reticuloendothelial cells (macrophages and monocytes) found in the liver, spleen and bone marrow.

Its incidence is high in Ashkenazi Jews (1 in 2000) and it usually presents in childhood with splenomegaly, hepatomegaly, anaemia, and elevated levels of serum aminotransferase.

Liver failure is rare and treatment includes splenectomy, bone marrow transplantation, and replacement enzyme therapy (with alglucerase). If there is neurological involvement, then the outlook is poor.

Infectious and inflammatory disease

Viral hepatitis

Viral hepatitis is a common cause of liver injury and it may be caused by:

- Hepatitis virus A, B, C, D, E, or G.
- Cytomegalovirus (CMV).
- Epstein–Barr virus (EBV).
- Arboviruses (e.g. in yellow fever).
- Herpes viruses 1, 2, and 6.
- Adenovirus.
- Parvovirus.

Hepatitis may occur as an unusual complication of non-hepatitis viruses. CMV, EBV, and yellow fever may cause general illness, but only subclinical hepatitis. However, liver function tests will be abnormal.

CMV, herpes simplex virus, and varicella-zoster virus may cause hepatitis in the immunocompromised.

Rubella and CMV acquired *in utero* may lead to hepatitis. Enteroviruses and herpes simplex virus are causes of perinatal hepatitis. Acute viral hepatitis may be asymptomatic or symptomatic with or without jaundice and itching.

Asymptomatic infection is common particularly in hepatitis A acquired by children and more than 50% of those suffering from hepatitis B and C.

Symptoms are similar, regardless of the infecting virus and present as a non-specific influenza-like illness, or with symptoms of gastroenteritis. Hepatitis B infection may lead to arthritis or arthralgia with a rash (caused by immune complexes). Occasionally, fulminant hepatic failure may occur.

Infection with hepatitis A and E do not result in chronic infection. Hepatitis A, C, D, and E are all RNA viruses; hepatitis B is a DNA virus (Fig. 5.6).

Hepatitis A

This is an RNA virus found worldwide, especially where there is poor sanitation and hygiene, and it is spread by the faecal–oral route through contaminated food and water. It may cause outbreaks, and it is very resistant to heat and disinfectant.

The incubation period is 2–3 weeks and infection may be asymptomatic (as in most childhood infections) or cause gastroenteritis-like illness followed by jaundice for 1–3 weeks. Diagnosis is by virus-specific IgM. Neither carrier states nor chronic infections occur (Fig. 5.7).

Hepatitis B

Infection with hepatitis B may lead to a chronic carrier state, liver cancer, or cirrhosis.

Transmission is through contaminated blood or blood products, body fluids, sexual contact, and vertical transmission from mother to baby.

It is also secreted in breast milk.

It is found worldwide, especially in South East Asia, China, and tropical Africa (areas of high endemicity).

Eastern Europe, Central and South America, and the Mediterranean are areas of intermediate endemicity.

Areas of low endemicity include Northern Europe, North America, and Australia. Infection in these areas is associated with high-risk activities such as intravenous drug use, unprotected male homosexual contact, tattoo and acupuncture practices, and the use of blood products by haemophiliacs.

Incubation is 2–6 months and over 50% of cases are asymptomatic.

Of infected adults, 90–95% recover completely and become immune, the remaining 5–10% become carriers, but infants infected perinatally have a worse prognosis: 70–90% become carriers.

Complications of chronic carriage include chronic, active hepatitis, cirrhosis, and hepatocellular carcinoma.

Carriers may have high, intermediate or low infectivity, depending on their serum antigens (Fig. 5.8). All carriers have surface antigen and anti-core

				Viral hepatitis				
Type	Virus	Spread	Incubation period	Carrier state/ chronic infection	Diagnosis of acute infection	Specific prevention	Treatment
A	Hepatovirus	Faecal–oral	2–3 weeks	No	HAV IgM	Vaccine HNIG	N/a
B	Hepadnavirus	Contaminated blood and body fluids: • percutaneous • sexual • mother to baby	2–6 months	Yes Adults 5–10% Neonates 70–90%	HBsAg HBeAg HBcIgM	Vaccine, HBIG	α-interferon
C	Pestivirus-like	Contaminated blood and body fluids: • percutaneous • sexual • mother to baby	6–8 weeks	Yes Adults 60–90%	Anti-HCV PCR	N/a	α-interferon
D	Defective RNA virus coated with HBsAG	Contaminated blood and body fluids: • percutaneous • sexual Note: requires HBsAg for propagation and hepatotropism	N/a	Yes	HD Ag HDV IgM (up to 6 wks) HDV IgG (after 6 wks)	Prevent HBV	N/a
E	Calicivirus	Faecal–oral	2–9 weeks	No	HEV IgG	N/a	N/a

Fig. 5.6 Viral hepatitis. (HAV IgM, hepatitis A immunoglobulin M; HBsAg, hepatitis B surface antigen; HBeAg, hepatitis B e antigen; HBcIgM, hepatitis B core immunoglobulin M; anti-HCV, anti-hepatitis C virus; PCR, polymerase chain reaction; HD Ag, hepatitis D antigen; HDV IgM, hepatitis delta virus immunoglobulin; HEV IgG, hepatitis E virus immunoglobulin G; HBIG, hepatitis B immunoglobulin; HNIG, human normal immunoglobulin.) (Data courtesy of Dr Tilzey, St. Thomas's Hospital, London.)

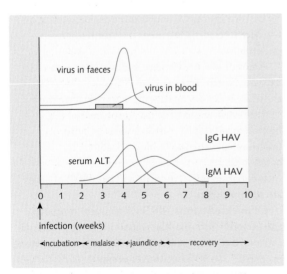

Fig. 5.7 The sequence of events in hepatitis A infection. (ALT, serum alanine aminotransferase; IgG HAV, IgM HAV, antibodies to hepatitis A virus—immunoglobulin G and M.)

antibody. Immune people have anti-surface and anti-core antibodies. The e-antigen determines infectivity: highly infectious carriers have e-antigen, carriers without e-antigen are intermediately infective, and anti-e antibody means a person has low infectivity. Carriers are defined as people in whom hepatitis B surface antigen has been detected for more than 6 months.

The risk of contracting hepatitis B from a needle contaminated with e-antigen positive (i.e. highly infectious) blood following a needlestick injury is 30%.

Those who should receive hepatitis B vaccination are:

- All healthcare workers.
- Members of emergency and rescue teams.
- Haemophiliacs.
- Homosexual and bisexual men and prostitutes.
- Long-term travellers.
- Children in high-risk areas.
- Morticians/embalmers.

Hepatitis C

This is the major cause of post-transfusional non-A, non-B hepatitis.

It may be transmitted parenterally, from mother to baby or through sexual contact, but because blood viral titres are much lower, these routes of transmission are uncommon (unlike hepatitis B). It has a low incidence rate at sexually transmitted disease (STD) clinics, suggesting that transmission via sexual contact is uncommon.

It is found worldwide, particularly in Japan, parts of South America, the Mediterranean, Africa, and the Middle East.

The UK, Northern Europe, and North America are areas of low seroprevalence, and most infection is associated with high-risk activity (intravenous drug abuse or multiple blood transfusions).

The incubation period is 6–8 weeks and infection is asymptomatic in about 90% of cases. However, 60–90% of people become chronic carriers with a risk of developing chronic, active hepatitis, cirrhosis, or hepatocellular carcinoma.

Hepatitis D

This is a defective RNA virus that can only cause infection and replicate in conjunction with hepatitis B.

It has a worldwide distribution, and it is particularly prevalent in the Middle East, parts of Africa, and South America.

Infection in Northern Europe is mainly confined to high-risk behaviour (intravenous drug abuse and multiple blood transfusions). Transmission is mainly parenteral. Hepatitis D may infect at the same time as hepatitis B or infect someone already chronically infected with hepatitis B.

Hepatitis E

This is especially common in Asia, Africa, and the Middle East.

The first documented outbreak was in New Delhi in 1955 when 29 000 people became infected through faecal contamination of water. It is spread by the faecal–oral route. The incubation period is 2–9 weeks (usually 6 weeks).

High-risk age groups include those aged 15–40 years, and it has a 15–20% mortality rate in pregnant women. It does not lead to chronic infection.

The treatment for viral hepatitis depends on the specific infecting virus. Prophylactic vaccines are available for hepatitis A and B viruses.

There is no vaccine for hepatitis viruses C, D, and E, although the hepatitis B vaccine may be given to help reduce the chance of hepatitis D infection.

Treatment is supportive and the use of alcohol must be avoided. Alpha-interferon is useful against hepatitis B and C. The antiviral drugs lamivudine and ribavirin can be used for hepatitis B and C respectively. All sexual and household contacts of the infected person with hepatitis B should be vaccinated, if possible.

Autoimmune hepatitis

This form of chronic hepatitis affects predominantly young and middle-aged women, and it is associated with the HLA alleles HLA-B8, HLA-DR3 and HLA-DR4.

It is also associated with other autoimmune diseases, such as pernicious anaemia and thyroiditis. The patient may be asymptomatic, present with

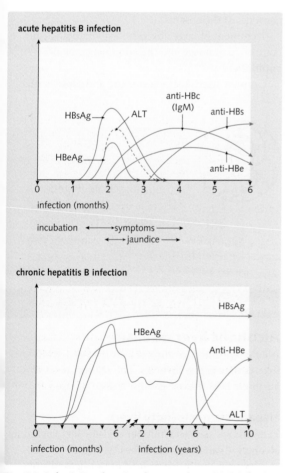

Fig. 5.8 Infectivity of carriers for acute hepatitis B infection and chronic hepatitis B infection. (ALT, serum alanine aminotransferase; HBc, hepatitis B core; HBs, hepatitis B surface.) (Redrawn with permission from Kumar and Clarke, 1994.)

91

fatigue, or present with acute hepatitis (25% of cases) displaying jaundice.

On examination, the patient may have hepatosplenomegaly, bruises, cutaneous striae, acne, and hirsutism and possibly ascites. Extrahepatic manifestations may be present, such as glomerulonephritis, fever, or pleurisy.

The liver biochemistry shows elevated serum aminotransferases, alkaline phosphatases and bilirubin (to a lesser degree). Serum α-globulins are usually twice the normal titre.

There are two types of autoimmune hepatitis, classified by the autoantibodies detected:

- Type I has antinuclear and anti-smooth muscle autoantibodies.
- Type II has anti-liver and kidney microsomal autoantibodies and anti-liver cytosolic autoantibodies.

Type I autoimmune hepatitis affects women, whereas type II mainly affects girls (aged 5–20 years), and it is generally less common.

Primary biliary cirrhosis is another form of autoimmune liver disease and mitochondrial antibodies are found in the serum. Patients present with itching and jaundice, and slowly progress to cirrhosis.

Treatment for autoimmune hepatitis involves steroids (prednisolone) and immunosuppressants (azathioprine). The therapy is given indefinitely, and it can bring remission to 90% of the cases. Liver transplantation is also an option if the drug therapy fails.

Fulminant hepatitis

Fulminant means developing suddenly (from the Latin for 'lightning') and fulminant hepatitis is the development of hepatic encephalopathy within 2–3 weeks of the first symptoms of hepatic insufficiency. Viral infection is the most common cause.

The prognosis depends on the health and age of the patient, as in many other diseases.

Symptoms include those of liver failure, described in Fig. 5.4. However, some of these (e.g. spider naevi and loss of body hair) take time to develop and may not be evident.

Hepatic encephalopathy that takes longer to develop (2–12 weeks) is called subfulminant hepatitis.

Liver abscess

Liver abscesses are more common in developing parts of the world.

In the past, they were relatively common complications of appendicitis or perforation of the gastrointestinal tract, but improved management of these conditions has seen a decrease in the formation of abscesses.

They usually result from the spread of infection through the biliary tree (ascending cholangitis) carried from the gut in the portal system, from a penetrating injury to the liver, direct extension from a perinephric or other abscess, or infection carried in branches of the hepatic artery.

Amoebic abscesses must be considered in travellers, as *Entamoeba histolytica* causes abscesses as well as amoebic dysentery.

Symptoms vary from general malaise to febrile jaundice with right upper quadrant pain and tender hepatomegaly.

Diagnosis is by ultrasonography, chest radiography, serological tests, and analysis of the aspirated contents of the abscess.

Treatment of large abscesses is by radiologically controlled drainage and the administration of antibiotics.

Complications include rupture and septicaemia.

Abscesses are collections of pus, caused by an inflammatory reaction, often as a result of bacterial infection. In general, 'if there is pus about, let it out' treatment of abscesses in accessible parts of the body is usually by surgical drainage or aspiration.

Alcohol, drugs, and toxins

Alcoholic liver disease

Alcohol produces a range of liver diseases, from fatty liver (steatosis) to cirrhosis. The pathogenesis of alcoholic liver disease is summarized in Fig. 5.9.

Hepatic steatosis (fatty liver)

Fatty liver is seen in a number of disorders, including alcoholic liver disease and obesity.

Normally, lipids from the diet or released from adipose tissue are transported to the liver where they are metabolized.

Alcohol is toxic and when it is drunk in excess, its metabolism becomes a priority (Fig. 5.10). Cellular

Fig. 5.9 Pathogenesis of alcoholic liver disease.

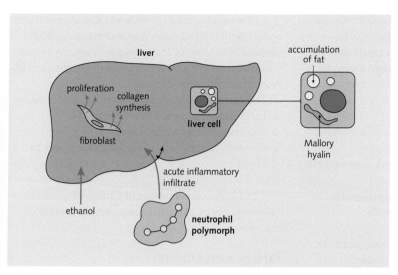

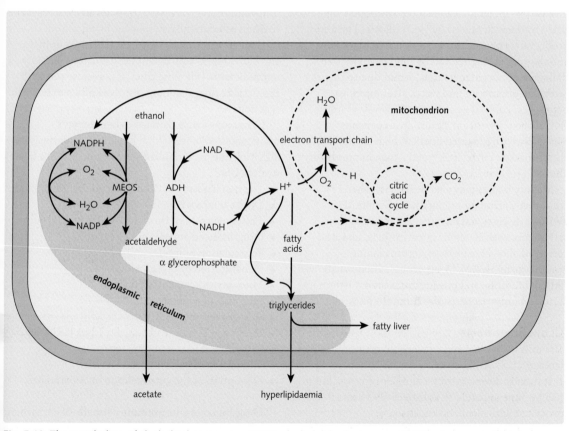

Fig. 5.10 The metabolism of alcohol in hepatocytes. (ADH, alcohol dehydrogenase; MEOS, microsomal ethanol oxidizing system.) (From MacSween RNM, Whaley K. *Muir's Textbook of Pathology*, 13th edn. London: Edward Arnold, 1992. Reproduced by permission of Hodder/Arnold Publishers.)

energy is diverted towards this and away from other essential metabolic pathways, including the metabolism of fat in the liver.

Fat then accumulates in the cytoplasm of liver cells, particularly in zone 3, the area adjacent to the central vein and furthest from the arterial supply.

In chronic ingestion of alcohol, the liver becomes a large greasy organ weighing as much as 5–6 kg.

If alcohol abuse continues, fibrosis and cirrhosis may occur but fatty change is reversible if alcohol intake is stopped.

Alcoholic hepatitis

This is inflammation of the liver caused by alcohol ingestion.

Alcohol is directly cytotoxic at high concentration and cells swell with granular cytoplasm.

Intracytoplasmic aggregates of intermediate filaments (Mallory bodies) appear in the hepatocytes.

Neutrophils accumulate around damaged liver cells (especially those with Mallory bodies), and lymphocytes and macrophages enter the lobule.

Necrosis is found in zone 3 (centrilobular zone) aided by damage caused by free radicals. These are produced by phagocytes in response to cytokines, and they are also generated by lipid peroxidation. Ballooning of hepatocytes can occur, due to the retention of proteins and water after injury to organelles.

Collagen deposition almost always ensues, especially with repeated bouts of high alcohol intake, and the risk of cirrhosis is greater than in purely fatty change.

Mallory bodies may also be seen in other conditions including primary biliary cirrhosis, Wilson's disease, and hepatocellular carcinoma.

Patients with alcoholic hepatitis have elevated serum alkaline phosphatase, serum alanine aminotransferase (ALT), aspartate aminotransferase (AST), bilirubin, and prothrombin time. Often a low serum albumin accompanies these findings.

Alcoholic cirrhosis

Cirrhosis is the final and irreversible result of alcohol damage.

It usually develops over a number of years, but it may become apparent in as little as 2–3 years if associated with alcoholic hepatitis.

In the early stages, the liver is usually large and fatty but later it shrinks to become small, brown, and almost non-fatty.

The hepatocytes attempt to regenerate but the normal architecture is disturbed and nodules form, separated by fibrous septa.

This disrupts the normal blood flow through the liver, and it becomes less efficient at performing its functions.

Cirrhosis may result from a number of causes and is classified into micronodular and macronodular cirrhosis. Both forms may coexist, in which case the cirrhosis is described as mixed. Alcohol abuse usually causes micronodular cirrhosis.

The nodular surface of the liver can vary in colour:
- Fatty changes give it a pale appearance.
- Cholestasis causes bile stains.
- Congestion causes the liver to look red, due to blood.

The major complications of cirrhosis include liver failure, portal hypertension, and hepatocellular carcinoma.

Drugs and toxins

The liver is vital in the metabolism and excretion of drugs and toxins. At least 10% of all adverse reactions to drugs affect the liver.

Drug reactions may be predictable (occur in any individual if a sufficient dose is given) or unpredictable (idiosyncratic, or non-dose related). Predictable drug reactions are also known as intrinsic reactions.

Drugs may cause damage to hepatocytes, indistinguishable from viral hepatitis, cholestasis by affecting bile production or excretion, or other liver dysfunction.

The mechanisms of drug-induced damage include:
- Direct toxicity to cells.
- The conversion of the drug to a toxic metabolite.
- Drug-induced autoimmune reaction.
- Peroxidation of lipids.
- Denaturation of proteins.
- Mitochondrial dysfunction.
- Free radical generation.
- ATP depletion.
- Binding or blockage of transfer RNA (tRNA).
- Attachment to membrane receptors.
- Disruption of calcium homeostasis.
- Disruption of the cytoskeleton in hepatocytes.

Drug-induced autoimmunity usually occurs when the drug, or one of its metabolites, acts as a hapten (a small molecule that is not immunogenic on its own, but which can bind to another molecule and produce an immune response).

A careful drug history should be taken from anyone with signs or symptoms of liver disease, including drugs taken many months before, as there may be a long delay between the administration of the drug and signs of any injury becoming apparent.

Injury may also be immediate, depending on the drug or toxin and the type of damage caused.

Diagnosis is made on the history and clinical signs, the fact that improvement should occur if the patient stops taking the offending drug, and by excluding other causes of liver damage.

A summary of hepatotoxins and their effects is given in Fig. 5.11.

Circulatory disorders

Liver infarction

Liver infarction is rare, because of the dual blood supply of the liver.

It may occur if an intrahepatic branch of the hepatic artery is occluded. If the main hepatic artery

Hepatotoxins and their effects on the liver	
Disorder	**Hepatotoxic agents**
Acute disorders	
Hepatitis-like syndromes (acute necroinflammatory liver disease)	Dapsone, isoniazid, indometacin, phenytoin
Fulminant hepatic failure	Paracetamol, halothane, isoniazid, methyldopa, nicotinic acid, nitrofurantoin, propylthiouracil, valproic acid
Cholestatic syndromes	Amitriptyline, ampicillin, carbamazepine, chlorpromazine, prochlorperazine, cimetidine, ranitidine, captopril, oestrogens, trimethoprim-sulfamethoxazole
Mixed necroinflammatory	Carbimazole, naproxen, phenytoin, thioridazine
Granulomatous hepatitis	Allopurinol, benzylpenicillin, dapsone, diazepam, diltiazem, phenytoin
Macrovesicular steatosis	Alcohol, glucocorticoids, methotrexate, minocycline, nifedipine, total parenteral nutrition
Microvesicular steatosis	Alcohol, amiodarone, aspirin, zidovudine (AZT), piroxicam, sodium valproate, tetracyclines
Budd–Chiari syndrome	Oral oestrogens
Ischaemic necrosis	Cocaine, methylenedioxymethamfetamine
Chronic disorders	
Chronic active hepatitis	Alpha-methyldopa, isoniazid, nitrofurantoin
Fibrosis/cirrhosis	Alcohol, alpha-methyldopa, isoniazid, methotrexate
Peliosis hepatis	Anabolic/androgenic steroids, azathioprine, hydroxyurea, oral contraceptives, tamoxifen
Phospholipidosis	Amiodarone, diltiazem, nifedipine
Primary biliary cirrhosis	Chlorpromazine, haloperidol, prochlorperazine
Sclerosing cholangitis	Floxuridine FUDR via hepatic artery infusion
Steatohepatitis	Amiodarone, total parenteral nutrition
Veno-occlusive disease	Azathioprine, busulfan, cyclophosphamide, daunorubicin, tioguanine, X-irradiation
Oncogenic effects	
Cholangiocarcinoma	Thorotrast
Focal nodular hyperplasia	Oestrogens, oral contraceptives
Hepatic adenoma	Oestrogens, oral contraceptives
Hepatoma	Alcohol, anabolic/androgenic steroids
Hepatoblastoma	Oestrogens
Angiosarcoma	Arsenic, vinyl chloride, Thorotrast

Fig. 5.11 Hepatotoxins and their effects on the liver. (From Friedman and Keefe, 1997.)

is occluded, blood flow through the portal venous systems is usually sufficient to prevent necrosis, except in the case of a transplanted liver when occlusion usually leads to complete necrosis (in which case another transplant is needed).

Occlusion of an intrahepatic branch of the portal vein causes an infarct of Zahn (or 'red infarct'). This is a well-demarcated area that looks red–blue because of stasis of blood in the sinusoids, which become distended. Despite its name, an infarct of Zahn is not a true infarct (necrosis does not occur), but hepatocellular atrophy may occur secondarily to it.

 An infarct is the death of tissue caused by an insufficient blood supply.

Portal vein obstruction and thrombosis

Portal vein obstruction may occur outside the liver (extrahepatic) or inside (intrahepatic). Extrahepatic obstruction is by thrombosis. Intrahepatic obstruction is most commonly caused by cirrhosis, but it can also be caused by congenital hepatic fibrosis and metastases, or primary carcinoma of the liver.

It may lead to portal hypertension, with abdominal pain, ascites, and oesophageal varices.

Passive congestion and centrilobular necrosis and cardiac sclerosis

Passive congestion may be acute or chronic, and it is usually due to right-sided heart failure. It causes the classic 'nutmeg appearance' when looking at the cut surface of the liver. Centrilobular necrosis is usually due to left-sided heart failure or shock causing hypoperfusion of the liver. As might be expected, zone 3 of the acini (being furthest from the portal triad) is most badly affected (Fig. 5.12).

Where both hypoperfusion and congestion occur together, centrilobular haemorrhagic necrosis may occur.

Cardiac sclerosis

Fibrosis of the liver is seen in cardiac sclerosis and also in cirrhosis. The fibrosis of cardiac sclerosis is less severe than that in cirrhosis, however, and the fibrosis is principally found in zone 3.

It is caused by chronic congestive heart failure causing hypoperfusion and venous congestion.

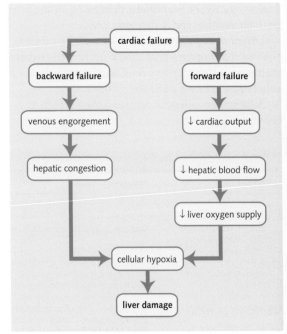

Fig. 5.12 Pathophysiology of liver dysfunction in cardiac failure. (Redrawn with permission from Friedman and Keefe, 1997.)

 Sclerosis is the hardening of a tissue, usually caused by the production of abnormal amounts of collagen.

Peliosis hepatis

Peliosis hepatis is a rare, and usually reversible, dilatation of hepatic sinusoids. It is most commonly caused by anabolic steroids, the contraceptive pill, danazol (an antioestrogenic and antiprogestrogenic drug), and azathioprine (an immunosuppressant).

Improvement occurs if the offending drug is stopped.

Hepatic vein thrombosis (Budd–Chiari syndrome)

Budd–Chiari syndrome is a rare condition where occlusion (due to thrombosis) of the hepatic vein results in blockage of the flow of venous blood out of the liver. This may be acute or chronic. Acute presentation is usually with sudden onset of abdominal tenderness, epigastric pain, nausea (and vomiting), and shock.

Chronic thrombosis results in hepatomegaly, portal hypertension (and its associated signs and symptoms), jaundice, and cirrhosis. Ascites can be found in both acute and chronic forms of the disease.

It may be caused by any condition that predisposes to the formation of thrombi, most notably:

- Polycythaemia.
- Pregnancy.
- Post partum states.
- Oral contraceptive.
- Hepatocellular carcinoma.
- Other intra-abdominal cancers.

Surgical treatment is often required. Creation of an anastomosis can considerably improve the problem. However, liver transplantation is often the treatment of choice. Mortality is higher in acute cases but, even in its chronic form, 5-year survival is only about 50%.

Veno-occlusive disease

Veno-occlusive disease is similar to Budd–Chiari syndrome in its presentation. It is believed to be caused where damage to the endothelium of the sinusoids allows red blood cells into the space of Disse, which activates the coagulation cascade. The products of coagulation are then swept into the central vein, occluding it.

The incidence is higher in those receiving marrow transplants (25% in allogenic recipients), probably because chemotherapy and radiotherapy, given as part of transplant therapy, damage the endothelium.

Treatment of this disease is aimed at controlling hepatocellular failure and ascites formation.

Hepatic disease in pregnancy

Pregnancy-induced hypertension and eclampsia

Pregnancy-induced hypertension (pre-eclamptic toxaemia) is a serious condition affecting about 7% of pregnancies, most commonly in primigravidas (women pregnant for the first time) and women under 25 or over 35 years of age.

Other risk factors include smoking, diabetes, hypertension, short stature, and kidney disease.

It is characterized by hypertension, oedema, and proteinuria. Symptoms include headache, nausea, vomiting, abdominal pain, and visual disturbances, usually in the 2nd and 3rd trimesters. The cause of eclampsia is poorly understood, but there may be a failure of invasion of the trophoblast in the 2nd trimester so that the spinal arteries are obstructed and the abnormal placenta is inadequately perfused.

Vascular endothelial damage leads to platelet and fibrin deposition in sinusoids. The resultant ischaemia leads to hepatocellular necrosis in zone 1 (the periportal zone).

In severe pre-eclampsia, investigations reveal *h*aemolysis, *e*levated *l*iver enzymes, and *l*ow *p*latelet count—the HELLP syndrome. This occurs in 5% of all patients.

Untreated, it may lead to eclampsia (seizures) and maternal death, fetal death, or both.

Caesarean section or induction of labour may be necessary if the pregnancy is close to term. Seizures of eclampsia may be treated with anticonvulsants.

Acute fatty liver of pregnancy

Acute fatty liver of pregnancy is a rare condition, usually occurring in late pregnancy. The cause is unknown and treatment involves early delivery and management of acute liver failure. Liver transplantation may rarely be necessary.

Fatty degeneration of centrilobular liver cells occurs, which may lead to liver failure, coma, and death of the mother or fetus. Diagnosis is by liver biopsy.

Intrahepatic cholestasis of pregnancy

Intrahepatic cholestasis of pregnancy is often a benign condition caused by excess oestrogen.

However, malabsorption, gall stones, fetal distress, prematurity, or stillbirth may result.

It may arise from changes in bile acid metabolism and enterohepatic recirculation, decreased inactivation of oestrogens by the liver, and an alteration of the secretory function of hepatocytes.

The urine is dark, the stools pale, and there is pruritus. Spontaneous recovery occurs after delivery.

Disorders of the biliary tract

Anomalies of the biliary tree

Anomalies of the biliary tree are characterized by changes in the architecture of the biliary tree within the liver.

In normal development, embryonic bile ducts involute (spiral and roll inwards at the edges), and anomalies of the biliary tree are thought to be caused by remnants that have not involuted completely.

Anomalies vary in severity. They may be clinically insignificant or be severe enough to cause hepatosplenomegaly and portal hypertension. They are often inherited.

von Meyenburg's complexes (bile duct microhamartomas)

Microhamartomas are benign tumour-like malformations. They are composed of two or more types of mature tissue that are present in the structure from which the hamartomas arise. Bile duct hamartomas are usually clinically insignificant, but they may be mistaken for liver metastases on a radiograph!

The complexes are small clusters of slightly dilated bile ducts surrounded by a fibrous stroma, and they may communicate with the biliary tree.

They occur sporadically, are slightly more common in females, and may present in pregnancy.

Polycystic liver disease

In polycystic liver disease, the liver has numerous cysts, lined with flattened or cuboidal biliary epithelium and containing straw-coloured fluid. This is an autosomal dominant condition.

The cysts are not connected to the biliary tree, and they do not contain pigmented bile.

The number of cysts varies from just a few to several hundred, and the cysts themselves vary in diameter from 0.5 cm to 4.0 cm.

They may cause discomfort or pain if the patient stoops, and rupture of a cyst may cause acute pain.

Asymptomatic cysts do not need treatment; painful ones may require aspiration.

Polycystic liver disease may be associated with polycystic kidney disease, which may lead to renal failure, in which case the prognosis is worse.

The childhood version of this disease is autosomal recessive. It presents in the first months of life, and it is usually connected with polycystic kidney disease.

Congenital hepatic fibrosis

Congenital hepatic fibrosis is inherited as an autosomal recessive disorder. It may present with complications of portal hypertension and, perhaps most importantly, with bleeding varices (a medical emergency).

The liver is divided into irregular islands by bands of collagenous tissue that enlarge the portal tracts and form septa.

Abnormally shaped bile ducts are scattered throughout the fibrous tissue and the septal margins contain bile duct remnants.

Associated conditions include polycystic kidneys and medullary sponge kidneys.

Diagnosis is by wedge biopsy. This will allow differentiation between fibrosis and cirrhosis.

Caroli's disease

Caroli's disease is inherited as autosomal recessive, and it is characterized by segmental dilatations in the larger intrahepatic bile ducts.

The dilated sections may contain inspissated (thickened) bile and stones, and they may become infected.

Caroli's disease rarely occurs on its own. It is usually found in association with congenital hepatic fibrosis.

Diagnosis is by ultrasonography, percutaneous transhepatic cholangiography, or endoscopic retrograde cholangiopancreatography (ERCP).

Complications include cholangitis, hepatic abscesses, and intrahepatic cholelithiasis.

Disorders associated with biliary cirrhosis
Primary biliary cirrhosis

Primary biliary cirrhosis (PBC) is an autoimmune disorder and, like other autoimmune diseases, affects women (40–50 years of age) more than men. It can occur in conjunction with other autoimmune diseases (e.g. Sjögren's syndrome, rheumatoid arthritis, and scleroderma).

The epithelium of the bile ducts (especially that of the smaller intrahepatic ducts) is destroyed by an autoimmune reaction and the damaged areas become surrounded by lymphocytes. Granulomas may also be present. All patients with PBC have anti-mitochondrial autoantibodies.

An attempt at regeneration then takes place in the form of a proliferation of small bile ductules, and fibrosis occurs, disturbing the normal architecture of the liver.

Eventually, diffuse and irreversible cirrhosis occurs, and this may be complicated by liver failure, portal hypertension, and, rarely, hepatocellular carcinoma.

Elevated serum alkaline phosphatase, IgM and the presence of anti-mitochondrial autoantibodies are diagnostic for PBC. The patient will also have pruritus, jaundice, and xanthelasma.

Xanthelasma are deposits of cholesterol-laden macrophages around the eyes, and they are easily visible to the naked eye.

The course and prognosis of the disease is slow but variable and there is no effective medical treatment although ursodeoxycholate (a bile acid substitute) is of benefit in some patients, improving liver function and survival. Cholestyramine lessens pruritus.

Cholestasis results in malabsorption of the fat-soluble vitamins, therefore supplements are given. Treatment of PBC is difficult and often ineffective, so liver transplantation should be considered when the bilirubin levels rise above 100 µmol/L.

Secondary biliary cirrhosis

Secondary biliary cirrhosis is caused by prolonged obstruction of extrahepatic bile ducts, often as a result of gall stones, biliary atresia, strictures caused by previous surgery, or carcinoma of the head of the pancreas.

Bile remains in the obstructed ducts and inflammation and periportal fibrosis may result, eventually leading to cirrhosis.

Bile duct proliferation may occur and secondary bacterial infection (ascending cholangitis) may complicate biliary strictures and gall stones.

Diagnosis is by ultrasonography, ERCP, or percutaneous transhepatic cholangiography.

Primary sclerosing cholangitis

Primary sclerosing cholangitis (PSC) is a chronic inflammatory disease often associated with inflammatory bowel disease. Seventy per cent of cases occur in association with ulcerative colitis.

Male patients outnumber females by 2:1, and they usually present at around 39 years of age.

Intrahepatic, and sometimes extrahepatic, bile ducts become surrounded by a mantle of chronic inflammatory cells.

Eventually onion skin fibrosis occurs (concentric fibrosis around the ducts) and the lumens become obliterated.

Patients vary from being asymptomatic to suffering from chronic liver disease, with pruritus, jaundice, fatigue, and eventually portal hypertension.

Elevated serum alkaline phosphatase and myeloperoxidase ANCA antibodies in 80% of cases

suggest diagnosis. However, liver biopsy is the best diagnostic tool.

Treatment is not satisfactory and patients may later develop a cholangiocarcinoma. Smoking has been found to be associated with a decrease in the development of PSC!

Gall stones

Gall stones (cholelithiasis) are a common complaint in the West. They occur twice as often in women than in men. However, the incidence of gall stones increases with age in both sexes.

 With gall stones, do not be fooled by 'fair, fat females in their forties'. They have the same chance of having gall stones as the rest of the population (10–20%).

Obese people and those with diabetes mellitus are more 'at risk'. Gall stones are rare in children.

Most gall stones are composed of cholesterol (80%). The rest are composed of bile pigment and calcium. (They can be a mix of all three components!)

Eighty per cent of all gall stones are asymptomatic. These remain in the gall bladder, but gall stones that impact in the neck of the cystic duct can cause biliary pain and acute cholecystitis.

If gall stones impact in the common bile duct, this can lead to obstruction of bile and cause pain and cholestatic jaundice. This sometimes gives rise to bacterial infections resulting in cholangitis.

The clinical presentations and complications are summarized in Figs 5.13 and 5.14.

Treatment varies according to the location of the gall stones and how they are presenting, for example, whether inflammation or a bacterial infection is present.

Fig. 5.13 Causes and clinical presentation of gall stones.

Clinical presentation and causes of gall stones	
Clinical presentations	Cause
Biliary pain (in epigastrium and right hypochondrium)	Impacted in the cystic duct
Biliary pain, cholestatic jaundice, and cholangitis	Impacted in the common bile duct
Asymptomatic	Located in the gall bladder

Complications of gall stones
Acute cholecystitis
Pancreatitis
Gall stone ileus
Biliary enteric fistula
Ileum obstruction
Carcinoma of the gall bladder

Fig. 5.14 The complications of gall stones.

Cholecystectomy (surgical removal of the gall bladder) is often performed laparoscopically, with good effect. If gall stones are only present in the common bile duct then they can be removed via ERCP.

Cholesterol gall stones may be dissolved or disrupted by giving bile acids to increase their solubility in bile. Dissolution of gall stones can take up to 2 years and 50% of the stones recur. This treatment is not suitable for calcified stones.

For inflammation (cholecystitis and cholangitis), antibiotics are administered.

Neoplasms of the liver and biliary tract

Metastatic tumours are the most common form of neoplasm found in the liver. These are mainly derived from the gastrointestinal tract, the breast, or the lung. Malignant liver tumours are more common than benign.

Hepatocellular carcinoma

Hepatocellular carcinoma (HCC) can develop following hepatitis B and C infections, alcoholic cirrhosis, and haemochromatosis. Aflatoxin (a fungal metabolite), androgens, and the contraceptive pill are all associated with HCC.

It affects men more than women, and it usually presents before 50 years of age. The signs and symptoms include:

- Fever.
- Pain in the right hypochondrium.
- Hepatomegaly.
- Weight loss.
- Anorexia.
- Ascites.
- Elevated serum α-fetoprotein.

Treatment usually involves surgical resection or transplantation. The prognosis is not good and survival is usually less than 6 months, but in a few cases, surgical resection is possible with palliation by percutaneous ethanol injection.

Cholangiocarcinoma

Cholangiocarcinomas are classified as intrahepatic and extrahepatic. These adenocarcinomas cause jaundice and they are not associated with hepatitis B virus or cirrhosis.

The prognosis is poor.

Primary adenocarcinoma of the gall bladder

Primary adenocarcinoma of the gall bladder occurs mostly in women and in those over 70 years of age. It presents with jaundice and right hypochondrial pain, and it is usually palpable. Cholecystectomy is a possible treatment, but again, prognosis is poor. Carcinoma of the ampulla has a 5-year survival rate of 40% due to surgical resection.

- Describe the different patterns of necrosis found in the liver.
- What is cirrhosis, how is it classified, and what causes it?
- What can cirrhosis lead to?
- How are the causes of portal hypertension classified, and what are the complications that can occur?
- Why might ascites form, and how is it diagnosed and managed?
- Where in the body do portosystemic anastomoses occur, and what are their consequences?
- Briefly describe the classification, causes, and clinical signs of jaundice.
- How does hepatic encephalopathy occur? What are the symptoms associated with it? How is it treated?
- What causes hepatorenal syndrome? How is it treated?
- What are the indications, contraindications, and possible outcomes of liver transplantation?
- Briefly describe the causes of primary and secondary haemochromatosis. What are their signs and symptoms?
- How is iron overload treated?
- What is Wilson's disease? How does it present, and how is it treated?
- Describe the factors predisposing to hyperlipidaemia. What treatments are available for this disease?
- Briefly compare and contrast glycogen and lysosomal storage diseases, stating aetiology, site of disorder, symptoms, and treatment.
- List the aetiological factors leading to neonatal hepatitis.
- Give a brief account of the viruses that can cause hepatitis, stating how they spread, the incubation period, the carrier status, and whether they cause chronic infection.
- What treatments are available for viral hepatitis?
- What is fulminant hepatitis? What are the consequences of liver failure?
- How do liver abscesses come about? What are the symptoms of and treatments for liver abscesses?
- How is alcoholic liver disease classified?
- Briefly describe the pathogenesis and clinical course of alcoholic liver disease.
- List the mechanisms by which drugs and toxins cause liver damage.
- Briefly describe the mechanisms that may impair hepatic blood flow.
- What are pre-eclampsia, eclampsia, and HELLP syndrome?
- Briefly describe the changes seen in acute fatty liver in pregnancy.
- What causes intrahepatic cholestasis of pregnancy? What are the diagnostic symptoms, and what consequences could occur?
- Describe the main anomalies of the biliary tree.
- What causes primary and secondary biliary cirrhosis? What is the pathogenesis in each disorder?
- What are gall stones? Where can they impact, and what are the consequences at each site?
- Briefly describe the tumours found in the liver and biliary tract.

6. The Pancreas

Organization of the pancreas

The pancreas is both an endocrine and an exocrine gland.

Most of the pancreas consists of exocrine tissue, in which are embedded islands of endocrine cells (islets of Langerhans). The exocrine cells produce enzymes that play an important role in digestion. The hormones produced by the islets are essential for the regulation of blood glucose.

Regional anatomy

The pancreas is a soft elongated digestive gland, which is grey–pink and 'feather-like' in appearance. It is approximately 15 cm in length, lobular, and weighs about 80 g.

It is retroperitoneal and extends transversely across the posterior abdominal wall from the curve of the duodenum to the hilus of the spleen.

The right side lies across the vertebral bodies of L1–L3. It is posterior to the stomach, and the transverse mesocolon is attached to its anterior margin. It is located in the left hypochondriac and epigastric regions.

The pancreas has a head, with an uncinate process (from the Latin meaning 'hook'), a neck, a body, and a tail (Fig. 6.1):

- The head is the expanded right portion, and it nestles in the curve of the duodenum, anterior to the inferior vena cava and the left renal vein. In a groove on the posterior surface of the head lies the common bile duct.
- The uncinate process is a small portion of the head tucked beneath the superior mesenteric vessels.
- The neck joins the body to the head, and it overlies the superior mesenteric vessels and the portal vein. The anterior surface of the neck is covered with peritoneum, and it is adjacent to the pylorus.
- The body is triangular in cross-section, and it extends as far as the hilum of the left kidney. It overlies the aorta, the left renal vein, the splenic vessels, and the termination of the inferior

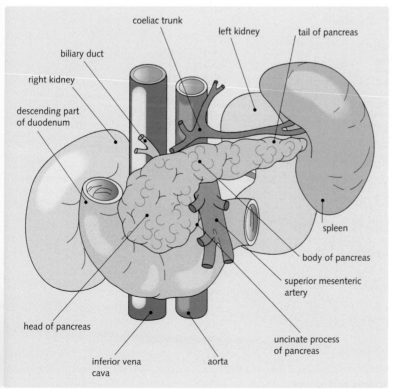

Fig. 6.1 The relations of the pancreas.

coeliac trunk
left kidney
tail of pancreas
biliary duct
right kidney
descending part of duodenum
spleen
body of pancreas
superior mesenteric artery
head of pancreas
uncinate process of pancreas
inferior vena cava
aorta

mesenteric vein. It is crossed anteriorly by the attachment of the transverse mesocolon.

- The tail lies in the lienorenal ligament and ends at the hilum of the spleen.

The main pancreatic duct traverses the gland from left to right and, together with the bile duct, opens into the second part of the duodenum at the ampulla of Vater.

An accessory duct may drain part of the head and, if present, it has a separate opening into the duodenum above the ampulla of Vater.

Blood supply

The pancreas is an endocrine organ and, therefore, it has a rich blood supply. The superior and inferior pancreaticoduodenal arteries supply the head. Branches of the splenic artery supply the remainder of the pancreas. Venous drainage is to the portal, splenic, and superior mesenteric veins.

Lymphatic drainage and innervation

Lymphatic drainage is to pancreaticosplenic or suprapancreatic nodes alongside the splenic artery, and to preaortic nodes around the coeliac and superior mesenteric arteries.

The innervation of the pancreas is from the splanchnic nerves and the vagi through the coeliac and superior mesenteric plexuses.

Development

The pancreas develops from two buds (the dorsal and ventral pancreatic buds) that originate from the endodermal lining of the duodenum in weeks 4–6 (Fig. 6.2).

The duodenum rotates to form a C shape and, in doing so, the ventral pancreatic bud migrates around the back of the duodenum to lie caudal and dorsal to the dorsal pancreatic bud. This allows fusion of the ventral and dorsal pancreatic buds.

The distal part of the dorsal pancreatic duct joins with the duct of the ventral pancreatic bud, to become the main pancreatic duct.

The proximal part of the dorsal pancreatic duct either regresses and disappears, or becomes an accessory pancreatic duct (duct of Sartorini). The pancreatic islets of Langerhans develop from pancreatic parenchyma tissue in month 3, and they are scattered throughout the gland.

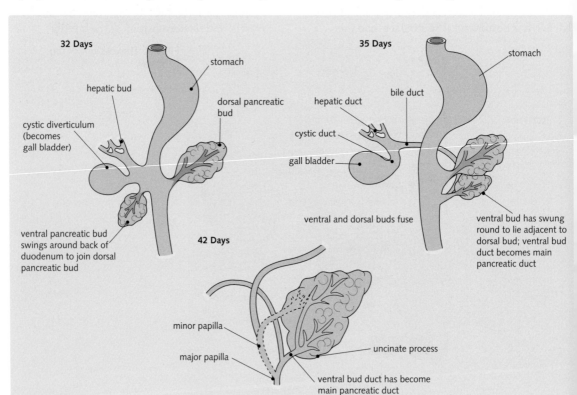

Fig. 6.2 Development of the liver, gall bladder, and pancreas.

Insulin secretion begins during the 5th month of embryonic development and fetal levels of insulin are independent of those of the mother. Insulin does not cross the placenta.

Tissues

The pancreas is covered with a thin capsule of fibrocollagenous connective tissue, from which septa extend into the gland, dividing it into lobules. Nerves and larger blood vessels travel within the septa.

The exocrine pancreas

The exocrine cells secrete digestive enzymes into a network of ducts that meet to form the main pancreatic duct, which joins the common bile duct and opens into the duodenum at the ampulla of Vater (see Fig. 7.2).

The exocrine units or acini are tubuloacinar glands similar to salivary glands in their organization. They are called 'acinar' (latin for 'berry') because the secretory portion is similar to a grape, with the duct resembling a stalk (Fig. 6.3). The acini consist principally of pyramidal epithelial cells, which produce the digestive enzymes of the pancreas. The intercalated ducts begin within the acini where the duct cells are called centroacinar cells. The nuclei of the acinar cells are characteristically found at the cell base along with a large quantity of rough endoplasmic reticulum (RER). The apical portion contains zymogen granules containing enzyme precursors, which are numerous in the resting gland.

Microvilli extend from the apical surface into the lumen of the acini. The intercalated ducts are lined with squamous epithelium, and they lead into intralobular ducts lined with cuboidal or low columnar epithelium.

Larger ducts in the interlobular connective tissue are lined by columnar epithelium and the larger ducts also contain goblet and enteroendocrine (APUD) cells.

The endocrine pancreas

The islets of Langerhans (the endocrine cells of the pancreas) are most prevalent in the tail, and they are surrounded by many blood vessels into which they secrete the hormones insulin, glucagon, and somatostatin (Fig. 6.4).

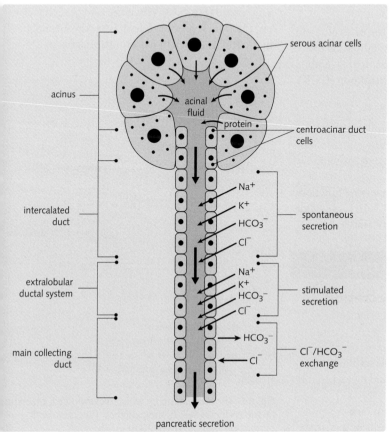

Fig. 6.3 A pancreatic acinus. The secretion of alkaline fluid and proenzymes is regulated separately, and pancreatic fluid rich in one or the other can be produced depending on the stimulus. Secretin initiates production of alkaline-rich fluid, and cholecystokinin initiates production of an enzyme-rich fluid.

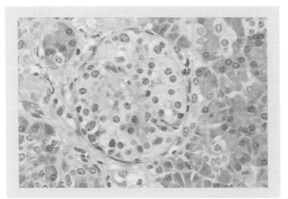

Fig. 6.4 High-power micrograph showing the α and β cells in the islets of Langerhans (in the endocrine pancreas). α cells produce glucagon and β cells produce insulin. Note that each cell is in contact with the capillary network. (Reproduced with permission from Stevens and Lowe, 1996.)

- Insulin is produced by pancreatic β (or 'B') cells. It acts on all cells in the body to increase the uptake of glucose from the blood into the cells.
- Glucagon is produced by pancreatic α (or 'A') cells, and it acts mainly on the liver. It increases glycogenolysis and gluconeogenesis to raise the blood glucose concentration.
- Somatostatin is secreted from δ (or 'D') cells, and it acts locally as a paracrine agent, inhibiting the production of insulin and glucagon. It also inhibits the gut peptides secretin, cholecystokinin (CCK), gastrin, and motilin.

Other cell types include vasoactive intestinal polypeptide (VIP) secreting cells and enterochromaffin cells, which secrete serotonin, motilin, and substance P.

A more detailed account of the endocrine function of the pancreas may be found in the *Crash Course* title on *Endocrinology and Reproductive Systems*.

Exocrine pancreatic function

Overview of pancreatic secretion

The pancreas has two functions: exocrine and endocrine.

It secretes about 1.5 L of fluid a day (over 10 times its own weight!), and this fluid contains cations, anions, albumin, globulin, and digestive enzymes.

The bulk of the fluid is the sodium- and bicarbonate-rich juice secreted by cells of the small

ducts, which neutralizes acid entering the duodenum from the stomach.

The acinar cells secrete a small volume of fluid rich in digestive enzymes, which break down carbohydrates, fats, proteins, and nucleic acids.

Most of these enzymes are secreted in an inactive form, to protect the pancreas from autodigestion, and they are activated in the duodenum.

Alkaline secretion

The pancreas secretes a fluid rich in bicarbonate, which, together with secretions from the gall bladder and the intestinal juices, neutralizes gastric acid in the duodenum, raising the pH to 6 or 7.

Secretion in the pancreas takes place in a similar way to that in the salivary glands. The acini secrete a slightly hypertonic fluid, rich in bicarbonate, which is modified as it travels through the ducts (Fig. 6.3). Chloride is actively exchanged for bicarbonate as the fluid travels through the main collecting ducts (Fig. 6.5) and concentrations of bicarbonate and chloride are reciprocal.

When the pancreas is stimulated to increase its rate of secretion, there is less time for chloride and bicarbonate to be exchanged and the fluid is richer in bicarbonate (Fig. 6.6). When the rate of secretion is low, the fluid is produced mainly by the intralobular ducts. However, when secretin stimulates an

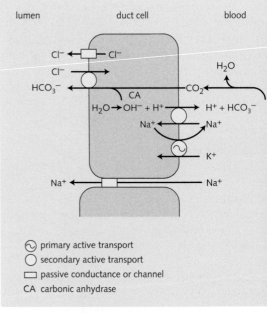

primary active transport
secondary active transport
passive conductance or channel
CA carbonic anhydrase

Fig. 6.5 The mechanism by which bicarbonate is taken up by the epithelial cells of the pancreas. (Redrawn with permission from Johnson, 2000.)

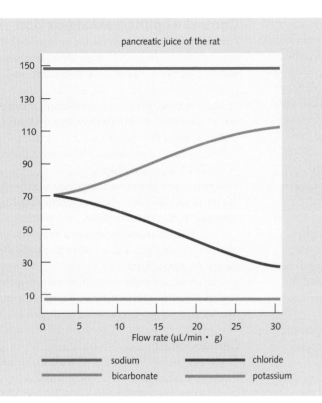

pancreatic juice of the rat

Fig. 6.6 The variation in composition of pancreatic juice with rate of flow. (Redrawn with permission from Mangos JA, McSherry NR. *Am J Physiol* 1971; **221**: 496.)

ncreased rate of production, most of the additional fluid is produced by the extralobular ducts.

The bicarbonate in pancreatic juice is derived from the blood and its concentration in the juice and the rate of production of juice are both proportional to the concentration of bicarbonate in the blood.

The mechanism by which it is taken up by the epithelial cells of the extralobular ducts is summarized in Fig. 6.5. H^+ ions, which are pumped out of the duct cells in exchange for K^+ and Na^+, neutralize bicarbonate in the blood, by forming carbonic acid. This dissociates to form CO_2 and H_2O.

The dissociation is catalysed by carbonic anhydrase, and it is a similar reaction to that occurring in the kidney.

The carbon dioxide diffuses across the basolateral membrane into the duct epithelial cell. Here, it is combined with water by carbonic anhydrase, to make carbonic acid (H_2CO_3), which then dissociates to form H^+ and HCO_3^- (bicarbonate) ions.

The H^+ ions are actively eliminated at the basolateral membrane (which helps drive the reaction to produce more CO_2 in the blood and, therefore, HCO_3^- ions).

Na^+ ions are thought to move through a paracellular junction from the interstitial fluid into the fluid in the duct.

Enzyme secretion

The main enzymes secreted by the pancreas are summarized in Fig. 6.7.

Several of the pancreatic enzymes are capable of damaging the tissues of the pancreas, and so they are secreted as proenzymes, which are activated by substances in the duodenum.

Enteropeptidase (enterokinase) in the brush border of the duodenum (secreted in response to cholecystokinin) converts trypsinogen to trypsin.

Trypsin then activates other pancreatic enzymes (Fig. 6.7) including its own proenzyme trypsinogen, resulting in an autocatalytic chain reaction.

To protect the pancreas from the chain reaction and autodigestion (that would result from even a small amount of trypsin in the pancreas), the pancreas contains a trypsin inhibitor called the kazal inhibitor. This forms a complex with trypsin and prevents it acting.

Other mechanisms are involved to prevent autodigestion of the pancreas by its enzymes. These include an enzyme called enzyme Y, which destroys zymogens (proenzymes) before they can be activated.

Also, the maintenance of an acid pH in the zymogen granules prevents the proenzymes being exposed to their optimal pH.

In acute pancreatitis, phospholipase A_2 is activated by trypsin in the pancreatic duct, and it acts on lecithin (a normal constituent of bile) to form lysolecithin, which damages cell membranes and causes disruption of pancreatic tissue and necrosis of surrounding fat.

Circulating levels of pancreatic α-amylase also increase in acute pancreatitis and measurement of levels in the blood are used as a diagnostic tool.

The fate of enzymes in the duodenum

The digestive enzymes survive for differing periods of time, once they enter the intestines.

Measurements have shown that around 75% of amylase and 20% of trypsin were present in the distal ileum, but only 1% of lipase secreted actually reached this part of the small intestines. Different mechanisms are thought to be involved, and the small intestines are thought to be permeable to several digestive enzymes.

It has been found that chymotrypsinogen and amylase are capable of crossing the basolateral membranes of pancreatic cells.

Some foods contain inhibitors of the digestive enzymes. For example, soy beans contain the Bowman–Birk inhibitor, which stops trypsin and chymotrypsin activities.

Control of pancreatic secretion

Pancreatic exocrine secretion is controlled by neuroendocrine signals, which are hormones and substances released from nerve terminals (Fig. 6.8).

Vagal stimulation (parasympathetic) enhances the rate of secretion of both enzyme and aqueous components of pancreatic juice.

Sympathetic stimulation inhibits secretion, probably by decreasing blood flow.

Secretin and cholecystokinin (released from the duodenal mucosa) stimulate secretion of the aqueous component of pancreatic fluid.

Separate control of the aqueous and enzymatic components explains the variation in composition of pancreatic juice (Fig. 6.6).

The control of secretion can be split up into the cephalic, gastric, and intestinal (duodenal) phases, like the control for gastric secretions.

Cephalic phase

This is very minor in humans. Gastrin is released from the mucosa of the antrum in response to vagal stimulation (via acetylcholine—ACh—and VIP). This causes the release of a small amount of pancreatic juice with a high protein content.

Pancreatic enzymes		
Enzyme	**Activator**	**Substrate**
Trypsin	Secreted as trypsinogen, activated by enteropeptidase (and by trypsin)	Proteins and polypeptides
Pancreatic lipase		Triglycerides
Pancreatic α-amylase	Activated by Cl^-	Starch
Ribonuclease		RNA
Deoxyribonuclease		DNA
Elastase	Activated by trypsin	Elastin and some other proteins
Phospholipase A_2	Activated by trypsin	Phospholipids
Chymotrypsins	Secreted as chymotrypsinogen, activated by trypsin	Proteins and polypeptides
Carboxypeptidase A and B	Activated by trypsin	Proteins and polypeptides
Colipase	Activated by trypsin	Fat droplets

Fig. 6.7 Pancreatic enzymes.

Gastric phase

Gastrin is released in response to gastric distension (via the vago-vagal reflex) and the presence of amino acids and peptides in the antrum. This continues to stimulate release of pancreatic juice.

Vago-vagal reflexes elicited by distension of the fundus or antrum also cause the release of small amounts of pancreatic juice with a high enzyme content (by acting on receptors on the acinar cells in the pancreas).

Intestinal phase

This is the largest and most important phase. It involves the secretion of two hormones. Chyme in the duodenum and upper jejunum stimulate pancreatic secretion.

Secretin is released from the duodenal and upper jejunal mucosa cells in response to acid in the lumen. Secretin acts on the pancreatic ducts, and it stimulates the secretion of a large volume of HCO_3^--rich fluid (but with low levels of pancreatic enzymes).

It also stimulates bile production in the liver.

Cholecystokinin (CCK; also called pancreozymin) is secreted from duodenal and upper jejunal mucosal cells in response to peptides, amino acids, and fatty acids in the lumen. It has two actions:

- It acts on pancreatic acinar cells to stimulate enzyme synthesis and release.
- It acts on the gall bladder, and stimulates contraction of the gall bladder and relaxation of the sphincter of Oddi. This allows release of bile into the duodenum.

Therefore, CCK induces the secretion of a pancreatic juice that is rich in enzymes and which is accompanied by concentrated bile for fat absorption. The substances that stimulate pancreatic secretin are summarized in Fig. 6.8.

CCK has little direct effect on ductular epithelium but potentiates the effect of secretin, which is a weak agonist of acinar cells.

Vagal stimulation is important and vagotomy reduces the response to chyme in the duodenum by 50%.

Somatostatin has the opposite effect and by inhibiting adenylate cyclase and decreasing cyclic AMP, it inhibits the secretion of acinar and duct cells.

Insulin, insulin-like growth factors, and epidermal growth factor potentiate enzyme synthesis and secretion, through the activation of receptor-associated tyrosine kinase.

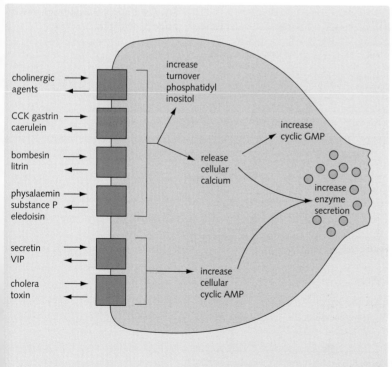

Fig. 6.8 Summary diagram of all the stimulating substances of pancreatic secretion. (CCK, cholecystokinin; VIP, vasoactive intestinal peptide; AMP, adenosine monophosphate; GMP, guanosine monophosphate.)

Disorders of the exocrine pancreas

Congenital abnormalities
Agenesis and hypoplasia
As with other organs, the pancreas may fail to develop at all (agenesis) or develop incompletely (hypoplasia).

Annular pancreas and pancreas divisum
In normal development, the duodenum rotates and the ventral pancreatic bud migrates around the back of the duodenum to lie caudal and dorsal to the dorsal bud. This allows fusion of the ventral and dorsal pancreatic buds (Fig. 6.2).

Sometimes, migration of the ventral bud is incomplete, or the left portion migrates in the opposite direction to the right portion, so that a ring of pancreatic tissue surrounds the duodenum. This is called an annular pancreas, and it may cause constriction or complete obstruction of the duodenum.

Pancreas divisum may occur where fusion of the two pancreatic buds does not take place, and it is found in 5% of patients undergoing endoscopic retrograde cholangiopancreatography.

Ectopic pancreatic tissue
Heterotopic pancreatic tissue is sometimes found in the mucosa of the stomach and in Meckel's diverticulum. More rarely, it may be found between the distal end of the oesophagus and any point proximal to the remnant of the attachment of the vitelline duct (the position at which Meckel's diverticulum would be found, if present). The pancreatic tissue is normal (although in an abnormal place), and it may produce substances normally made by the pancreas.

Pancreatitis
Pancreatitis (inflammation of the pancreas) is classified as acute or chronic, but it is sometimes difficult to separate the two.

Acute pancreatitis
Acute pancreatitis may lead to rapid death (mortality 5–10%). Ranson's criteria are used to assess the severity. If more than seven of his criteria are present, mortality approaches 100%.

Different agents cause acute pancreatitis by different mechanisms (Fig. 6.9) but all lead to the release of lytic enzymes, which are then activated and cause damage.

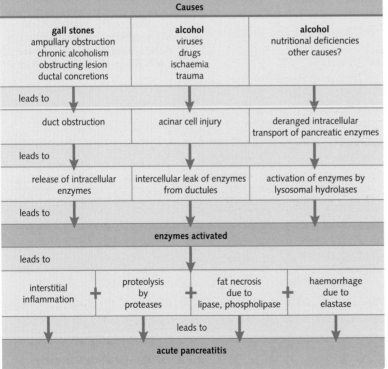

Fig. 6.9 Causes and pathogenesis of acute pancreatitis.

Pancreatic enzymes, in particular trypsin, lipase, and phospholipase A, digest blood vessel walls causing extravasation of blood and fat necrosis. These are known as ecchymoses. This may be extensive enough to discolour the skin of the flanks (Grey Turner's sign) or around the umbilicus (Cullen's sign).

Ecchymoses are bruises found on the skin caused by release of blood into the tissues. These are found in acute pancreatitis and called Grey Turner's sign (on the flanks) and Cullen's sign (around the umbilicus).

Calcium ions bind to the released fatty acid to form white precipitates. In severe cases this causes hypocalcaemia and tetany. Proteolytic enzymes may destroy the islets of Langerhans so that insulin and other hormones, are not produced, leading to hyperglycaemia.

The consequences of acute pancreatitis may be divided into early and late.

Diagnosis is by measurement of serum amylase. It is normally greatly elevated in acute pancreatitis (other conditions such as perforated peptic ulcer may cause a smaller increase).

Radiography shows characteristic findings in the abdomen.

The psoas shadow will be absent because of retroperitoneal fluid and an air-filled dilatation of the proximal jejunum will be seen, i.e. a sentinel loop.

The typical presentation is with severe abdominal pain of sudden onset that may radiate into the back, together with nausea and vomiting. The upper abdomen is usually tender to palpation.

Patients with acute pancreatitis are classified as 'nil-by-mouth', and they are given water and electrolyte replacement with opiate analgesia (not morphine). Mild pancreatitis responds well to this treatment, but if other complications have occurred then they must be treated specifically.

For example, peritoneal lavage may be required. If the pancreatitis is severe, the patient must receive intravenous nutrition.

Patients with cholangitis or jaundice and biliary pancreatitis may benefit from gall stone removal via ERCP from the bile duct.

It is easy to remember the causes of acute pancreatitis—'GET SMASHHHED': Gall stones; Ethanol; Trauma; Steroids; Mumps; Autoimmune; Scorpion bites; Hyperlipidaemia; Hyperthyroidism; Hypothermia; ERCP (or Emboli); Drugs (especially azathioprine and diuretics)!!

Chronic pancreatitis

Chronic pancreatitis is an on-going inflammation of the pancreas accompanied by irreversible architectural changes. It causes a great deal of pain and often permanent loss of pancreatic function.

This may or may not be preceded by acute pancreatitis.

Alcohol consumption causes more than 85% of cases, and it is the most common cause of pancreatitis in developed countries. High fat and protein diets amplify the damage done by alcohol.

The other causes include:
- Tropical malnutrition: this is found in young people in areas with fat and protein deficient diets.
- Hereditary: this is caused by a mutation in the cationic trypsinogen gene, resulting in the formation of calcifying plugs. This is very rare.
- Trauma and scar formation: this can lead to the obstruction of the main pancreatic duct.
- Hypercalcaemia: causing the formation of calcified plugs, which obstruct the pancreatic duct.
- Idiopathic.
- Cystic fibrosis in children.

Patients normally present with a history of:
- Prolonged ill-health.
- Steatorrhoea (lipase deficiency prevents complete breakdown and absorption of fat in the diet).
- Weight loss from malabsorption.
- Recurrent abdominal pain.
- Diabetes mellitus (as a result of destruction of pancreatic islets).

Deficiency of the fat soluble vitamins A, D, E, and K also occurs.

Damage to pancreatic tissue is followed by fibrosis and this may distort the pancreatic ducts.

Diagnosis is by plain abdominal radiography, showing speckled calcification of the pancreas (caused by the binding of calcium ions to necrosed fat), elevated blood glucose (particularly in advanced disease), and endoscopic retrograde cholangiopancreatography, or ERCP (showing distortion of pancreatic ducts caused by fibrosis).

Ultrasonography and computed tomography (CT) scans may also be useful.

Treatment involves stopping consumption of alcohol and control of pain with narcotics. Surgery is an option in some cases, but only in those who are committed to stop drinking.

Pancreatic supplements and a low fat diet help the steatorrhoea, and diabetes mellitus is treated with insulin or diet control and oral hypoglycaemic agents.

Pseudocysts

Pseudocysts are a complication of both acute and chronic pancreatitis. They are localized collections of pancreatic secretions, formed 3–4 weeks after the onset of an acute attack of pancreatitis.

They are usually solitary, 5–10 cm in diameter, and lie in the lesser sac.

They may produce abdominal pain and, more rarely, haemorrhage, infection, and peritonitis. They may also be mistaken for a tumour in the pancreas.

Pseudocysts differ from true cysts in that true cysts have an epithelial lining and are often congenital. Pseudocysts are surrounded by granulation tissue.

Treatment is either by aspiration, with the aid of ultrasound, or surgical removal.

Pancreatic insufficiency

Cystic fibrosis is an autosomal recessive disorder (with a carrier rate of 1 in 25 amongst Caucasians), and it is characterized by pancreatic insufficiency and a tendency to chronic lung infections. The underlying defect is an abnormality in the chloride ion transporter.

The incidence of the disease is 1 in 2000 live births amongst Caucasians, but lower amongst Jewish, Asian, and African populations.

Pancreatic enzymes are absent, or secreted in lower amounts than normal, and fat malabsorption occurs. A deficiency in the fat-soluble vitamins A, D, E, and K may also be found.

The cells lining the bronchial tubes are also affected, secreting thick, viscous mucus (predisposing to lung infections). The sweat contains abnormally high concentrations of sodium chloride.

Pancreatic insufficiency also occurs in chronic pancreatitis, which may be due to gall stones, alcoholism, or hyperparathyroidism, or may be hereditary.

Neoplasms of the pancreas

Tumours, wherever they arrive, are classified as benign or malignant and named according to the tissue from which they arise.

Carcinoma of the pancreas

About 6500 new cases of carcinoma of the pancreas occur in England and Wales every year, and it accounts for about 5% of all cancer deaths in the USA and UK.

It is particularly common in diabetic males, and it is most common over the age of 50 years. It is associated with smoking. Of all pancreatic carcinomas, 60% occur in the head of the pancreas, 15–20% in the body, and 5% in the tail.

Those arising in the head are likely to produce symptoms earlier than those arising elsewhere. They may obstruct the ampulla of Vater causing obstructive jaundice.

The gall bladder may be dilated and easily palpable (Courvoisier's sign).

Carcinomas arising in other parts of the pancreas are less likely to produce symptoms, are discovered late, and therefore have a worse prognosis, often having metastasized before diagnosis.

Most are adenocarcinomas and almost all begin in the ductal epithelium. Less than 1% begin in the acinar cells.

Weight loss usually occurs and some individuals develop thrombophlebitis migrans (flitting venous thromboses).

The carcinoma may be felt as a firm lump during surgery (similar to a pseudocyst).

The treatment for carcinoma of the pancreas is surgical and only 13% of patients are suitable. Whipple's procedure is performed, which consists of a partial gastrectomy, duodenectomy, and a partial pancreatectomy. It may or may not include the removal of the gall bladder and distal common bile duct.

Surgery to relieve or bypass obstructions may be performed.

There is a high risk of mortality associated with surgery (up to 20%). The median survival time, after bypass surgery is 24 weeks, and after Whipple's procedure, it is 40 weeks. Survival is only 9 weeks without any treatment. Palliative care is very important and analgesia should be used liberally.

Cystic tumours

Cystic tumours may be benign (cystadenoma) or malignant (cystadenocarcinoma). They comprise only 5% of neoplasms of the pancreas, and they are usually found in the body or tail.

112

- Briefly describe the anatomy of the pancreas, stating its relation to other organs, its blood supply, lymphatic drainage, and innervation.
- How does the pancreas develop in the embryo? At what stage of embryonic life is it functioning as an endocrine gland?
- What is the histology involved in the exocrine and endocrine functions of the pancreas? What do both secrete?
- What components make up pancreatic juice?
- What are the functions of the pancreatic juice in digestion?
- Give a detailed account of the production of the alkaline solution.
- What are the pancreatic enzymes, and what are their functions?
- Describe how pancreatic secretion is controlled.
- Describe the most common congenital abnormalities of the pancreas and how they arise.
- What are the causes and complications of acute and chronic pancreatitis?
- What is a pseudocyst, and how is it formed? What are the complications of pseudocysts?
- How does cystic fibrosis lead to pancreatic insufficiency? What other conditions lead to pancreatic insufficiency?
- Briefly describe the different types of neoplasms and where they are located.
- What treatments exist for carcinoma of the pancreas?

7. The Intestine

Organization of the intestine

The intestines have the same basic structure as the rest of the gastrointestinal tract: mucosa, submucosa, muscularis externa, nerve plexuses, and serosa (see Fig. 1.2). Absorption takes place in the intestine and its mucosa is specially adapted for this.

Regional anatomy
Small intestine

The small intestine extends from the stomach to the colon and is about 6–7 m in length.

It consists of the duodenum, jejunum, and ileum, and it is responsible for the absorption of most nutrients (Fig. 7.1).

Duodenum

The duodenum is about 25 cm in length, and it extends from the pylorus to the duodenojejunal flexure. It is C-shaped and snakes around the pancreas beginning 2–3 cm on the right side of the median plane and ending (at the jejunum) an equal distance from the median plane, but to the left. It lies in the umbilical region and except for the first 2.5 cm, it is retroperitoneal.

The duodenum receives the openings of the bile and pancreatic ducts. It is divided into four parts (D1–4).

- The first (superior) part—D1. This is 5 cm in length and starts at the pylorus.
- The second (descending) part—D2. This is 8 cm in length and descends to the right side of L3. The

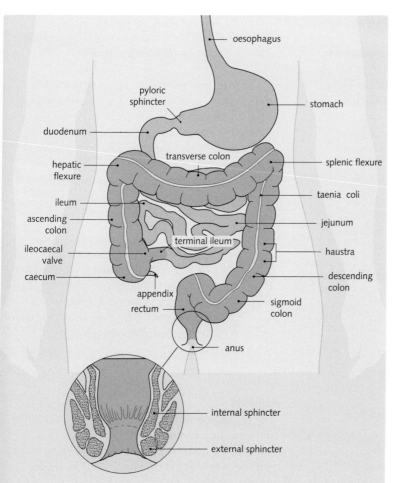

Fig. 7.1 The position of the small and large intestines.

115

ampulla of Vater lies halfway down its posteriomedial wall (Fig. 7.2).

- The third (horizontal) part—D3. This is 10 cm in length and passes to the left anterior to L3, before turning upwards to become the fourth part.
- The fourth (ascending) part—D4. This is 3 cm in length and ascends to the duodenojejunal flexure to the left of L2. The duodenum becomes the jejunum at the ligament of Treitz, a fibromuscular band, which is also called the suspensory muscle of the duodenum.

The first part of D1 is called the ampulla (or cap, or bulb) of the duodenum. The proximal half has mesentery, which allows mobility. The greater omentum and hepatoduodenal ligament are attached proximally. The distal half has no mesentery, and it is not mobile.

- Anterior to D1, lie the peritoneum, gall bladder, and quadrate lobe of the liver.
- Posterior to D1, lie the gastroduodenal artery, inferior vena cava, portal vein, and bile duct.
- Inferiorly, lies the neck of the pancreas.

D2 lies retroperitoneal and has no mesentery. The common bile duct and pancreatic duct enter the posteriomedial wall at the ampulla of Vater (hepatopancreatic ampulla), about two thirds along its length.

- Anterior to D2, lie the transverse colon, mesocolon, and coils of the small intestine.

- Posterior, lie the hilus of the right kidney, its renal vessels, the right ureter, and the psoas major muscle.
- The head of the pancreas and the bile and pancreatic ducts lie medially to D2.

The third part has no mesentery, and it lies retroperitoneally. It is adherent to the posterior abdominal wall.

- Posterior to D3, lie the right psoas major muscle, right ureter, the abdominal aorta, and inferior vena cava.
- Anteriorly, lie the coils of the small intestine and the superior mesenteric artery.
- Superior to D3, lie the superior mesenteric vessels and the head of the pancreas.

The distal end of the duodenum (D4) is covered with peritoneum.

- Anteriorly to D4, lie the coils of jejunum and the beginning of the root of the mesentery.
- Posterior to D4, lie the left psoas major muscle and the left margin of the aorta.
- The head and body of the pancreas lie medially and superiorly to D4, respectively.

The main pancreatic duct opens with the bile ducts at the ampulla of Vater. The ampulla opens in to the duodenum at the top of the major duodenal papilla. The pancreatic duct sphincter controls the terminal end of the duct. The sphincter of Oddi controls the ampulla opening.

The duodenal luminal surface is thrown into folds called plicae circulares.

 An accessory pancreatic duct is sometimes present, formed by the proximal end of the dorsal pancreatic duct, which normally disappears. It opens into the minor duodenal papilla.

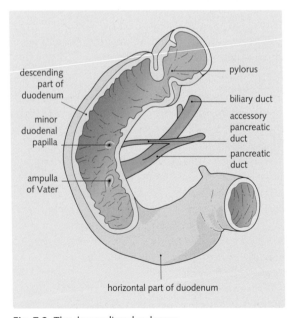

descending part of duodenum

minor duodenal papilla

ampulla of Vater

pylorus

biliary duct

accessory pancreatic duct

pancreatic duct

horizontal part of duodenum

Fig. 7.2 The descending duodenum.

Jejunum
The jejunum begins at the duodenojejunal flexure and makes up about two fifths of the small intestine (it is about 2.5 m long). It is often empty and this is how it got its name! (Jejunus means empty in Latin.)

In life, it is thicker, redder, and more vascular than the ileum. It mostly lies in the umbilical region. The jejunum has large and well developed mucosal plicae circulares (circular folds) and these can be felt in a living person. It has no prominent Peyer's patches, but diffuse lymphoid tissue.

Ileum

The ileum constitutes the remaining three fifths of the small intestine (about 3.5 m long), but there is no clear demarcation between the jejunum and ileum.

It is situated in the hypogastric and inguinal regions. Its terminal part lies in the pelvis major, ascending over the right psoas muscle and the right iliac vessels to join with the caecum at the ileocolic junction.

The plicae circulares are small in the superior part of the ileum and absent in the terminal end. The ileum is thinner walled, and it has more Peyer's patches than the jejunum.

Mesentery

The small intestine has a fan shaped mesentery, which suspends it from the posterior abdominal wall and allows the jejunum and ileum to be mobile. The root of the mesentery is about 15 cm long and this moves from left to right in an oblique and inferior direction.

It begins on the left side of L2 and crosses:
- The horizontal part (D3) of the duodenum.
- The aorta.
- The inferior vena cava.
- The right psoas major muscle.
- The right ureter.
- The right testicular (or ovarian) vessels.

The root of the mesentery ends at the right sacroiliac joint.

Blood supply

The duodenum is supplied by the coeliac and superior mesenteric arteries. Its main supply comes from the superior pancreaticoduodenal artery (a branch of the gastroduodenal artery) and the inferior pancreaticoduodenal artery (a branch of the superior mesenteric artery).

The superior pancreaticoduodenal artery supplies the proximal half and the inferior supplies the distal half of the duodenum. The vessels form an anastomosis called the anterior and posterior arcades. These lie in between the duodenum and the pancreas.

The supraduodenal arteries all supply the superior part of the duodenum. They anastomose with one another.

The arterial supply for the jejunum and ileum arise from the superior mesenteric artery, which arises from the abdominal aorta at the level of L1.

The superior mesenteric artery gives rise to many branches that supply the intestines. There are 15–18 jejunal and ileal branches (arising from the left side of the superior mesenteric artery) that pass between the two layers of the mesentery, to form arches or loops called arcades.

Straight arteries called vasa recta branch off from the arcades and do not anastomose in the mesentery. Many blood vessel anastomoses are found within the walls of the intestines.

The jejunum is more vascular than the ileum, and it has longer arterial arcades, with straighter and less complex vasa recta. The arterial supplies of the jejunum and ileum are compared in Fig. 7.3.

The last ileal branch from the superior mesenteric artery anastomoses with a branch of the ileocolic artery.

Venous drainage

The venous drainage follows the arterial supply of the small intestine. From the duodenum, blood drains into the portal venous system, via the superior mesenteric vein.

Drainage to these occurs in three ways:
- Direct drainage to the portal vein.
- Indirect drainage, via small veins, to the pancreaticoduodenal veins.
- Indirect drainage, via the prepyloric veins, to the right gastric vein.

In the jejunum and ileum, all the tributaries of the superior mesenteric vein run alongside the branches of the superior mesenteric artery.

Lymphatic drainage

In the duodenum, the anterior and posterior surface lymphatics anastomose. The anterior vessels drain to the pyloric and pancreaticoduodenal lymph nodes, which then drain to the coeliac lymph nodes. The posterior vessels drain to the superior mesenteric nodes.

In the jejunum and ileum, the lymphatics are present in the villi as lacteals. The lymph vessels drain in to the mesenteric lymph nodes close to the intestinal wall, along the arterial arcades and along the proximal section of the superior mesenteric artery.

The terminal ileal lymph vessels drain to the ileocolic lymph nodes, which run with the ileal branch of the ileocolic artery.

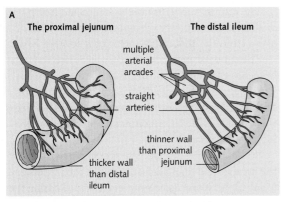

A

The proximal jejunum

The distal ileum

multiple arterial arcades

straight arteries

thinner wall than proximal jejunum

thicker wall than distal ileum

Fig. 7.3 (A) The proximal jejunum and distal ileum. Note that the arterial arcades in the ileum are more complex and the vasa recta are shorter than in the jejunum. (B) Arteries to the gastrointestinal tract.

Innervation

Duodenal innervation comes from the vagus and sympathetic nerves via nerve plexuses on the pancreaticoduodenal arteries.

The jejunum and ileum are also supplied by the vagus and splanchnic nerves. These travel through the coeliac ganglion and they have plexuses around the superior mesenteric artery.

The superior mesenteric nerve plexus, supplying the small intestine, receives a sympathetic and parasympathetic supply from the superior mesenteric ganglion and coeliac division of the vagal trunk, respectively.

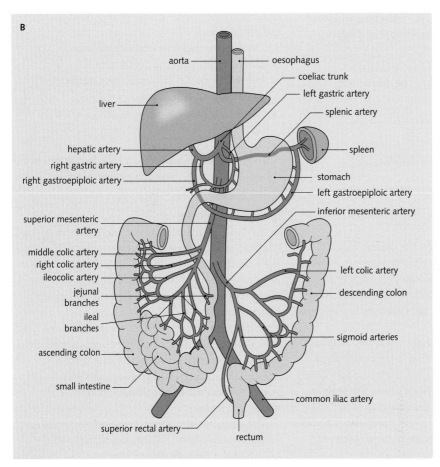

B

aorta

oesophagus

coeliac trunk

left gastric artery

liver

splenic artery

hepatic artery

spleen

right gastric artery

right gastroepiploic artery

stomach

left gastroepiploic artery

inferior mesenteric artery

superior mesenteric artery

middle colic artery

right colic artery

ileocolic artery

left colic artery

jejunal branches

descending colon

ileal branches

ascending colon

sigmoid arteries

small intestine

common iliac artery

superior rectal artery

rectum

Large intestine

The large intestine extends from the ileocaecal junction to the anus, and it is about 1.5 m in length. It can be divided into eight sections:

- The caecum.
- The appendix.
- The ascending colon.
- The transverse colon.
- The descending colon.
- The sigmoid colon.
- The rectum.
- The anal canal.

The outer, longitudinal muscle forms three distinct bands visible at dissection called taenia coli, from the Latin for 'flat band'.

These bands are shorter than the circular muscle layer and gather the caecum and colon into a series of pouch-like folds called haustrations, or sacculations.

The haustra are visible on radiographs when an opaque medium is introduced through the rectum. They do not extend across the entire width, and this distinguishes the large intestine from the small intestine, which has plicae circulares (Kerckring's valves or valvulae conniventes) visible across the whole width on radiographs.

The outer surface of the large intestine has appendices epiploicae projecting from it. These are sacs of omentum distended with fat.

Caecum

The caecum lies in the right iliac fossa and is a sac, continuous with the ascending colon.

It communicates with the ileum through the ileocaecal sphincter or valve (Fig. 7.4).

It is covered entirely in peritoneum, but has no mesentery. The caecum is often attached by peritoneal caecal folds to the iliac fossa to form the retrocaecal recess, a small peritoneal cavity. The appendix lies in this cavity.

 The ileocaecal valve is an incompetent valve! This is good, because it prevents the build-up of wind or stools in the colon and allows for the easing of pressure.

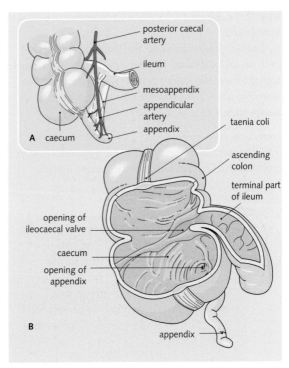

Fig. 7.4 The ileocaecal valve (exterior view [A] and cutaway view [B]) and the appendix.

Blood supply

The caecum is supplied by the ileocolic artery, a branch of the superior mesenteric artery. Venous blood from the caecum drains via the ileocolic vein into the superior mesenteric vein.

Appendix

The appendix, or vermiform appendix (from the Latin for 'worm') is about 8 cm in length, and it protrudes from the posterolateral wall of the caecum (Fig. 7.4).

It is a blind-ending sac that may become obstructed and inflamed (appendicitis), requiring surgical removal to prevent rupture and peritonitis. The appendix is mobile and, because of the way that it develops (described below), its position is variable. It usually lies behind the caecum or in the pelvis.

Blood supply and lymphatics

It is covered in peritoneum and supplied by the appendicular artery (a branch of the ileocolic artery), which lies in the mesentery (the mesoappendix) that connects the appendix to the terminal ileum.

The ileocolic vein drains the appendix.

It has aggregations of lymphatic tissue and the three taenia coli of the caecum come together at the base of the appendix, forming an outer longitudinal muscle coat.

The lymphatic drainage and innervation for the caecum and appendix is the same. The lymph drains into the ileocolic lymph nodes (which lie along the ileocolic artery) and the lymph nodes in the mesoappendix.

Innervation

The innervation to the caecum and appendix comes from the coeliac and superior mesenteric ganglia.

The base of the appendix is usually constant and can be located deep to McBurney's point. This is found at the junction of the lateral and middle thirds of the line between the ASIS (anterior superior iliac spine) and the umbilicus.

Ascending colon

The ascending colon is between 12 and 20 cm in length and fixed to the posterior abdominal wall by peritoneum.

It ascends from the ileocaecal valve to the under surface of the liver where it turns to the left, forming the hepatic (right colic) flexure (Fig. 7.5).

It has no mesentery, and it lies retroperitoneally. However, it has peritoneum covering the lateral and anterior surfaces, which attaches it to the posterior abdominal wall. The peritoneum on the lateral side of the ascending colon forms the right paracolic gutter.

Anterior to the ascending colon lie the coils of the small intestine, the greater omenum, and the anterior abdominal wall.

Posterior to the ascending colon lie the iliacus, transverse abdominus and quadratus lumborum muscles, and the right kidney.

Blood supply and lymphatics

The ascending colon is supplied by the right colic artery and ileocolic artery. Both are branches of the superior mesenteric artery. Its venous drainage is via the right colic and ileocolic veins, which drain into the superior mesenteric vein.

Lymph from this region drains to the paracolic and epicolic lymph nodes. These drain into the superior mesenteric lymph nodes.

Innervation

Innervation to the ascending colon comes from the coeliac and superior mesenteric ganglia.

Transverse colon

The transverse colon is not actually transverse, but extends from the hepatic (right colic) flexure to the splenic (left colic) flexure. It is the largest part of the large intestine and is about 45–50 cm in length.

The transverse colon is mobile, and its mesentery is called the mesocolon. This double layer of peritoneum allows it to hang from the posterior abdominal wall, and it is attached to the inferior border of the pancreas and greater omentum.

The splenic flexure is slightly more superior than the hepatic flexure, due to the spleen being smaller than the liver.

The splenic flexure is attached to the diaphragm by the phrenicocolic ligament, a fold of peritoneum.

Blood supply and lymphatics

The arterial blood supply is from the middle, right, and left colic arteries (Fig. 7.3). The middle colic artery is the major arterial supply, and it is a branch of the superior mesenteric artery, along with the right colic artery.

The left colic artery is a branch of the inferior mesenteric artery.

The superior mesenteric vein drains the transverse colon, and its lymph drains to the lymph nodes along the middle colic artery. These then drain into the superior mesenteric lymph nodes.

Innervation

Innervation to the transverse colon comes from the superior mesenteric plexus, which follows the path of the middle and right colic arteries. The nerves from the inferior mesenteric plexus follow the path of the left colic artery. Both sympathetic and parasympathetic (vagal) nerves supply the transverse colon.

Descending colon

The descending colon is about 30 cm in length, and it is the narrowest part of the colon.

It extends from the splenic flexure to the left iliac fossa at the pelvic brim where it becomes the sigmoid colon.

The descending colon has no mesentery, and it lies retroperitoneally, but it is attached to the posterior abdominal wall.

The lateral border of the left kidney, the transversus abdominus, and quadratus lumborum muscles lie posterior to the descending colon.

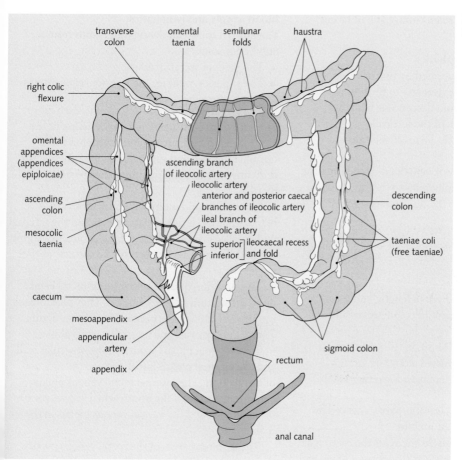

Fig. 7.5 The large intestine.

Blood supply and lymphatics

The left colic and superior sigmoid arteries supply the descending colon. Both are branches of the inferior mesenteric artery. Venous drainage is via the inferior mesenteric vein, and the lymph drains to the intermediate colic lymph nodes, which lie along the left colic artery.

Innervation

Parasympathetic innervation comes from the pelvic splanchnic nerves and sympathetic innervation is derived from the lumbar part of the sympathetic trunk and the superior hypogastric plexus.

Sigmoid colon

The sigmoid colon is so called, because of its S-shape. It is about 40 cm in length.

It lies in the left iliac fossa and extends from the pelvic brim to join the rectum at the level of S3. The sigmoid colon has a long mesentery called the sigmoid mesocolon, which has a V-shaped root

It is easy to tell the difference between the large and small intestines on X-rays. The small intestine, being small, has plicae circulares that extend across its entire width. The large intestine, being large, has haustra that only reach part of the way across.

attachment. Therefore, the sigmoid colon is very mobile.

It lies anterior to the left external iliac vessels, the left sacral plexus and the left piriformis muscle. It also resides in the retrouterine (in females) or retrovesical (in males) pouches.

Long appendices epiploicae hang from the external wall of the sigmoid colon. The position, size, and shape of the sigmoid colon depend on how full of

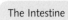

faeces it is. This is the main storage site of faeces, prior to defecation.

Blood supply and lymphatics

The sigmoid colon is supplied by two or three sigmoid arteries. These descend to the left and divide into ascending and descending branches. The descending branch of the left colic artery anastomoses with the most superior sigmoid artery.

The inferior mesenteric vein drains blood from the sigmoid colon, and lymph drains to the intermediate colic lymph nodes, as in the descending colon.

Innervation

The innervation is the same as that to the descending colon.

Rectum

The rectum is about 12 cm in length, and it is continuous with the sigmoid colon proximally and the anus distally.

It starts at the level of S3, in the posterior part of the pelvis and curves along the sacrum and coccyx, before widening to form the rectal ampulla.

It has no mesentery, but it is partly covered by peritoneum, and it is not mobile.

The puborectalis muscle encircles the rectum at the junction with the anal canal to form a 'sling' and produce a 90° anorectal angle, or the anorectal flexure.

The relations of the rectum are different in the male and female. In the male, the bladder, prostate, seminal vesicles, and ducti deferentia lie in front of it, in the female it is related anteriorly to the uterus and vagina.

Posterior to the rectum lie:
- The three inferior sacral vertebrae.
- The coccyx.
- The anococcygeal ligament.
- The median sacral vessels.
- Branches of the superior rectal artery.
- The inferior ends of the sympathetic trunks and sacral plexuses.

The rectal ampulla is very distendable, and it is supported by the levator ani muscles.

The rectum is S-shaped in coronal section, and it has three transverse folds, which are formed by infoldings of the bowel wall. They are maintained by the taeniae coli. These three rectal folds partly close the lumen.

Blood supply and lymphatics

The arterial supply to the rectum comes from a number of sources:
- The median sacral arteries.
- The superior, middle, and inferior rectal arteries.

The rectal arteries anastomose with each other. The superior rectal artery is a continuation of the inferior mesenteric artery, and it supplies the terminal sigmoid and superior region of the rectum. It divides into left and right branches posterior to the rectum.

The middle and inferior rectal arteries are branches of the internal iliac arteries and the internal pudendal arteries, respectively. These arteries supply the middle and inferior parts of the rectum, as their names suggest!

The superior, middle, and inferior rectal veins drain the rectum of venous blood. They anastomose to form a rectal venous plexus around the rectum. There is an external and internal venous plexus.

The external plexus is outside the muscular wall and the internal plexus is just deep to the mucosa of the rectum. The internal rectal venous plexus communicates with the uterovaginal venous plexus in the female and the vesical venous plexus in the male.

The different areas of the rectal venous plexus drain into the different vessels:
- The superior part drains into the superior rectal vein, then into the inferior mesenteric vein.
- The middle part drains into the middle rectal vein, then into the internal iliac vein.
- The inferior part drains into the internal pudendal vein.

The superior rectal veins drain into the portal system and the inferior rectal veins drain into the systemic circulation.

The superior part of the rectum drains lymph into the pararectal lymph nodes, which then drain to the sigmoid mesocolon lymph nodes and inferior mesenteric lymph nodes. The inferior part of the rectum drains lymph into the internal iliac lymph nodes.

Innervation

The rectum receives sympathetic and parasympathetic innervation. The inferior hypogastric plexus provides between four and eight nerves to make up the middle rectal plexus. Parasympathetic innervation is derived from S1, S3, and S4 nerves, which run with the pelvic splanchnic nerves, finally joining up with the inferior hypogastric plexus.

Sensory fibres follow the sympathetic fibres, and they are stimulated by rectal distension.

Anus

The anal canal is continuous with the rectum and is about 4 cm long. It begins at the anorectal angle and it is surrounded by the levator ani muscles, ending at the anus.

The anal canal descends between the perineal body and the anococcygeal ligament. The ischioanal fossae are two wedge shaped spaces on either side of the anal canal.

The anus has an internal and external sphincter. The external sphincter surrounds the lower two thirds of the anal canal and is under voluntary control. For example, it allows delay of defecation until a convenient time. It is made up of striated muscle.

The internal sphincter surrounds the upper two thirds of the anal canal and is made up of involuntary circular muscle. This is a thickened continuation of the circular muscle layer of the rectum.

In the male, the anal canal lies behind the prostate and the bulb of the penis. The perineal body separates the anal canal from these structures, but a digital rectal examination can give important information about the prostate.

In the female, the perineal body separates the anal canal from the vagina.

In the superior half of the anal canal are six to twelve longitudinal ridges in the mucosal membrane. These ridges are called anal columns, and they contain the terminal branches of the superior rectal artery and vein.

The superior ends of the anal columns mark the anorectal junction. Folds of epithelium, called anal valves, connect the inferior ends of the anal columns.

Just superior to the anal valves are the anal sinuses, which release mucus to aid defecation.

The pectinate line is found between the superior and inferior parts of the anal canal. It is the boundary between the columnar epithelium of the superior part and the stratified squamous epithelium of the inferior part.

Structures associated with the superior part of the anal canal (above the pectinate line) have developed from the endodermal hindgut.

Structures below the pectinate line have developed from the ectodermal anal pit, or proctodeum. Therefore, the differences in blood, lymphatic and nerve supply above and below the pectinate line are due to embryological development.

To learn the details of Meckel's diverticulum, just remember 2-2-2. It is present in about 2% of the population, is roughly 2 inches long, and found approximately 2 feet from the caecum.

Blood supply and lymphatics

The superior and inferior parts of the anal canal are supplied by the superior and inferior rectal arteries, respectively. There are two inferior rectal arteries.

The terminal branches of the superior rectal artery anastomose in the anal valves. The middle rectal arteries anastomose with the superior and inferior rectal arteries.

Venous drainage both superior and inferior to the pectinate line occurs via the internal rectal venous plexus. The plexus drains into the superior rectal vein, superior to the pectinate line and into the inferior rectal veins, inferior to the line.

The veins in the wall of the anal canal provide a cushion for the passage of faeces and help close the anus, but they can enlarge to form haemorrhoids.

In the superior part of the anal canal, the lymph drains to the internal iliac lymph nodes and then into the common iliac and lumbar lymph nodes. In the inferior part of the anal canal, lymph drainage is to the superficial inguinal nodes.

Innervation

Superior to the pectinate line, the sympathetic nerve supply is derived from the inferior hypogastric plexus. The parasympathetic supply comes from the pelvic splanchnic nerves.

Inferior to the pectinate line, the nerve supply comes from the inferior rectal nerves, which are branches of the pudendal nerve.

The lower part of the anal canal is sensitive to touch, temperature, and pain.

The pelvic splanchnic nerves (parasympathetic) and the aortic and pelvic plexuses (sympathetic) innervate the internal anal sphincter.

The inferior rectal nerve, a branch of the pudendal nerve (S2 and S3) and the perineal branch of S4 innervate the external anal sphincter.

Development of the intestine

The proximal portion of the small intestine (from the pylorus to the duodenal papilla) develops from the foregut. The remainder of the intestine develops from the midgut and hindgut (see Fig. 1.6). Rapid elongation of the midgut, to form the primary intestinal loop, occurs from 5 weeks of embryonic life.

The midgut gives rise to the remainder of the duodenum (that part distal to the duodenal papilla) and to the proximal two thirds of the transverse colon.

The duodenum is, therefore, supplied by branches of the artery of the foregut (the coeliac artery) and the superior mesenteric artery (which supplies the midgut).

The midgut is suspended from the dorsal abdominal wall by a mesentery, and it communicates with the yolk sac through the vitelline duct.

A small portion of the vitelline duct persists in 2% of individuals, and it forms an outpouching of the ileum known as Meckel's diverticulum.

During development, the liver and primitive gut grow so rapidly that there is not enough room in the fetal abdominal cavity, and the midgut herniates outside the abdominal cavity at about the 6th week. It develops in the umbilical cord until the end of the 3rd month, when it begins to return to the abdominal cavity.

While outside the abdomen, the primary intestinal loop rotates approximately 270° around the superior mesenteric artery. Viewed from the front, the rotation is anticlockwise (Fig. 7.6).

The jejunum and ileum form a number of coiled loops, but the large intestine remains uncoiled, and the jejunum is the first portion of gut to return to the abdominal cavity.

The caecal bud appears on the caudal limb of the primitive gut tube at about week 6, and it develops into the caecal swelling, which is the last part of the developing tube to re-enter the abdominal cavity.

The appendix develops from the distal end of the swelling during the descent of the colon, and it may come to lie in a variety of positions. However, it is usually found posterior to the large intestine.

Failure of the intestinal loops to return to the abdominal cavity results in exomphalos, the protrusion of abdominal contents through the abdominal wall at the site of insertion of the cord. The contents of this hernia are covered by amnion (which distinguishes them from gastroschisis, described in Chapter 8).

The distal third of the transverse colon and the upper part of the anal canal arise from the hindgut. They are supplied by the inferior mesenteric artery.

The distal part of the hindgut grows into the cloaca, an endodermal lined cavity, which is in contact with the surface ectoderm.

During the 9th week of development, the anal membrane ruptures to open up the rectum to the external environment.

In the anal canal, the pectinate line indicates the junction between the endodermal and ectodermal parts. It is also the point at which the columnar

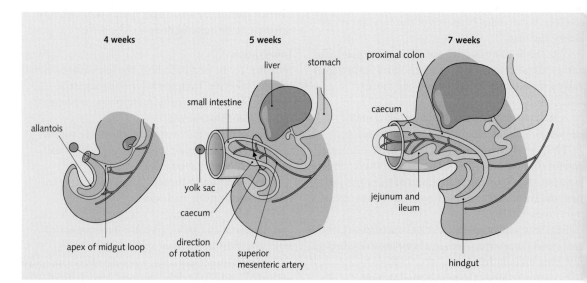

Fig. 7.6 Rotation and herniation of the developing gut.

epithelium in the upper part of the anal canal changes to stratified squamous epithelium in the lower part.

Tissues of the small intestine
Tissue layers
The tissue layers are essentially the same as those found elsewhere in the gastrointestinal tract (see Fig. 1.2), consisting of a mucosa, submucosa, muscularis externa, and serosa. The mucosa consists of:
- An epithelium.
- Lamina propria.
- Muscularis mucosae.

The submucosa contains the submucosal (Meissner's) plexus. The muscularis externa is made up of two layers of muscle, an inner circular muscle layer and an outer longitudinal one. The myenteric (Auerbach's) plexus is located between the muscle layers. A large amount of GALT (gut-associated lymphoid tissue) is present in the submucosa of the small intestine.

Mucosa of the small intestine
The mucosa of the small intestine is the main site of absorption for digestion products, such as amino acids, fats, and sugars. The mucosa and submucosa are specialized to allow maximum absorption.

The mucosa has a much greater surface area than other parts of the gastrointestinal tract due to the presence of:
- Plicae circulares.
- Numerous villi.
- A striated border of microvilli.

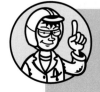

Villi are projections consisting of a series of epithelial cells, microvilli are smaller protrusions from individual epithelial cells.

These factors together produce a 600-fold increase in the absorptive area of the small intestine. Plicae circulares are folds in the mucosa and submucosa, arranged on a circular fashion around the lumen of the small intestine. They are most prominent in the jejunum, but absent in the distal part of the small intestine.

Intestinal glands (crypts of Lieberkühn) are found throughout the length of the small intestine. They are simple tubular glands extending through the thickness of the mucous membrane and opening into the intestinal lumen at the base of the villi (Fig. 7.7).

Villi
The villi change in shape along the length of the small intestine. In the duodenum they are broad, but they become leaf-like further down the tract. In the terminal ileum, villi are finger-like projections.

They consist of an epithelial cover and a lamina propria with a centrally placed lymphatic capillary (lacteal) that drains into the large lymphatic vessels in the submucosa (Fig. 7.8). Lacteals dilate after a meal, but they are collapsed in the fasting state.

In coeliac disease, the surface of the jejunum is flattened and there is extensive loss of villi. This

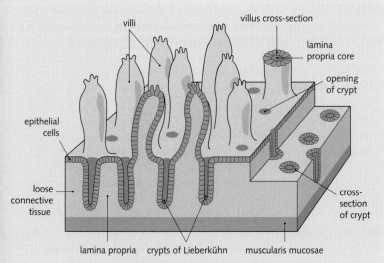

Fig. 7.7 Villi and crypts of Lieberkühn.

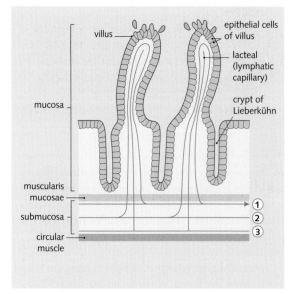

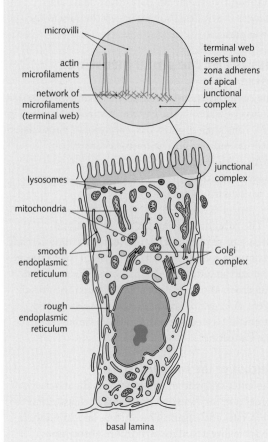

Fig. 7.8 Villi of the small intestine. Drainage is to: 1 hepatic portal vein; 2 branch of superior mesenteric artery; 3 lymphatic system.

results from an allergy to the wheat protein, gluten. This immune-mediated inflammation causes malabsorption, due to the loss of villi. A gluten-free diet can restore normal absorption by regeneration of villi.

Cell types of the mucosa
Enterocytes (intestinal absorptive cells)
Enterocytes are the most numerous cells. They are found chiefly on the villi and surface of the small intestine and, in lesser numbers, in the intestinal glands. They are tall columnar cells with striated microvilli borders and irregular outlines (Fig. 7.9).

The cells absorb water from the lumen of the gut, and the paracellular spaces contain ATPases that transport sodium from the cell into the spaces, drawing the water absorbed from the lumen from the cell by osmosis.

The ultrastructure of these cells is indicative of their absorptive role. They contain large quantities of rough endoplasmic reticulum (RER), mitochondria, and golgi. Many ribosomes are present.

The glycocalyx of the microvilli contain many enzymes (e.g. lactase, alkaline phosphatase, lipases), which are involved in digestion and transport.

Microvilli are destroyed by the flagellate parasite *Giardia lamblia*, but they regenerate if the organism is eradicated.

Fig. 7.9 Enterocyte.

Goblet cells
Goblet cells (Fig. 7.10) in the intestine produce mucus, as they do in other epithelia.

They are interspersed between the enterocytes, and they are most numerous on the villi and in the superior two thirds of the crypts.

Goblet cells are least numerous in the duodenum, but they increase in frequency along the length of the small intestine. They are most numerous in the terminal ileum.

Paneth cells
Paneth cells are found in the deepest part of the intestinal glands. They are typical of cells that synthesize and secrete large amounts of protein, and their cytoplasm is rich in RER.

They are phagocytic and contain granules of lysozyme, an enzyme that digests the walls of certain bacteria. Paneth cells are thought to play a role in the regulation of intestinal flora.

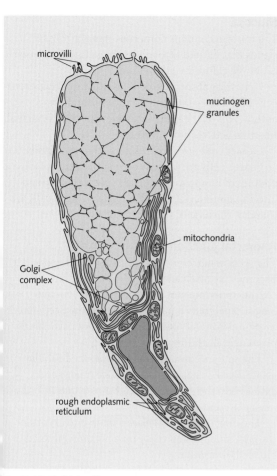

Fig. 7.10 Goblet cell.

M cells

Membranous microfold 'M' cells are epithelial cells that overlie the organized lymphoid tissue, called Peyer's patches.

They are flattened cells, which allows for entry of antigen.

Undifferentiated (stem) cells

Stem cells are located in the lower third of the crypts of Lieberkühn. They give rise to the enterocytes, goblet cells and enteroendocrine (APUD) cells.

Approximately 1.7 billion enterocytes are shed from the adult intestine each day, and they are replaced by undifferentiated cells migrating up from the bases of the crypts. The turnover of enterocytes takes about 5 days.

The protein content of the cells lost from the gut each day is approximately 30 g. It accounts for a substantial amount of the daily protein loss from the body.

Enteroendocrine cells

The enteroendocrine (APUD) cells situated in the crypts of the small intestine are very similar to those found in the stomach. They are triangular-shaped cells with the luminal apex displaying microvilli.

They secrete hormones and neuropeptides, including somatostatin, 5-hydroxytryptamine (5-HT; serotonin), secretin, gastrin, motilin, and vasoactive intestinal polypeptide (VIP).

Peyer's patches

Peyer's patches are present in the mucosa of the ileum, extending into the submucosa, and they are characteristically found opposite the attachment of the mesentery.

They consist of aggregations of lymphoid nodules and form part of the mucosa-associated lymphoid system (MALT).

The Peyer's patches contain three types of cell:
- Membranous microfold 'M' cells, which allow antigen to enter.
- Dome cells, which are rich in MHC class II and present antigen to lymphocytes.
- Lymphocytes (B and T) found in the follicular zone.

Cells of the small intestinal mucosa are summarized in Fig. 7.11.

Lamina propria

The lamina propria of the small intestine is made up of a glycosaminoglycan (GAG) matrix, fibroblasts, collagen, reticulin, and smooth muscle fibres.

It also contains capillaries, lymphatics, nerves, and diffuse lymphoid tissue.

Submucosa

The submucosa contains blood vessels, lymphatics, and the submucosal nerve plexus (Meissner's plexus). It contains GALT and Brunner's glands. Compound tubular Brunner's glands are only present in the duodenum.

They secrete mucus, bicarbonate, and growth factors such as epidermal growth factor. The last of these promotes the growth and regeneration of tissues.

Brunner's glands also secrete urogastrone, an inhibitor of acid secretion.

Tissues of the large intestine
Tissue layers

The layers of the large intestine are essentially the same as those in the rest of the gastrointestinal tract (see Fig. 1.2).

At the microscopic level, it is easy to tell the three sections of the small intestine apart. The duodenum has submucosal Brunner's glands. The jejunum has the most complex and numerous plicae circulares and villi (it is the main site of absorption) and the ileum has the most developed Peyer's patches and GALT, extending into the submucosa.

However, the walls are thicker, the lumen is larger, and the outer longitudinal muscle layer forms three bands (taeniae coli) visible on the outside of the intestine (Figs 7.1 and 7.2). The large intestine has no villi or plicae circulares.

Most nutrients have already been absorbed by the time the intestinal contents reach the large intestine, but the large intestine is responsible for most of the reabsorption of water and electrolytes, and it plays an important role in electrolyte homeostasis.

Approximately 90% of the water in the faeces is reabsorbed by the colon, and faeces become more compact as they travel through the large intestine. The other function of the large intestine is mucus secretion.

Mucosa

The mucosa contains numerous straight tubular glands that extend through its thickness and consist of simple columnar epithelium.

Columnar absorptive cells are the most numerous cells of the large intestine. They are similar to enterocytes of the small intestine, but their principal function is to reabsorb water.

Goblet cells are also present within the glands.

Paneth cells are present only in the young. Isolated nodules of lymphatic tissue are found that extend into the submucosa. Undifferentiated stem cells are found at the base of the tubular glands.

Anorectal junction

The rectum narrows towards its terminal end and it becomes the anal canal (Fig. 7.12).

The upper portion of the anal canal contains longitudinal folds (anal or rectal columns) separated by depressions (anal sinuses). They are particularly prominent in children.

The sinuses contain straight, branched tubular glands (anal glands) which produce mucus and extend into the submucosa and sometimes into the muscularis externa.

The ducts of the anal glands open into crypts in the anal mucosa, and these may become infected or blocked, forming a cyst.

The mucosa of the upper anal canal is similar to that of the large intestine but the lower portion

Fig. 7.11 Cells of the small intestinal mucosa and their functions.

Cells of the small intestinal mucosa	
Cell type	Function
Enterocytes	Intestinal absorptive cells. These tall columnar cells have microvilli and absorb water and nutrients from the lumen of the gut
Goblet cells	These produce mucus and are found on the villi. They are least numerous in the duodenum and most numerous in the terminal ileum
Paneth cells	These are phagocytic cells and contain lysozyme granules. They are found deep in the intestinal glands
Membranous microfold 'M' cells	Epithelial cells, which overlie Peyer's patches and allow for entry of antigen
Undifferentiated (stem) cells	These give rise to enterocytes, goblet cells and enteroendocrine cells. They are located in the lower thirds of the crypts
Enteroendocrine (APUD) cells	These cells secrete hormones and neuropeptides, such as somatostatin, 5-HT, secretin and gastrin. They are found in the crypts of the small intestine and have microvilli at their luminal apices

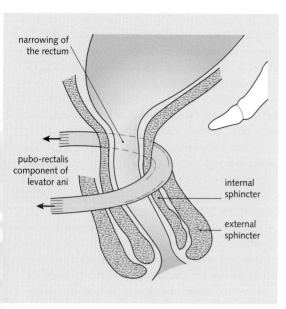

Fig. 7.12 The ano-rectal junction.

consists of stratified squamous epithelium, continuous with the skin surrounding the anal canal. The middle portion contains stratified columnar epithelium.

The anus contains two sphincters, an internal (involuntary) and an external (voluntary) one, described below.

The anal columns contain terminal branches of the rectal veins in the submucosa. The venous branches may enlarge to form haemorrhoids. Small folds of mucosa (anal valves) are present at the lower end of the anal canal.

Cellular functions of the small intestine

Overview of small intestine function

The small intestine has a very large surface area, and it is specially adapted to digest and absorb nutrients, salt, and water. Enzymes and hormones produced in the small intestine complete the digestion that began in the mouth and stomach.

The small intestine has immunological defences against antigens that have been ingested consisting of solitary lymph nodules and Peyer's patches (aggregations of lymphatic nodules).

Gastrointestinal hormones produced in the small intestine play an important role in gastrointestinal secretion and motility.

Defence against antigens is both mechanical, by the production of mucus, and immunological, principally through gut-associated lymphoid tissue, described below.

Epithelial cell turnover

The cells of the intestinal epithelium are described in the 'Organization of the intestine' section above. They have a high rate of turnover and are replaced by undifferentiated (stem) cells, which migrate up from the bases of the crypts of Lieberkühn (Fig. 7.13). The cells become partially differentiated and they continue to divide as they migrate upwards from the bottom of the crypts (Fig. 7.13).

The average lifespan of an enterocyte is about 2–3 days, but this is reduced in coeliac disease and as a side effect of some drugs (e.g. prolonged anticancer therapy). The undifferentiated cells cannot keep up with the increased loss, resulting in a flattening of the villi and malabsorption.

Radiotherapy may have a similar effect (radiation enteritis) depending on the dose and the site at which it is administered. Symptoms usually resolve within 6 weeks of the final dose of radiotherapy, but some patients experience chronic radiation enteritis (symptoms persisting for more than 3 months). Radiation damage causes ulceration due to ischaemia, muscle fibre atrophy, and fibrosis, which may result in stricture formation and obstruction.

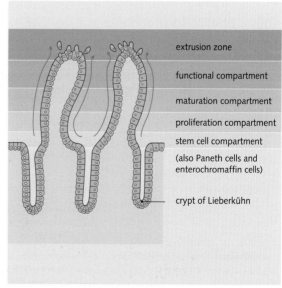

Fig. 7.13 The migration and shedding of cells in the small intestine.

Secretions of the small intestine

The small intestine secretes mucus and gastrointestinal hormones.

- Mucus is produced by the goblet cells (Fig. 7.10), which are most numerous on the villi. The mucus lubricates the mucosal surface and protects it from trauma as particles of food pass through it.
- Gastrointestinal hormones found in the small intestine are summarized in Fig. 7.14.

The epithelial cells secrete an aqueous solution during the course of digestion but, under normal conditions, they absorb slightly more than they secrete.

Under certain conditions, e.g. cholera infection, secretion greatly exceeds absorption and secretory diarrhoea occurs.

The immune system in the small intestine

T lymphocytes are made in the thymus, a bilobular organ found in the thorax, and they migrate into peripheral tissues such as the spleen and lymph nodes (encapsulated organs). T lymphocytes also migrate to non-encapsulated lymphoid tissue known as mucosa-associated lymphoid tissue (MALT). This gives protection against antigens entering the body through mucosal epithelial surfaces (Fig. 7.15).

The majority of MALT is present as gut-associated lymphoid tissue (GALT); smaller amounts are present as bronchial-associated lymphoid tissue (BALT), skin-associated lymphoid tissue (SALT), and in the genitourinary tract.

B lymphocytes are made in the bone marrow and, in the fetus, in the liver. They also migrate to peripheral tissues, including MALT.

T cells are divided into:

- Helper (CD4) cells, which enhance the reaction of the immune system following the presentation of antigen to T helper cells by antigen presenting cells, via MHC class II.
- Cytotoxic (CD8) cells are capable of killing other cells (e.g. cancer cells and cells that have been infected with viruses), and they can also downregulate the immune response. They are activated via an endogenous antigen and MHC class I complex.

CD4 and CD8 cells together make up approximately 75% of all lymphocytes.

B cells produce antibody and, once they have encountered a particular antigen, form memory cells, which can undergo clonal expansion (multiply rapidly to form large numbers of identical B cells). B cells then differentiate to form plasma cells, which have a relatively short half-life but which produce

Main actions of the principal gastric hormones			
Hormone	Gastrointestinal source	Signal for release	Action
CCK	Enteroendocrine (APUD) cells in upper intestine	Peptides and amino acids and fats, elevated serum Ca^{2+} in duodenum	Contracts gall bladder and relaxes sphincter of Oddi; causes secretion of alkaline enzymatic pancreatic juice, inhibits gastric emptying, exerts trophic effect on pancreas acts as a satiety hormone, stimulates glucagon secretion and contracts the pyloric sphincter
Secretin	S cells in upper small intestine	Acid and products of fat digestion in duodenum	Increases secretion of HCO_3^- by the pancreas and biliary tract, decreases acid secretion, contracts the pyloric sphincter and augments CCK's production of pancreatic secretions
Gastrin	G cells in antrum	Peptides and amino acids, distension, vagal stimulation, blood-borne calcium and adrenaline	Acid and pepsinogen secretion, trophic to mucosa of stomach and small and large intestines, increases gastric motility, may close LOS, stimulates insulin and glucagon secretion after protein meal. Inhibits gastric emptying
Somatostatin	D cells of pancreatic islets, intestinal cells	Glucose, amino acids, free fatty acids, glucagon and β-adrenergic and cholinergic neurotransmitters	Inhibits secretion of insulin, glucagon, acid, pepsin, gastrin, secretin and intestinal juices, decreases gastric, duodenal and gall bladder motility

Fig. 7.14 Main actions of the principal gastric hormones. (CCK, cholecystokinin; LOS, lower oesophageal sphincter.)

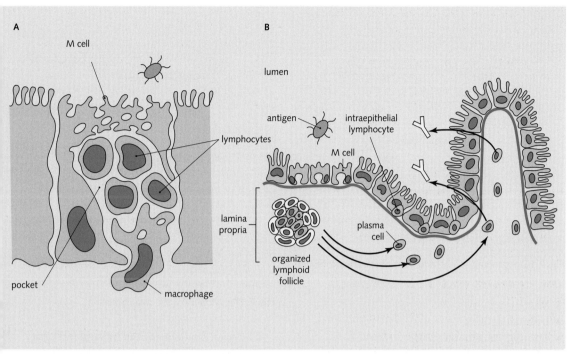

Fig. 7.15 The mucosal associated lymphoid tissue (MALT) of the gut. (A) M cells endocytose antigen in the lumen of the digestive tract, transport it across the cell, and release it into the basolateral pocket. (B) Antigen activates B cells, which differentiate into IgA-producing plasma cells. (Redrawn with permission from Kuby J. *Immunology*, 3rd edn. WH Freeman & Co.)

large numbers of specific antibody to particular antigens. Scattered lymphoid cells are also found in the mucosa of the small intestine.

Specialized M cells (so named because of the numerous microfolds on their luminal surface) overlie the Peyer's patches and they absorb, transport, process, and present antigens to the lymphoid cells lying between them.

Secretory IgA is produced by B cells. There are approximately 10^{10} plasma cells per metre of small intestine, the majority of which (70–90%) produce IgA.

IgA and smaller amounts of IgM are transported across the glandular epithelium into the gut lumen and prevent microorganisms from entering.

Dimers of IgA bind to a receptor on the membrane of the epithelial cells. The IgA–receptor complex is endocytosed and transported across the cell into the lumen. Part of the receptor (the secretary component) remains attached to the IgA and protects IgA from proteolytic enzymes in the lumen.

Motility of the small intestine
Functions of intestinal motility
Motility in the small intestine facilitates three main functions:

- Mixing of intestinal contents.
- Bringing the contents into contact with the absorptive surfaces of the small intestine.
- Forward propulsion of the contents.

Chyme takes between 2 and 3 hours to pass through the small intestine, which is the site at which most digestion and absorption of nutrients takes place.

There are two main types of contraction seen in the fed state in the small intestine: segmentation and peristalsis.

Segmentation mixes the digested food and exposes it to the absorptive surfaces. It involves the progressive contraction and relaxation of the circular muscles. There is a slow net movement towards the anus (Fig. 7.16).

Peristaltic contraction brings about rapid propulsion of the intestinal contents towards the anus, at a rate of 2–25 cm/s. It involves contraction of the longitudinal muscles, and it is a reflex initiated by local distension, caused by the bolus of food. The reflex is always orad to anus in direction.

The functions of segmentation and peristalsis generally overlap.

The fasting state in the small intestine has a different sequence of motility. It involves three phases:

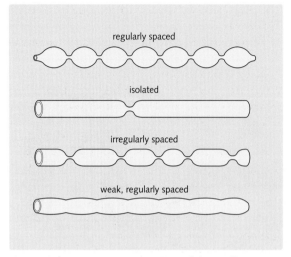

Fig. 7.16 Segmentation contractions of the small intestine.

- Motor inactivity.
- Irregular activity.
- The migrating motor complex (MMC).

Migrating motor complexes occur every 90–120 min, during fasting. The MMC involves high frequency bursts of powerful contractions, beginning in the stomach and moving towards the terminal ileum.

The pyloric sphincter is open wide during the MMC.

The MMC has a number of functions:
- It moves indigestible food (e.g. tomato skins, nuts, sweetcorn) into the lower bowel.
- It allows for the removal of dead epithelial cells.
- It prevents bacterial overgrowth.
- It prevents colonic bacteria entering the small intestine.

As soon as food is ingested, the MMC stops and motility switches to the fed-state pattern.

Control of intestinal motility

The motility of the small intestine is controlled by nervous, hormonal, and local factors (Fig. 7.17).

The vagus is required to maintain the fed motor pattern. Segmentation is coordinated by the myenteric plexus, and circular muscle contraction is brought about by acetylcholine and substance P.

The peristaltic reflex occurs by the simultaneous oral (proximal) contraction and anal (distal) relaxation, either side of the bolus. The contraction is mediated by vagal excitatory contractions, via substance P and acetylcholine.

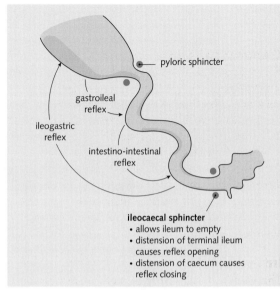

ileocaecal sphincter
- allows ileum to empty
- distension of terminal ileum causes reflex opening
- distension of caecum causes reflex closing

Fig. 7.17 Motility of the small intestine.

The relaxation is mediated by vagal inhibitory contractions, via nitric oxide (NO) and VIP. Movement of the bolus into the next section of the intestine triggers the next reflex.

In the fasting state, the MMC is coordinated by the enteric nervous system. It is initiated by vagal stimulation and motilin. During an MMC, plasma motilin concentrations increase, but they decrease on the arrival of food in the stomach.

The ileocaecal sphincter

The ileocaecal valve (sphincter) separates the terminal ileum from the colon and is normally closed. However, it opens in response to:
- Distension of the terminal ileum (by a reflex mechanism).
- Short-range peristalsis in the terminal ileum.
- Gastroileal reflex (which enhances emptying of the ileum after a meal).

When the ileocaecal valve opens, small amounts of chyme enter the colon at the rate at which the colon is able to reabsorb most of the salts and water contained in the chyme. It is an incompetent valve, which is useful as it stops the build-up of wind or stools in the colon.

Digestion and absorption in the small intestine

Digestion begins in the mouth and continues in the stomach, but most digestion and absorption takes place in the small intestine.

General concepts

For food to be absorbed, it must be broken down into small particles that can be transported across the epithelial cells of the gastrointestinal tract and into the bloodstream. Substances are then carried to the liver via the hepatic portal system.

As elsewhere in the body, molecules may be transported across the epithelial cells by simple diffusion, facilitated diffusion, and primary or secondary active transport. The properties of these different types of transport are shown in Figs 7.18 and 7.19.

Intestinal circulation

The intestinal circulation is part of the splanchnic circulation, which supplies the lower oesophagus, stomach, liver, gall bladder, pancreas, spleen, and intestines.

At rest, approximately 10–30% of the cardiac output flows to the digestive organs and three quarters of this is required by the mucosa and submucosa for facilitation of absorption and transport. The remaining quarter is utilized by the smooth muscle layer of the bowels.

The splanchnic circulation has a major role as a large reservoir that can be mobilized easily when required, such as during exercise.

Another function of this circulation, is the intestinal countercurrent system. In the mucosal villi, the blood vessels are arranged in a network of hairpin loops.

The arteriole enters at the base of the villus, and it divides into a capillary network at the tip of the villus, just deep to the epithelial lining of the villus. The arteriole and venule are only 20 μm apart and lipid permeable molecules, such as oxygen, can pass from one vessel to the other.

The blood flows are countercurrent, or opposite in direction.

This facilitates some of the dissolved oxygen in the plasma to move along its diffusion gradient from the arteriole to the venule, without entering the capillary network.

When intestinal blood flow is low, this shunting of oxygen can cause death to the epithelial cells at the villus tip. Necrosis of enterocytes at the villus tip is a sign of severe intestinal ischaemia.

The most important function of the countercurrent blood flow is to produce a region of hyperosmolarity in the villus tip by means of a countercurrent multiplier system (Fig. 7.20).

Hyperosmolarity is achieved by the following mechanisms:

- Na^+ ions are pumped into the subepithelial extracellular fluid by the enterocytes and taken up in the capillary network. As blood flows down into the venule, Na^+ ions diffuse across to the capillary, which returns the Na^+ ions to the villus tip. This results in a hyperosmolar region at the tip, which draws in water molecules from the intestinal lumen.
- Water molecules may also be drawn into the descending capillaries from the arterial vessel, if there is an increased Na^+ concentration. This also results in the delivery of hyperosmolar blood to the villous tip.

The countercurrent mechanism is very similar to that seen in the loop of Henle in the kidney.

The control of the intestinal circulation

Nerves, hormones, and local factors control the intestinal circulation.

Molecule transport mechanisms			
Type of transport	Proteins required	Transport against or with concentration gradient	Energy required
Passive diffusion	No	With	No
Facilitated diffusion	Yes	With	No
Primary active transport	Yes	Against	Yes: hydrolysis of ATP
Secondary active transport	Yes	Against	Yes: electrochemical gradient

Fig. 7.18 Molecule transport mechanisms. (Data courtesy of Dr MA Rattray, UMDS, London.)

133

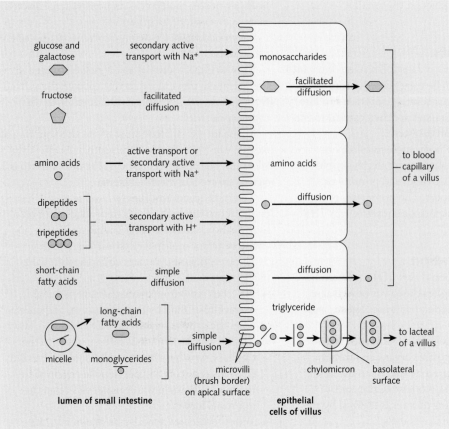

Fig. 7.19 Absorption in the small intestine. For simplicity, all digested foods are shown in the lumen of the small intestine, even though some are digested by brush-border enzymes. (Redrawn with permission from Berne and Levy, 2000.)

A change in the cardiac output, arterial pressure or blood volume will have the same effect on this circulation as on the general systemic circulation. For example, massive haemorrhage will result in a decreased venous return to the heart, decreased cardiac output, and a drop in arterial blood pressure.

This activates baroreceptors to bring about the sympathetic reflex of vasoconstriction in precapillary vessels. This is particularly marked in the intestinal circulation.

Autonomic nervous control regulates the blood flow by:
- Parasympathetic nerves, which are vasodilators, via acetylcholine and VIP.
- Sympathetic nerves, which are vasoconstrictors, via adrenaline and noradrenaline (acting on alpha$_2$-adrenoreceptors).
- Enteric nerves, which are vasodilators, via acetylcholine and VIP.

- Primary sensory nerves (C fibres), which are vasodilators, via NO, substance P and calcitonin gene related peptide (CGRP).

Endocrine and paracrine controls can also regulate the intestinal circulation. These are summarized in Fig. 7.21.

Metabolites in the gut after a meal can act as vasodilators. Glucose and fatty acids cause postprandial hyperaemia, which is mediated by VIP release from the enteric nervous system.

Factors that control absorption by the small intestine

A number of factors control absorption by the small intestine:
- Adequate blood supply.
- Carrier molecule density and availability at the brush border.
- Cell maturation rate.

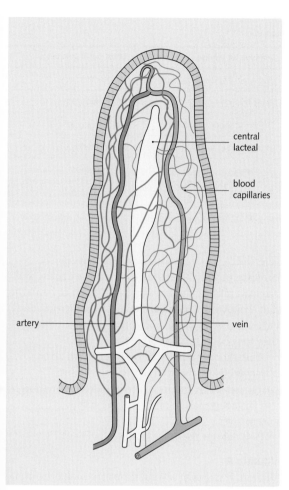

central
lacteal

blood
capillaries

artery

vein

Fig. 7.20 The countercurrent mechanism in the villi of the small intestine. This enables absorption of electrolytes and water.

- Number of transporting cells.
- Passive permeability and the intracellular concentrations of molecules.
- The electrochemical gradient for Na^+.
- Sympathetic innervation and adrenaline in the plasma both increase the absorption of Na^+ and Cl^- (and therefore water).
- Parasympathetic stimulation decreases the absorption of these substances.
- Aldosterone is a steroid hormone made from cholesterol in the zona glomerulosa of the adrenal glands. Aldosterone's main action is to increase the permeability of the collecting tubules of the kidney and the reabsorption of Na^+ and Cl^-. The excretion of potassium and hydrogen ions is increased. It also stimulates the absorption of Na^+ and water by the colon and the secretion of potassium. It is released in response to a decrease

in the Na^+ concentration of the plasma, an increase in the potassium concentration and by the activation of the renin–angiotensin system as a result of dehydration.
- Increased absorption of Na^+ and Cl^- in the kidney and gut (and the gastric, sweat, and salivary glands) causes retention of water and an increase in effective circulating volume.

Digestion and absorption of different components of the diet
Fat and fat soluble vitamins
Absorption of the fat soluble vitamins A, D, E, and K depend on the absorption of fat and any condition in which fat digestion and absorption is decreased will eventually lead to a deficiency of these vitamins.

Fat is not water soluble and its digestion and absorption is more complex than that of other substances.

Fat in the diet is principally in the form of triglycerides, and it is only released from the stomach into the duodenum at the rate at which it can be digested. The presence of fat in the duodenum, therefore, inhibits gastric emptying.

Lipase in the stomach (preduodenal lipase made up of gastric lipase produced in the fundus and, to a lesser extent, lingual lipase from the mouth), hydrolyses triglycerides in the stomach. These are then released into the duodenum. In the duodenum, bile acids form micelles (in much the same way as detergents in washing powder do). A minimum concentration of bile acids is needed to form micelles (the critical micelle concentration).

Micelles consist of 20–30 molecules, arranged so that lipid (non-polar) molecules lie in the centre, surrounded by conjugated bile acids and water-soluble molecules. Micelles are rather like a chocolate with a soft centre. The chocolate is the polar component, and the soft centre consists of the non-polar part of the bile acids together with lipids from the diet.

Lipase (glycerol esterhydrolase), cholesterol esterase and phospholipase 2, all of which are produced by the pancreas, act on fat droplets, which have been made smaller by the emulsifying action of bile acids and lecithin in the duodenum.

Pancreatic lipase is inactivated by acid, and it is ineffective if excess acid is produced by the stomach. This occurs in the Zollinger–Ellison syndrome, where fat malabsorption occurs.

Vasoactive hormones			
Hormone	Source	Stimulus for release	Effect on GI circulation
Catecholamines	Adrenal medulla	Oligaemic (hypovolaemic) shock	Vasoconstriction
Angiotensin II	Renal JGA	Heart failure	Vasoconstriction
Vasopressin	Posterior pituitary	Oligaemic shock	Vasoconstriction
Gastrin	GI mucosal G cells	Mealtimes	Vasodilatation
CCK	Intestinal mucosal I cells	Mealtimes	Vasodilatation
Secretin	Intestinal mucosal S cells	Mealtimes	Vasodilatation

Fig. 7.21 Control of the intestinal circulation by vasoactive hormones. (CCK, cholecystokinin; GI, gastrointestinal; JGA, juxtaglomerular apparatus.)

The products of fat digestion, being lipids, diffuse across the lipid membrane of the brush border of the small intestine.

Different components are absorbed at different rates. Free fatty acids diffuse across rapidly, cholesterol more slowly. The micelles, therefore, become more concentrated in cholesterol as they move along the small intestine.

Under normal conditions, most dietary fat is absorbed before the contents reach the end of the jejunum and any fat in the stools (in the absence of steatorrhoea) is from desquamated epithelial cells and from bacterial flora in the gut.

The surface of the normal small intestine is convoluted (providing a greater surface area for absorption). An unstirred layer is present on the surface, through which micelles must pass before dietary fat can be absorbed by the epithelial cells.

Once inside the epithelial cells, lipid is taken into the smooth endoplasmic reticulum where much of it is re-esterified.

Some lipid is also synthesized in the epithelial cells. Dietary and synthesized lipids are then incorporated into chylomicrons and, provided β-lipoprotein is present, the chylomicrons are exocytosed into lateral intercellular spaces to enter the lacteals. Having reached the lymphatic system, they travel up the thoracic duct and enter the venous circulation.

Apolipoproteins are an important constituent of chylomicrons, and they are made by hepatocytes and the epithelial cells of the intestine. Their absence leads to the accumulation of lipid in intestinal epithelial cells.

Chylomicrons consist mainly of triglyceride with a phospholipid coat studded with apolipoproteins (Fig. 7.22). They contain small amounts of cholesterol and cholesterol esters in the centre, and their overall size depends on the amount of fat in the diet. Following a high fat intake, chylomicrons may have a diameter of up to 750 nm, in low fat diets they may be as small as 60 nm.

Abetalipoproteinaemia is a rare inborn error of metabolism inherited as a recessive trait, characterized by failure of chylomicron formation and an accumulation of dietary fat within enterocytes.

Cellular uptake of fat is shown in Fig. 7.23.

Vitamin A
Vitamin A exists in several forms (retinol, β-carotene and retinal) with retinol being best absorbed.

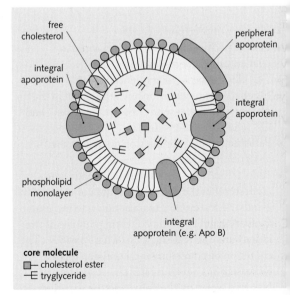

Fig. 7.22 The structure of a chylomicron.

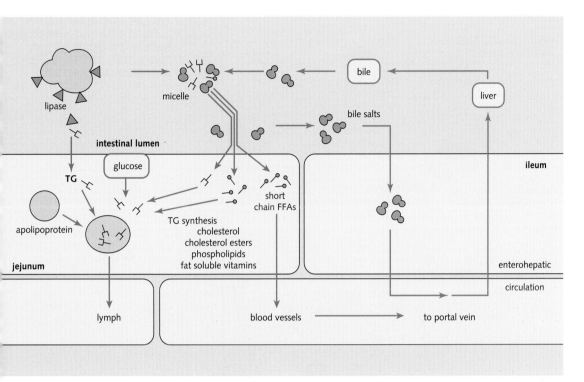

Fig. 7.23 Cellular uptake of free fatty acids and chylomicrons. (TG, triglyceride; FFA, free fatty acid)

Beta-carotene and retinal are both converted to retinol in the intestinal epithelial cells.

Vitamin D

This is absorbed mainly in the jejunum. It is transported to the liver or kidney for activation, by incorporation into chylomicrons.

Vitamin E

Vitamin E is incorporated into chylomicrons (provided micelles are formed) and enters the lymphatic system.

Vitamin K

Vitamin K exists in several forms. Vitamins K_1 and K_2 enter the lymphatic system, while vitamin K_3 enters the portal blood. The intestinal bacterial flora synthesizes most of the vitamin K we receive.

Carbohydrates

Carbohydrates provide most of the calories in the average diet, and the majority is in the form of starch (a polymer of glucose).

Starch contains α-1,4 and α-1,6 linkages: the former are hydrolysed by α-amylase in saliva (ptyalin) and in pancreatic secretions (pancreatic α-amylase).

This produces maltose and maltotriose (together known as malto-oligosaccharides), comprising 70% of the breakdown products, and α-limit dextrans (the remaining 30%).

Starch is, therefore, partially digested in the mouth (α-amylase is inactivated by gastric acid, so starch is not digested in the stomach) and its digestion continues in the duodenum.

Other enzymes exist in the brush border of the duodenum, and these complete the digestion of starch.

These enzymes further break down starch into glucose and galactose, which are actively taken up with sodium. Carbohydrates are only absorbed as monosaccharides through the gut mucosa. Glucose and galactose then cross the basal membrane into the capillaries by facilitated transport and simple diffusion (Fig. 7.24).

Another monosaccharide, fructose, is also produced and taken up by a sodium-independent mechanism.

A deficiency of enzymes in the digestive system can result in carbohydrate malabsorption. The most common deficiency is lactase deficiency, which

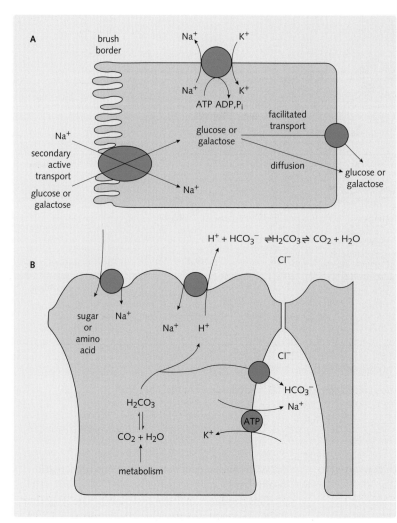

Fig. 7.24 (A) Sugar and (B) ion transport in the small intestine. ([A] Redrawn with permission from *Nature*, 1987; **330**: 379; London, Macmillan Magazines Ltd.)

results in lactose intolerance in about 50% of adults worldwide!

Lactase deficiency has a strong genetic component and its incidence varies in different races. Exclusion of milk and milk products relieves many of the symptoms.

Other, rarer deficiencies include congenital lactose intolerance (most cases are acquired), sucrase–isomaltase deficiency and glucose–galactose malabsorption syndrome.

Lactase deficiency is discussed in more detail in Chapter 8. The digestion of carbohydrates is summarized in Fig. 7.25.

Protein

The protein requirement of a normal healthy adult is about 40 g/day (to replace the 5–7 g/day nitrogen lost as urea, excreted in the urine).

In the Western world, meat eaters usually exceed this, but in the developing world the amount of protein in the diet is less.

We do not have a store of protein in the body (unlike, for example, glycogen). Every protein in the body performs a function and proteins are in a constant state of flux (1–2% of total body protein is turned over daily), being synthesized by ribosomes and then degraded in the body. We synthesize about 300 g/day protein.

Protein in the intestinal lumen comes from protein eaten in the diet and also from desquamated cells, almost all of which are digested and absorbed.

Digestion of dietary protein begins in the stomach (pepsin hydrolyses about 15% of dietary protein to amino acids and small peptides). It continues in the duodenum and small intestine where pancreatic proteases continue the process of hydrolysis (Fig. 7.26).

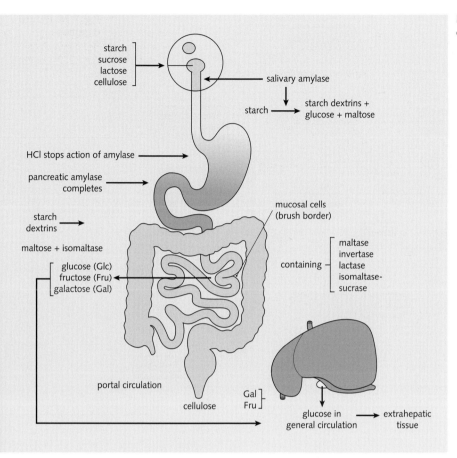

Fig. 7.25 Digestion of carbohydrates.

Absorption of the products of protein digestion

Small peptides, particularly dipeptides and tripeptides are absorbed more rapidly than amino acids. They are transported across the membrane by an active mechanism utilizing the electrochemical potential difference of Na^+.

There are a number of different amino acid carriers depending on the charge of the amino acid. Some of these require a Na^+ gradient for transport.

Amino acids enter the cells from the lumen and leave it to pass into the capillaries by three mechanisms: sodium-dependent transport, sodium-independent transport, and simple diffusion. The simple carrier systems for amino acid transport are summarized in Fig. 7.27.

Defects of amino acid absorption are rare but include Hartnup disease and prolinuria, neither of which on their own cause malnutrition.

Water and ions

The normal daily intake of water is about 1.5 L/day. However, up to 9 L water per day are absorbed from the gastrointestinal tract (through the reabsorption of secretions) under normal circumstances, most of it from the small intestine, especially the jejunum (Fig. 7.28).

Almost all of the Na^+ in the gastrointestinal tract is reabsorbed (about 99%), mostly from the jejunum in association with glucose, galactose, and certain amino acids.

Na^+ is transported across the epithelial cell membrane down its electrochemical gradient and pumped into the intercellular spaces in exchange for K^+. Na^+ is absorbed against its electrochemical gradient in the ileum and the colon.

Water follows the active pumping of Na^+ by Na^+/K^+ ATPases through a transcellular or paracellular (tight junctions) route.

Bicarbonate and chloride

Pancreatic secretions contain HCO_3^- (which neutralizes gastric acid reaching the duodenum from the stomach) most of which is reabsorbed from the

139

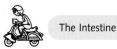

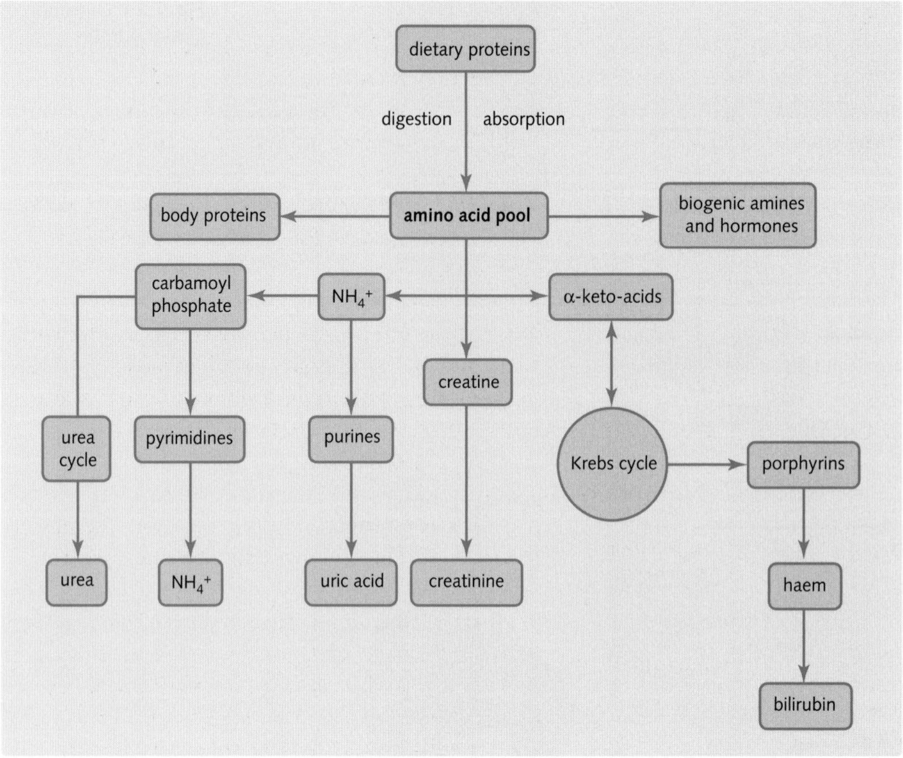

Fig. 7.26 Protein digestion.

```
                        ┌─────────────────┐
                        │ dietary proteins│
                        └─────────────────┘
                                 │
                    digestion    │    absorption
                                 ▼
┌──────────────┐        ┌─────────────────┐        ┌────────────────────┐
│ body proteins│◄───────│ amino acid pool │───────►│  biogenic amines   │
└──────────────┘        └─────────────────┘        │    and hormones    │
                                 │                  └────────────────────┘
      ┌──────────────┐   ┌──────────┐       ┌─────────────┐
      │  carbamoyl   │◄──│  NH₄⁺    │◄─────►│ α-keto-acids│
      │  phosphate   │   └──────────┘       └─────────────┘
      └──────────────┘        │                    
         │      │      ┌──────────┐                
         │      │      │ creatine │          ┌───────────┐
         │      │      └──────────┘          │           │
    ┌────────┐ ┌─────────────┐ ┌────────┐   │   Krebs   │──►┌───────────┐
    │  urea  │ │ pyrimidines │ │ purines│   │   cycle   │   │ porphyrins│
    │  cycle │ └─────────────┘ └────────┘   │           │   └───────────┘
    └────────┘                              └───────────┘         │
        │            │           │              │                 ▼
    ┌────────┐  ┌────────┐  ┌──────────┐  ┌────────────┐    ┌───────────┐
    │  urea  │  │  NH₄⁺  │  │ uric acid│  │ creatinine │    │   haem    │
    └────────┘  └────────┘  └──────────┘  └────────────┘    └───────────┘
                                                                  │
                                                                  ▼
                                                            ┌───────────┐
                                                            │ bilirubin │
                                                            └───────────┘
```

Fig. 7.27 Absorption of peptides and amino acids. (AA, amino acids.) (From Johnson, 2000.)

Carrier systems for the transport of amino acids		
Transport system	**Substrates**	**Dependence on Na⁺ gradient**
Brush border membrane		
Neutral	All neutral aromatic and aliphatic AA	Yes
PHE	Phenylalanine and methionine	Yes
Acidic	Glutamate, aspartate	Yes
Imino	Proline, hydroxyproline	Yes
y⁺	Basic AA	No
L	Neutral AA with hydrophobic side chains	No
Basolateral membrane		
A	Small neutral AA	Yes
ASC	Three and four carbon neutral AA	Yes
L	Neutral AA with hydrophobic side chains	No
y⁺	Basic AA	No

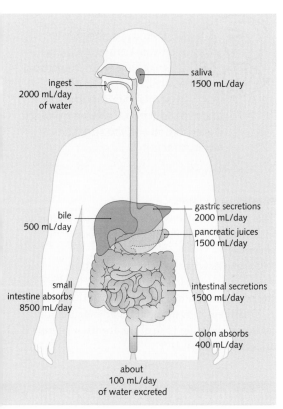

Fig. 7.28 Fluid secretion and absorption in the gastrointestinal tract.

jejunum. However, HCO_3^- is again secreted in the ileum and colon (partly in exchange for Cl^-).

Cl^- is absorbed in the jejunum, ileum, and colon.

Potassium

K^+ is absorbed in the jejunum and ileum. It is secreted into the colon when K^+ concentrations in the lumen are less than 25 mmol/L.

Calcium

This is absorbed throughout the small intestine (especially in the duodenum and jejunum) although absorption is disrupted in vitamin D deficient states.

The percentage of Ca^{2+} absorbed on a low Ca^{2+} diet is higher than that absorbed from a high Ca^{2+} diet.

Ca^{2+} passes across the luminal membrane and into the cytoplasm, where it is bound to a protein and then transported across the basal lateral membrane, some of it in exchange for Na^+.

Ca^{2+} deficiency is seen in vitamin D deficiency, for example in rickets. Vitamin D helps regulate Ca^{2+} absorption and metabolism in the body.

Iron

Iron deficiency is relatively common, particularly in women of childbearing age.

The total amount of iron in the body is only about 3–4 g (about enough to make one 3-inch nail), of which about two thirds is in haemoglobin.

An average Western diet contains about 20 mg of iron a day, of which only about 10% can be absorbed.

Both males and females lose almost 1 mg of iron a day in the urine and desquamated cells and females lose about 50 mg of iron a month in the menstrual flow. Women of reproductive age therefore lose an average of 3 mg of iron a day and iron deficiency anaemia is relatively common.

Growing children, pregnant women, and people who have bled are able to absorb increased amounts of iron to compensate for their greater need.

Absorption is increased in iron deficiency and by increased erythropoeitic activity.

Most dietary iron is in the form Fe^{3+}, which is reduced to Fe^{2+} by ascorbic acid or ferrireductase and then absorbed. Anything that prevents this reduction decreases the absorption of iron (e.g. the production of an insoluble complex with other dietary compounds such as tannin (present in tea), phytate, and certain fibres). Fe^{2+} is taken across the enterocyte membrane of the small intestinal villi by a divalent metal transporter. In the enterocyte, Fe^{2+} is oxidized to Fe^{3+} and then either released into the plasma where it binds to a transferrin molecule or stored in the epithelial cells, bound to ferritin.

 Iron absorption is increased by vitamin C and decreased by tea. Tannin in tea forms an insoluble complex with iron, preventing its reduction to Fe^{2+} and subsequent absorption.

The proportion of iron released depends on the body's requirement. A larger amount remains in the cell bound to ferritin when dietary intake exceeds the body's requirement. This iron is then shed when the epithelial cell is desquamated and prevents iron overload.

Excessive amounts of iron are absorbed in haemochromatosis, an autosomal recessive condition leading to deposition of iron in the liver, heart, pancreas, and pituitary. This results in damage to those organs. The disease is more common in men because premenopausal women are protected by menstruation and childbirth.

Stem cells in the crypts of Lieberkühn can be programmed to absorb more iron, e.g. following haemorrhage. An increase in absorption may be seen 3–4 days after trauma, and in response to other events causing blood loss (the time taken for stem cells to mature and reach the tips of the villi where most iron absorption takes place).

Water soluble vitamins

At the concentrations present in a normal diet, most of these are taken up by specific transport mechanisms, many of which are sodium dependent.

Vitamin B_{12}

Vitamin B_{12} is bound to R protein found in saliva and in gastric secretions, which protects it from digestion in the stomach.

The gastric parietal cells secrete intrinsic factor (IF) and, once vitamin B_{12} has been separated from R proteins in the duodenum by the action of pancreatic proteases, vitamin B_{12} binds to IF.

Receptors for the IF–vitamin B_{12} dimer are present in the membranes of the ileal epithelial cells, which bind the complex and allow uptake of vitamin B_{12}.

Vitamin B_{12} is then transported across the basal membrane of the epithelial cells into the portal blood (Fig. 7.29). It is then bound to transcobalamin II and taken up by the liver, kidney, spleen, heart, placenta, reticulocytes, and fibroblasts.

Vitamin B_{12} deficiency is relatively common after a gastrectomy or ileal resection, as well as in pernicious anaemia. It is important to understand the mechanism by which it is absorbed and the function of intrinsic factor.

Pernicious anaemia

This results from antibodies against IF, leading to malabsorption of vitamin B_{12} and macrocytic anaemia.

Diagnosis is by the Schilling test, the demonstration of low-serum vitamin B_{12} levels and the presence of anti-IF antibodies in the plasma.

Treatment is by intramuscular injections of hydroxocobalamin (one of the forms of vitamin B_{12}) at 2-month intervals.

The flora of the gastrointestinal tract

The intestinal flora

The body contains about 10^{13} human cells and 10^{14} bacterial cells!

Bacteria may be commensal (from the Latin for 'sharing the same table') or pathogenic (capable of causing disease), and aerobic or anaerobic.

In health, most of these bacteria are commensal and many of them have important functions. Flora that are harmless or even beneficial in one site may become pathogens in another part of the body.

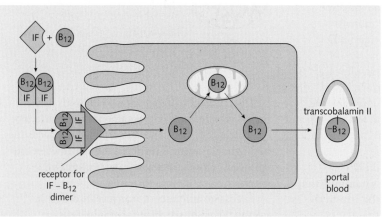

Fig. 7.29 Vitamin B_{12} absorption in the terminal ileum. (IF, intrinsic factor.)

A baby's gut is sterile at birth, but the baby picks up flora from its mother's rectum during delivery. This colonizes the baby's gut over the next 12–18 hours.

Most of the gastrointestinal tract is heavily colonized with flora (Fig. 7.30). Relatively sterile sites include the stomach (where the acid conditions are too hostile to support much flora), the gall bladder, and the salivary glands.

There are 10^{10} organisms per gram of tissue in the mouth and saliva is rapidly contaminated once it reaches the mouth.

The skin, including that around the oral and anal orifices, supports:

- Coagulase-negative staphylococci (mainly *Staphylococcus epidermidis*).
- Diphtheroids (including *Propionibacterium acnes* and Corynebacteria).

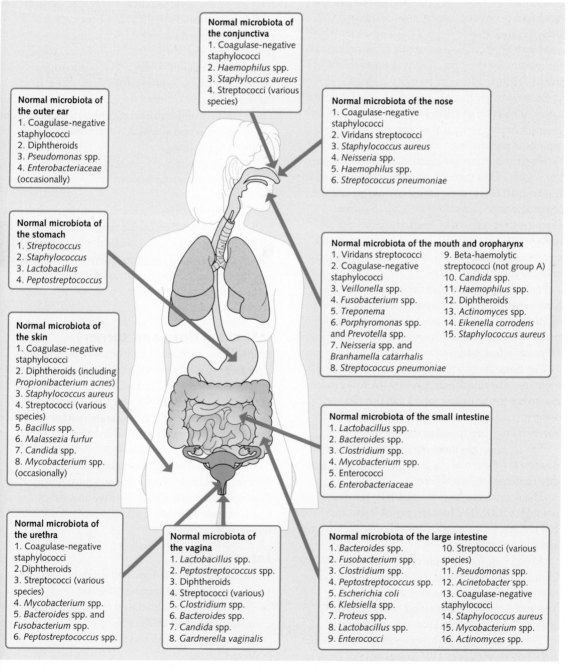

Normal microbiota of the conjunctiva
1. Coagulase-negative staphylococci
2. *Haemophilus* spp.
3. *Staphyloccus aureus*
4. Streptococci (various species)

Normal microbiota of the outer ear
1. Coagulase-negative staphylococci
2. Diphtheroids
3. *Pseudomonas* spp.
4. *Enterobacteriaceae* (occasionally)

Normal microbiota of the nose
1. Coagulase-negative staphylococci
2. Viridans streptococci
3. *Staphylococcus aureus*
4. *Neisseria* spp.
5. *Haemophilus* spp.
6. *Streptococcus pneumoniae*

Normal microbiota of the stomach
1. *Streptococcus*
2. *Staphylococcus*
3. *Lactobacillus*
4. *Peptostreptococcus*

Normal microbiota of the mouth and oropharynx
1. Viridans streptococci
2. Coagulase-negative staphylococci
3. *Veillonella* spp.
4. *Fusobacterium* spp.
5. *Treponema*
6. *Porphyromonas* spp. and *Prevotella* spp.
7. *Neisseria* spp. and *Branhamella catarrhalis*
8. *Streptococcus pneumoniae*
9. Beta-haemolytic streptococci (not group A)
10. *Candida* spp.
11. *Haemophilus* spp.
12. Diphtheroids
13. *Actinomyces* spp.
14. *Eikenella corrodens*
15. *Staphylococcus aureus*

Normal microbiota of the skin
1. Coagulase-negative staphylococci
2. Diphtheroids (including *Propionibacterium acnes*)
3. *Staphylococcus aureus*
4. Streptococci (various species)
5. *Bacillus* spp.
6. *Malassezia furfur*
7. *Candida* spp.
8. *Mycobacterium* spp. (occasionally)

Normal microbiota of the small intestine
1. *Lactobacillus* spp.
2. *Bacteroides* spp.
3. *Clostridium* spp.
4. *Mycobacterium* spp.
5. Enterococci
6. *Enterobacteriaceae*

Normal microbiota of the urethra
1. Coagulase-negative staphylococci
2. Diphtheroids
3. Streptococci (various species)
4. *Mycobacterium* spp.
5. *Bacteroides* spp. and *Fusobacterium* spp.
6. *Peptostreptococcus* spp.

Normal microbiota of the vagina
1. *Lactobacillus* spp.
2. *Peptostreptococcus* spp.
3. Diphtheroids
4. Streptococci (various)
5. *Clostridium* spp.
6. *Bacteroides* spp.
7. *Candida* spp.
8. *Gardnerella vaginalis*

Normal microbiota of the large intestine
1. *Bacteroides* spp.
2. *Fusobacterium* spp.
3. *Clostridium* spp.
4. *Peptostreptococcus* spp.
5. *Escherichia coli*
6. *Klebsiella* spp.
7. *Proteus* spp.
8. *Lactobacillus* spp.
9. Enterococci
10. Streptococci (various species)
11. *Pseudomonas* spp.
12. *Acinetobacter* spp.
13. Coagulase-negative staphylococci
14. *Staphylococcus aureus*
15. *Mycobacterium* spp.
16. *Actinomyces* spp.

Fig. 7.30 Summary of the gut flora. (Redrawn with permission from Prescott L et al. *Microbiology*. McGraw-Hill.)

- Bacillus species.
- Streptococci.

The perioral and perianal skin reflect the flora of the mouth and anus respectively. The oropharynx supports 'viridans' streptococci, bacteria of the *Neisseria* genus, corynebacteria (diptheroids) and anaerobes (but not *Bacteroides fragilis*, which is only found below the diaphragm). Anaerobes are especially prevalent between the teeth and in crevices where they are protected from oxygen.

Mouth flora can be pathogenic in places outside the mouth, for example, if they get into the bloodstream. Human bites can be nasty injuries!

Bacteria in the mouth are responsible for dental caries. Inhalation of saliva and gastric contents (for example, under general anaesthesia) can cause aspiration pneumonia.

The stomach has very little bacterial flora due to the acidity of the gastric secretions (there are usually less than 10 organisms per mL of fluid). However, *Streptococcus*, *Staphylococcus*, *Lactobacillus*, *Peptostreptococcus*, and *Candida* species can all survive in the stomach. Numbers of bacteria rise immediately after a meal, but fall rapidly once the acidic secretions take over.

Helicobacter pylori may be present and can have a pathogenic role, causing peptic ulcers. For eradication, triple therapy (two antibiotics and a proton pump inhibitor) is required for patients with *H. pylori* infections.

The flora changes along the length of the small intestine. The duodenum has few microorganisms, due to the acidic gastric juices and the alkaline biliary and pancreatic secretions. Mostly Gram-positive cocci and rods are found in the duodenum.

The jejunum has more bacteria than the duodenum. *Enterococcus faecalis*, lactobacilli and diphtheroids are found here.

The ileum has a large flora of 10^4–10^8 organisms per mL of fluid. The bacteria are obligate anaerobes and include Bacteroides, Clostridia, Bifidobacteria and Enterobactericeae.

Anaerobes, for example *Bacteroides fragilis*, are found in the large intestine, and they may produce vitamin K. The large intestine also supports 'coliforms' such as *Escherichia coli* and 'faecal' streptococci, including *Enterococcus faecalis*.

There are at least 400 species of bacteria in the large bowel, with over 10^{10} organisms per gram of stool. *Escherichia coli* makes up less than 1% of the bowel flora! Approximately one quarter of the weight of stool is bacteria.

Commensal bacteria keep pathogenic bacteria at bay by competing with them for space and nutrients. The value of this becomes apparent during antibiotic administration. Antibiotics disrupt the normal flora and predispose to clostridia and other gut infections.

Many patients taking broad spectrum antibiotics develop diarrhoea. This normally resolves on stopping the drug, but it may persist, with loss of epithelial cells and the formation of a pseudomembrane composed of mucin, polymorphs, and fibrin. This condition is called pseudomembranous colitis, and it is due to an overgrowth of *Clostridium difficile* resulting from the suppression of normal flora.

The intestinal flora convert conjugated bilirubin to urobilinogen, some of which is reabsorbed and excreted in the urine.

The flora also convert the remainder of the urobilinogen to stercobilinogen which is excreted in the faeces.

Suppression of the normal flora of the mouth may lead to its colonization by the fungus *Candida albicans*, causing thrush. Candidal oesophagitis may also occur in severely immunocompromised patients, e.g. those with human immunodeficiency virus (HIV) infection, or those receiving steroids (e.g. prednisolone).

Intestinal flora and surgery

Prophylactic antibiotics may be given during and after surgery on the gastrointestinal tract to prevent infection as a result of operating on a 'dirty site'.

The antibiotic or antibiotics given, and the dose, depend on the site of the operation (and of course on the patient!). Commonly used antibiotics include cefuroxime and metronidazole.

Cefuroxime is effective against Gram-negative *Neisseria* and coliforms, and metronidazole against Gram-negative and Gram-positive anaerobes.

Most anaerobes are sensitive to metronidazole, but aerobes are not.

Intestinal gas

Air is swallowed with food and drink (aerophagia). Gas is produced in a number of ways:

- Carbon dioxide is liberated from the neutralization of acids in the gut.
- Diffusion of oxygen and nitrogen from the bloodstream.
- Gaseous products from bacterial activity.

Normal bacterial flora produce methane, carbon dioxide, and hydrogen from intestinal contents.

The gastrointestinal tract normally contains about 200 mL of air, 99% of which is odourless (oxygen, carbon dioxide, hydrogen, nitrogen, and methane).

The socially unacceptable constituent of flatus is mainly composed of hydrogen sulphide, ammonia, and volatile amino and fatty acids.

Some of the air in the tract is expelled through the mouth (belched) and some is absorbed. Most of it is passed on to the colon.

Excess gas may cause noise (borborygmi), bloating, cramps, and abdominal pain or discomfort. It may be seen in a number of disorders, including Crohn's disease, and in malabsorption and functional bowel disorders, in which excess air is involuntarily swallowed (flatulent dyspepsia).

Transport and secretion of the large intestine

Secretion of mucus

The colonic mucosa has many goblet cells in its crypts and surface epithelium. They secrete mucus in response to mechanical irritation of the mucosa caused by substances passing through it, and as a result of cholinergic stimulation.

Conversely, secretion of mucus is inhibited by sympathetic stimulation. Sympathetic stimulation throughout the body prepares it for 'fight or flight'. The body cannot perform all its functions at once and digestion of food can wait until later!

Mucus lubricates the colon, preventing trauma from the contents passing through it, which become increasingly solid as water is reabsorbed on the way through. The ratio of mucus to aqueous secretion is greater in the colon than elsewhere in the gastrointestinal tract.

The aqueous component contains bicarbonate, which plays an important role in buffering, and it is rich in potassium. Chloride is absorbed in exchange for bicarbonate.

Transport of urea and electrolytes

The main function of the colon is absorption. It absorbs over 90% of the water from the contents passing through it, reducing them from 1–2 L thick fluid to about 200 mL of semi-solid faecal matter.

By the time they reach the end of the gastrointestinal tract, faeces are about 75% water. The remainder is solid material, of which 30%

consists of bacteria. Desquamated mucosal cells also make up part of the bulk of stool and bacteria. Desquamated cells largely account for the fact that a starving person continues to produce stools.

The ion transport processes of the colon are shown in Fig. 7.31.

Na^+ in the lumen is exchanged for H^+ (Na^+ is pumped into the epithelial cells and H^+ pumped out of it). HCO_3^- is exchanged for Cl^- (Cl^- is reabsorbed, bicarbonate pumped out).

In addition, paracellular spaces exist into which Na^+ and Cl^- is pumped, and from which K^+ passes out into the lumen. K^+ is pumped into the cells in exchange for the Na^+ pumped out into the paracellular spaces.

The net result of this is the creation of a potential difference of about -30 mV across the colonic mucosa (a greater difference than that across the jejunal and ileal mucosa).

It is this potential difference that allows the passage of K^+ across the tight junctions from the paracellular space into the lumen and accounts for the potassium-rich secretions found in the colon.

Urea synthesis is greater than its excretion by about 20%. The excess is secreted into the colon for metabolism by bacteria. The products are then absorbed.

Metabolism occurs near the mucosa, rather than in the lumen. The NH_4^+ and HCO_3^- ions produced are converted into NH_3, CO_2 and water. These freely diffuse across the mucosal epithelium into the circulation. The NH_3 is transported to the liver for synthesis of amino acids.

Water absorption in the colon

Absorption of water in the colon is similar to the mechanism used to concentrate the contents of the gall bladder described in Chapter 4.

Na^+ and Cl^- are pumped into the paracellular (lateral intercellular) spaces and water follows by osmosis. Water molecules and Na^+ and Cl^- then flow through the lateral intercellular spaces, away from the lumen, and across the basement membrane of the epithelial cells of the colon.

Some Cl^- from the colonic lumen also crosses the tight junction into the intercellular space because of the potential difference. It travels in the opposite direction to K^+ and increases the concentration of Cl^- in the intercellular space and, therefore, the passage of water.

The concentration of ions in that part of the intercellular space closest to the lumen is hypertonic,

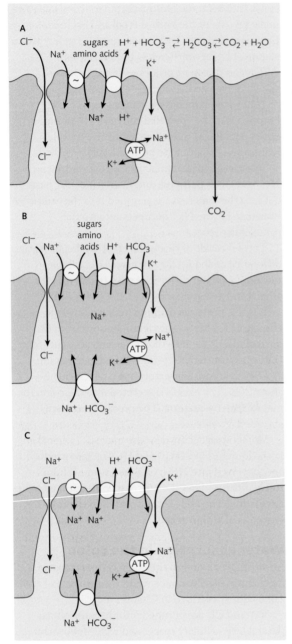

Fig. 7.31 Summary of electrolyte movement in the jejunum (A), the ileum (B), and the colon (C).

of water, excessive secretion or disorders of motility. Diarrhoea will be discussed in Chapter 8.

Motility of the large intestine and defecation

Motility of the large intestine

The movement of intestinal contents through the colon is slower than that seen in the rest of the gastrointestinal tract. This is partly due to the nature of the activity and partly due to its absorptive function of water and electrolytes.

The large intestine has four main activities.

- Storage.
- Segmental (or haustral) contractions.
- Peristalsis.
- Mass movement.

The proximal stomach and the colon are the only sites of storage within the gut. Storage is facilitated in the colon by non-adrenergic non-cholinergic (NANC) fibres, via NO and VIP release.

Segmental (or haustral) contractions are brought about by the contraction of the taeniae coli. These three bands of longitudinal muscles gather the colon into haustra. The haustra fill with intestinal contents and the distension stimulates contraction of the haustrum.

Contraction of adjacent haustra causes a mixing effect and allows the contents to be in contact with the mucosal surfaces, thus facilitating absorption.

Segmental contractions are initiated by acetylcholine and substance P release.

Peristalsis is slower in the large intestine than in the small intestine. It provides waves of propulsive contractions, slowly moving the intestinal contents towards the anus. As in the small intestine, distension initiates the contractions and vagal inhibitory and excitatory fibres control the movement.

Mass movement describes the intense contraction that begins halfway along the transverse colon and pushes the intestinal contents towards the rectum. This type of contraction only occurs a few times a day and is responsible for colonic evacuation.

It occurs shortly after a meal, and if faeces are present in the rectum, this stimulates the urge to defecate. This is called the gastro-colic reflex. It is partly neuronal and partly hormonal (via CCK). The gastro-colic reflex is particularly strong after breakfast.

but the fluid at the basement membrane end is isotonic. It is the isotonic fluid that crosses the basement membrane and moves into the intestinal capillaries.

Absorbed amino acids and sugars also increase the osmotic absorption of water.

Abnormalities in water absorption in the intestines can result in diarrhoea. Diarrhoea is an increase in volume and fluidity of faeces due to the malabsorption

As in other parts of the gastrointestinal tract, Auerbach's and Meissner's plexuses are present in the walls of the colon (see Fig. 1.2). Their activity is modulated by parasympathetic and sympathetic activity.

Parasympathetic stimulation is via branches of the vagus (X) and pelvic nerves from the sacral spinal cord. It increases contraction of the proximal colon, allowing greater absorption of salts and water.

Sympathetic innervation is via the superior and inferior mesenteric and hypogastric plexuses. It decreases colonic movements.

Colo-colonic reflexes occur (mediated in part by the sympathetic system) causing one part of the colon to relax if an adjacent part is distended (Fig. 7.32).

Dietary fibre

The importance of dietary fibre in maintaining regular defecation and in reducing the frequency and severity of symptoms in diverticular disease is well recognized.

The incidence of cancer of the colon is also lower in countries where a high fibre diet is normal.

Dietary fibre consists of those carbohydrates that humans are unable to digest, including cellulose, hemicellulose, lignin, and other carbohydrates with β-glycosidic linkages.

Bread, potatoes, fruit, and vegetables are all high in fibre, and they increase the bulk of the stools by about 5 g for every gram of fibre!

Low fibre foods are less filling and often eaten in greater quantities than high fibre foods, contributing to obesity.

Fibre has a number of important functions:

- It increases the rate of food transport, by giving bulk to the faeces.
- It holds water and forms a gel in the presence of water.
- Fibre can bind and hold cations, such as calcium, magnesium, iron and zinc; this aids their excretion.
- It is a substrate for bacterial metabolism and a major source of nutrients and energy for the bacteria.
- Fibre can alter digestion and absorption within the gut. For example, more bile acids and nitrogenous waste are excreted in the presence of fibre, due to the ability of fibre to bind these molecules.
- Fibre acts to decrease gastric emptying, thus increasing the digestion of food. It also decreases carbohydrate absorption.

Defecation

The anal canal has an internal and external sphincter (Fig. 7.33).

The internal sphincter is made up of a thickened continuation of the circular muscle of the colon, and it is under involuntary control. It relaxes as a reflex in response to distension of the distal rectum.

Intact Auerbach's and Meissner's plexuses are needed for this reflex relaxation to occur. In Hirschsprung's disease, there is a congenital absence of ganglion cells in these plexuses in the rectum and sometimes in the colon, with the result that the internal sphincter does not relax in response to stretching of the rectum. Faeces

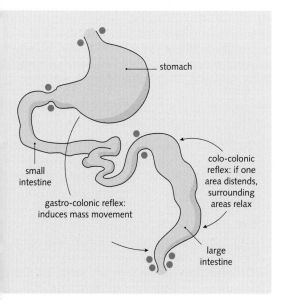

Fig. 7.32 Motility of the large intestine.

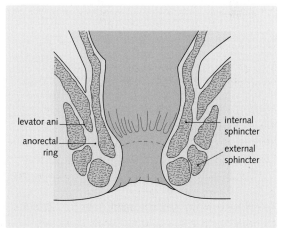

Fig. 7.33 The rectum and anal canal.

147

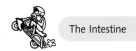

remain in the rectum and colon, causing distension of the lower gastrointestinal tract and the abdomen.

This relaxation is only temporary. If defecation does not take place the internal sphincter contracts again and the urge to defecate is lost (until the sphincter relaxes again later).

The urge to defecate is felt because stretching of the rectum causes impulses in cholinergic parasympathetic nerves of the pelvis. These are transmitted to a nerve centre in the sacral spinal cord. A pressure of about 18 mmHg in the rectum is needed.

Impulses are then conveyed to higher centres, allowing an individual to decide whether to defecate; i.e. whether voluntarily to relax the external sphincter or delay doing so. In the latter case, the internal sphincter will recontract and the urge to defecate will subside.

The external sphincter is made up of striated muscle and, like most other striated muscle, it is under voluntary control.

If there has been damage to the spinal nerves (and therefore to the control of the external sphincter), the external sphincter will relax when the pressure in the rectum reaches about 55 mmHg.

The anal canal is a remarkable structure. It can tell the difference between air, liquid, and solid contents, and allow the selective release of air as flatus.

Normally the rectum is distended as a result of mass movements filling it with faecal material. It may also be distended by a neoplasm or other mass, however, giving rise to tenesmus (the feeling of incomplete evacuation).

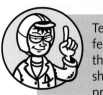

Tenesmus is an unpleasant feeling that 'something is still there' after defecation. It should be investigated promptly as it may be due to a potentially fatal neoplasm.

When the external sphincter is voluntarily relaxed for defecation, an increase in intra-abdominal pressure must be achieved to expel the faeces.

A breath is taken in and the glottis closes over the trachea. The respiratory muscles contract on lungs filled with air, which increases both the intra-thoracic and intra-abdominal pressures.

The pelvic floor muscles relax and the floor 'drops', thus straightening the rectum and preventing rectal prolapse. The faeces are then expelled from the anus.

- Briefly outline the general anatomy of the duodenum, jejunum, and ileum.
- What is the blood supply to each part of the small intestine?
- How can you tell the difference between the three sections of the small bowel?
- Give an overview of the anatomy of the large intestine.
- How is the large intestine supplied with blood?
- Describe the venous drainage of the rectum.
- Give a brief account of the anal sphincters.
- What is the pectinate line, and what is its relevance?
- Describe from which parts of the embryonic gut the intestines develop.
- Briefly, give an account of the structure of the small intestinal wall.
- What cell types are found in the small intestinal mucosa?
- Give a brief description of the structure of Peyer's patches.
- What do Brunner's glands do? Where are they found?
- How does the structure of the large intestinal mucosa compare to that of the small intestine?
- Describe the fed-state motility in the small intestines.
- What are the four main stages of motility during the fasting state in the small intestine?
- What controls the motility in the small intestine?
- How is digestion and absorption facilitated by the small intestinal mucosal cells?
- How does the countercurrent mechanism in the villi of the small intestine work?
- What factors control absorption in the small intestine?
- What are micelles and chylomicrons? What functions do they have?
- In what form are carbohydrates absorbed? How does the absorption occur?
- How are amino acids absorbed in the small intestine?
- Name four colonic bacteria that help to make up our flora, and the sites in which they are found.
- What functions do the bacterial flora serve?
- How does water enter the mucosal cells in the large intestine?
- What are the four main activities of the large intestine?
- What is the difference between segmental contractions and peristalsis?
- What is mass movement?
- Describe the process of defecation.

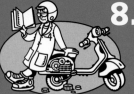

Congenital abnormalities

Meckel's diverticulum

Meckel's diverticulum is the remnant of the vitelline duct present in embryonic life. It connects the developing embryo with the yolk sac.

Meckel's diverticulum is:

- Present in 2% of the population.
- About 2 inches long.
- Found approximately 2 feet from the caecum (the rule of 2 s).
- Twice as common in males compared with females.

In the embryo, the vitelline duct is found at the apex of the primary intestinal loop that forms when the midgut rapidly elongates (see Fig. 7.6). The long sides of the loop are known as the cephalic limb (which forms the duodenum, jejunum, and part of the ileum) and the caudal limb (which forms the remainder of the ileum, the caecum, appendix, ascending colon, and the proximal two thirds of the transverse colon).

Meckel's diverticulum, therefore, marks the junction of the cranial and caudal limbs of what was the embryonic midgut.

Heterotopic gastric epithelium (normal tissue present in the wrong place) may sometimes be found in the diverticulum, including HCl-secreting oxyntic cells, resulting in peptic ulceration. Rarely, ulcers may perforate. Heterotopic pancreatic tissue may also be found there.

Acute inflammation of the diverticulum may occur, mimicking acute appendicitis. The mucosa at the mouth of the diverticulum may become inflamed and lead to intussusception, or the diverticulum may perforate and cause peritonitis. In most cases, however, diverticula are asymptomatic.

If the vitelline duct remains patent throughout its length, a fistula may form onto the umbilicus.

Hirschsprung's disease (congenital aganglionic megacolon)

Hirschsprung's disease is caused by an absence of ganglion cells in Auerbach's and Meissner's plexuses in the distal bowel as a result of the failure of neuroblasts to migrate during weeks 5–12 of gestation.

When these parasympathetic plexuses fail to develop, the circular muscle layer of the intestine goes into spasm, resulting in intestinal obstruction and, as in other causes of obstruction, dilatation of the intestine occurs, proximal to the area in spasm occurs (Fig. 8.1).

Hirschsprung's disease usually affects the rectum and distal colon but, in severe cases, it may also affect the small intestine. The colon may become distended with faeces resulting in megacolon and death from acute enterocolitis.

It is four times more likely to occur in males, and severe cases may become apparent shortly after birth with symptoms of obstruction. Less severe cases may simply result in chronic constipation.

The incidence is 1 in 5000 live births; it is ten times as likely to occur in children with Down syndrome (trisomy 21), and it is often found in association with other congenital abnormalities.

Diagnosis is by barium enema and biopsy showing an absence of ganglion cells.

Pressure studies show a failure of relaxation of the internal anal sphincter.

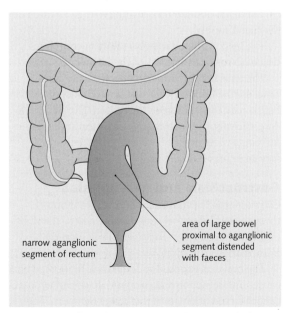

area of large bowel proximal to aganglionic segment distended with faeces

narrow aganglionic segment of rectum

Fig. 8.1 The effect of Hirschsprung's disease on the large bowel.

Acquired megacolon

Hirschsprung's disease is a congenital abnormality, but megacolon may also be acquired, usually as a result of chronic constipation in childhood. It may also be seen in the elderly.

Causes of acquired megacolon include Chagas' disease, inflammatory bowel disease, and bowel obstruction.

Acquired megacolon may be differentiated from Hirschsprung's disease by rectal examination. In patients with Hirschsprung's disease, a narrow empty segment of rectum can be felt, above which the colon is dilated and full of faeces. In patients with acquired megacolon, in contrast, no empty segment of rectum is felt and faeces are present in the distal rectum.

The definitive distinguishing test is a rectal biopsy. In acquired megacolon, ganglion cells are present in the rectal wall.

Atresia and stenosis

Atresia is a failure of canalization and it results in complete obstruction. Stenosis is a narrowing of the lumen and it results in partial obstruction.

Atresia and stenosis may occur anywhere along the length of the gastrointestinal tract, but they are found most often in the duodenum and least often in the colon.

The incidence is 1 in 5000 births, and they are diagnosed quickly after birth. The causes of atresia and stenosis range from lack of recanalization (in the proximal duodenum) to malrotation and gastroschisis (in the distal duodenum), leading to the cessation of the blood supply.

The loss of a blood supply results in complete tissue necrosis to that part of the bowel.

The anus may be imperforate, with the anal canal ending blindly at the anal membrane, or a fistula may form between the rectum and perineum. Alternatively, the rectum may empty into the vagina forming a rectovaginal fistula or into the urethra, forming a urorectal fistula.

Gastroschisis and exomphalos

Gastroschisis is a congenital herniation of bowel through the abdominal wall, usually just to the right of the umbilical cord. Treatment is by surgery, immediately after birth.

The bowel is exposed to fetal urine *in utero*, which causes inflammation and paralytic ileus, and neonates cannot be fed orally until the bowel recovers. The condition is not associated with other abnormalities and overall mortality is about 5%.

The incidence of gastroschisis is 1 in 10 000 live births. It is related to cocaine use by the mother.

Exomphalos occurs when the gut fails to return to the abdominal cavity after its physiological herniation and development outside the cavity during weeks 7–11 of gestation.

Affected children are born with gut and sometimes liver protruding through the umbilicus, covered by cord coverings. The gut is not exposed to fetal urine. The condition is associated with other congenital abnormalities, however, most commonly cardiac, renal, or chromosomal. Overall mortality is 25–50%.

Infections and enterocolitis

Diarrhoea and dysentery

Diarrhoea is an increase in volume and fluidity of faeces, or malabsorption of water. It is generally considered normal for bowels to be opened anything from once every three days to three times a day. The important thing for any individual is a change in bowel habits.

The small intestine and colon together absorb almost 9 L of water per day from the lumen of the gastrointestinal tract and more water is reabsorbed than is secreted. Clearly, if a failure of absorption takes place, faeces will contain abnormal amounts of water and diarrhoea will result.

Dysentery may be defined as painful, bloody, but low-volume, diarrhoea. The main categories and causes of diarrhoea are summarized in Fig. 8.2.

The main categories of diarrhoea
Osmotic diarrhoea Disaccharidase deficiencies Drug-induced Galactose Generalized malabsorption
Secretory diarrhoea Infectious Defects in intraluminal digestion and absorption Excess laxative use
Deranged motility Increased intestinal transit time Decreased motility
Malabsorption
Exudative diseases Infectious Inflammatory bowel disease

Fig. 8.2 The main categories of diarrhoea.

Reduced absorption may be due to one or more of a number of factors including:

- An increase in the number of osmotic particles in the lumen, resulting in a flow of water into the lumen (osmotic diarrhoea).
- An increase in the rate of flow of intestinal contents, leaving less time for the absorption processes to take place (deranged motility diarrhoea).
- An abnormal increase in secretions of the gastrointestinal tract (secretory diarrhoea).

 Amoebic dysentery is one of a number of diseases that UK law requires doctors to give notification of to the local medical environmental health officer at the Department of Health. Failure to notify is an offence for which a doctor may be fined. Notification is rewarded with a small fee!

Osmotic diarrhoea

Both electrolytes and absorbed nutrients (such as sugar and amino acids) contribute to osmosis. If the absorption of either of these is reduced (for example, due to the failure of ion transport or malabsorption of nutrients for whatever reason), osmotic diarrhoea will occur. These osmotic particles will remain in the lumen, keeping water with them.

Secretory diarrhoea

Normally, immature cells in the crypts of Lieberkühn in the small intestine are responsible for the secretion of water and electrolytes into the lumen. Mature cells near the tips of the villi are responsible for absorption. They are stimulated to increase their rate of secretion by a number of factors such as acetylcholine, substance P, 5-hydroxytryptamine (5-HT; also known as serotonin) and neurotensin, all of which increase intracellular calcium.

Increased stimulation by these substances can result in secretory diarrhoea.

Potentially fatal secretory diarrhoea can also be caused by cholera. Different strains of the causative organism *Vibrio cholerae* are endemic in developing parts of the world, and they cause profuse 'rice water' stools. Infection is spread by the faecal–oral route and pandemics are by no means unusual.

The organism can survive in the acid conditions of the stomach and multiplies in the small intestine where it produces an enterotoxin that binds to receptors on the immature cells in the crypts.

This causes an increase in adenylate cyclase, elevating cyclic AMP and increasing the secretion of sodium, chloride, and water into the lumen.

Bloody, exudate diarrhoea

Inflammation, infection, or neoplasms cause this type of diarrhoea. If the diarrhoea is very bloody then it is due to chronic disease, such as a neoplasm or ulcerative colitis. Inflammatory bowel disease can cause chronic exudative diarrhoea.

Deranged motility diarrhoea

Increased gut motility leads to lack of absorption (due to rapid transit), which can result in diarrhoea. Some agents may stimulate secretion as well as motility.

Gastrointestinal stasis may also cause diarrhoea by facilitating bacterial overgrowth.

Infectious enterocolitis

Enterocolitis is inflammation of the intestines. It may be caused by a variety of agents. In 40–50% of cases, no specific agent is isolated and an educated guess must be taken according to the age, circumstances, and degree of immunocompetence of the patient.

Improved sanitation has led to a decreased prevalence of infectious enterocolitis in the developed world, but infectious enterocolitis accounts for more than 50% of all deaths before the age of 5 years worldwide, and over 12 000 deaths each day amongst children in developing countries.

Viral gastroenteritis

Gastroenteritis is the inflammation of the stomach and intestines. The illness includes vomiting, fever, abdominal pain, and diarrhoea. The rapid loss of water and electrolytes can result in metabolic disturbances. This may be caused by rotaviruses, enteric adenoviruses, and small round viruses (caliciviruses, astroviruses, and featureless viruses) (Fig. 8.3).

Bacterial enterocolitis

The major causes of bacterial enterocolitis are summarized in Fig. 8.4.

The principal mechanisms by which bacterial infection may lead to gastroenteritis are:

Common causes of viral gastroenteritis		
Virus	Host age	Transmission method
Rotavirus (group A)	6–24 months	Person-to-person, food, water
Astroviruses	Child	Person-to-person, water, raw shellfish
Norwalk-like viruses	School age, adult	Person-to-person, water, cold foods, raw shellfish
Enteric adenoviruses	Child under 2 years	Person-to-person
Caliciviruses	Child	Person-to-person, water, cold foods, raw shellfish

Fig. 8.3 Common causes of viral gastroenteritis.

Major causes of bacterial enterocolitis	
Organism	Source of transmission
Campylobacter	Milk, poultry, animal contact
Clostridium difficile	Nosocomial environment
Clostridium perfringens	Meat, poultry, fish
Escherichia coli	Food, water, undercooked beef products, weaning foods, cheese, person-to-person
Mycobacterium tuberculosis	Contaminated milk, swallowing of coughed-up organisms
Salmonella	Milk, beef, eggs, poultry
Shigella	Person-to-person, low-inoculum
Vibrio cholerae, other vibrios	Water, shellfish, person-to-person
Yersinia enterocolitica	Milk, pork

Fig. 8.4 Major organisms and causes of bacterial enterocolitis.

- The ingestion of a bacterial organism that proliferates in the gut lumen and that is enterotoxic.
- Ingestion of a ready-made (preformed) toxin in contaminated food, which is heat stable (e.g. *Staphylococcus aureus*, *Vibrio cholerae*, and *Clostridium perfringens*).
- The ingestion of an enteroinvasive bacterial organism, which proliferates in the gut and destroys the mucosal epithelial cells.

The incubation period can give clues as to whether the food poisoning was due to bacterial contamination or preformed toxins. Usually, the incubation period of bacterial contamination is longer, as time is required to establish an enterotoxic colony in the gut.

Treatment consists of fluid replacement therapy with antibiotics. Sometimes intravenous fluids must be given if vomiting is severe.

Necrotizing enterocolitis

As the name suggests, this is a necrotizing inflammation of the small and large intestines (primarily the terminal ileum and ascending colon), and it is the most common acquired gastrointestinal emergency of neonates.

It is most common within the first few days of life (when infants start oral feeding), but it may occur at any time within the first 3 months, especially in premature or low birth weight babies being given formula milk rather than breast milk.

Symptoms vary from mild gastrointestinal upset to perforation of necrosed intestine leading to shock, and, if untreated, death.

Surgical resection of affected intestine may be necessary.

Pseudomembranous colitis

Pseudomembranous colitis is caused by an overgrowth of *Clostridium difficile* following antibiotic therapy. Any antibiotic may cause it, including penicillin, due to an alteration of intestinal flora.

It is so named because of the appearance of what looks like a membrane (a pseudomembrane) on the surface of the large bowel, formed by an eruption of mucin, polymorphs, and fibrin. Treatment is with vancomycin or metronidazole.

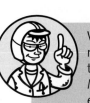

When prescribing metronidazole, advise patients to avoid alcohol. Metronidazole has a disulfiram effect and patients will feel severely ill if they drink alcohol at the same time. Unless they are warned, they will understandably think the illness is caused by the metronidazole and stop taking it.

Protozoa and other parasites

A number of different protozoa may be found in the faeces, which do not cause disease.

However, the protozoan organisms *Entamoeba histolytica* and *Giardia lamblia* commonly cause diarrhoea and both are transmitted by the faecal–oral route.

Infection may be asymptomatic or cause amoebic dysentery (a notifiable disease), which may have a gradual onset accompanied by systemic symptoms, such as anorexia and headache.

Treatment of acute amoebic dysentery is with metronidazole. Diloxanide is given in chronic disease.

Chagas' disease (South American trypanosomiasis)

This is caused by *Trypanosoma cruzi*, and it may present acutely or chronically after many years latency.

Hepatosplenomegaly may be present in acute disease, and many organs of the body may be invaded by the organism and damaged if the disease becomes chronic. The smooth muscle of the gastrointestinal tract is often involved, leading to megaoesophagus, a dilated stomach, and megacolon.

The organism may be isolated in acute disease but diagnosis of chronic disease is by Chagas' IgG ELISA (enzyme-linked immunosorbent assay).

Treatment of acute disease is with nifurtimox or benzimidazole (the parasite persists in 50% of cases). Treatment of chronic disease is symptomatic.

Inflammatory disorders of the bowel

There are two major non-specific inflammatory bowel diseases: Crohn's disease and ulcerative colitis.

Crohn's disease

Crohn's disease may affect any part of the gastrointestinal tract from the mouth to the anus. It is most common in the lower ileum.

Crohn's disease is more frequent in the Western world, particularly amongst Caucasians, where the incidence is approximately 5–6 per 100 000 and prevalence 50–60 per 100 000.

It commonly presents in adolescence, but the peak onset is between 20 and 40 years of age. Both sexes are equally affected.

There is a high rate of concordance in monozygotic twins, which suggests both a genetic and environmental cause.

There is a 3–4 fold increase in risk with smoking and Crohn's patients generally eat a diet higher in refined sugars and lower in fibre than those without Crohn's.

Macroscopically, the bowel appears bright red and swollen. Later, small, discrete aphthoid ulcers with a haemorrhagic rim form, so named because they look similar to aphthous ulcers in the mouth.

Later, deeper longitudinal ulcers form, which may develop into deep fissures involving the full thickness of the wall of the gastrointestinal tract.

Fibrosis may follow, with stricture formation visible as a narrow string-like area on contrast radiographs.

The mucous membrane of the gastrointestinal tract is often described as cobble-stoned. This occurs where longitudinal fissures are present in oedematous transverse mucosal folds. Aggregations of inflammatory cells and lymphocytes infiltrate the bowel wall. Mesenteric lymph nodes may be enlarged due to reactive hyperplasia. Granulomas may be present in the lymph nodes.

Damage to the gastrointestinal tract in Crohn's disease is often patchy (skip lesions) with normal areas of tissue found in between the patches.

Symptoms include diarrhoea, with or without malabsorption, abdominal cramps, fever, malaise, and weight loss. The signs include:

- Abdominal tenderness.
- Perianal lesions.
- Anaemia.
- Aphthous ulcers in the mouth.
- Weight loss.

Diagnosis involves sigmoidoscopy, rectal biopsy, and contrast radiography.

The aetiology of Crohn's disease is controversial. At present, three main organisms are being investigated as the possible aetiological agent:

- *Mycobacterium avium* (subspecies *paratuberculosis*).
- Paramyxovirus (measles virus).
- *Listeria monocytogenes*.

Complications of Crohn's disease

Complications depend on the site and extent of the lesions.

Malabsorption may occur where large areas of small intestine are affected (short bowel syndrome, following surgical resection). Fistulae may form because of deep fissuring. These may be internal (between loops of gut or from the gut to the bladder), perianal, or, following surgery, open onto the skin.

Acutely, perforation of ulcerated gut may occur.

A variety of lesions may be seen around the anus, most commonly skin tags, fissures, and fistulae in 60% of patients.

Treatment

All Crohn's disease patients require symptomatic relief and, for some, this is all the treatment they ever need. Diarrhoea is treated with anti-diarrhoeal drugs, such as loperamide and codeine phosphate.

Vitamin and nutrient supplements are given to overcome any deficiency from malabsorption. Other treatments include anti-inflammatory steroids (e.g. prednisolone) and immunosuppressive drugs (e.g. ciclosporin or azathioprine).

Antibiotics, such as metronidazole and cotrimoxazole, are useful in severe perianal disease.

However, 80% of patients will require surgery at some point in their life because of:

- Failure to thrive in children.
- Complications (e.g. perforation, obstruction, stricture or fistula formation).
- Failure or side effects of drug therapy.

Surgery is never curative. Remission is achievable, but almost all patients have significant relapses.

Granulomas are collections of epithelioid macrophages and giant cells surrounded by a cuff of lymphocytes.
Granulomas in Crohn's disease are not the same as those found in tuberculosis—tubercular granulomas are characterized by central caseous (cheese-like) necrosis.

Ulcerative colitis

Ulcerative colitis only affects the large intestine. The incidence of ulcerative colitis is 5–10 per 100 000 and the prevalence is 80–120 per 100 000.

Ulcerative colitis affects women more than men, and it is most common between the ages of 20 and 40 years, although it can occur at any age.

It usually starts in the rectum and it may extend proximally, although never beyond the colon. Occasionally, inflammation of the terminal ileum is seen (backwash ileitis) but this is a result of an incompetent ileocaecal valve rather than ulcerative colitis itself. Its aetiology is unknown, although possible causative agents include genetics, infection, and immunological factors. It has been suggested that ulcerative colitis is the result of an atypical immune response to an enteropathogenic *Escherichia coli*.

Unlike Crohn's, which commonly shows skip lesions, ulcerative colitis is continuous. Areas of normal gut are not found between lesions.

The disease is a chronic relapsing inflammatory disorder, and diffuse superficial inflammation is seen in the large bowel. The mucosa is granular and haemorrhagic (Fig. 8.5), rarely involving the muscle layer (unlike Crohn's, where deep fissure ulcers form).

Both acute and chronic inflammatory cells are found infiltrating the mucosa, and aggregates of polymorphs are seen in the crypts (crypt abscesses). Healing of ulcers leads to periods of remission but, in areas of healing, the normal large bowel epithelium may be replaced by a simple layer of mucus-secreting cells without crypts.

The major symptom in ulcerative colitis is bloody exudative diarrhoea. Often lower abdominal pain,

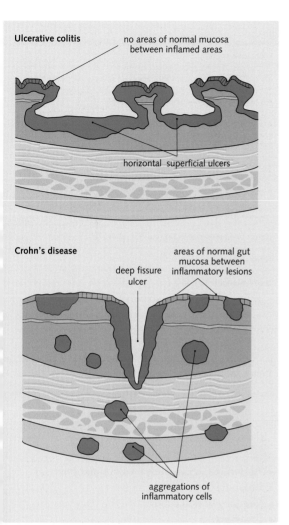

Ulcerative colitis

no areas of normal mucosa between inflamed areas

horizontal superficial ulcers

Crohn's disease

deep fissure ulcer

areas of normal gut mucosa between inflammatory lesions

aggregations of inflammatory cells

Fig. 8.5 Ulcerative colitis and Crohn's disease. Unlike Crohn's disease, ulcerative colitis is continuous; areas of normal gut are not found between lesions.

anorexia, and malaise accompany this. If the disease is confined to the rectum, urgency and tenesmus accompany the bloody diarrhoea.

Diagnosis requires rectal examination, sigmoidoscopy, and biopsy. A barium enema can show fine ulceration.

In the developed world, this is the most frequent cause of prolonged bloody diarrhoea and it should be suspected whenever bloody diarrhoea lasts for more than 7 days.

Complications of ulcerative colitis

The mucosa may haemorrhage, leading to blood loss and anaemia.

Distension and perforation of the colon (toxic megacolon) may occur in acute fulminating cases.

Ulcerative colitis is premalignant and carcinoma of the colon may develop after 10 years in people with total ulcerative colitis.

Extraintestinal complications include:

- Skin involvement.
- Liver disease.
- Eye inflammation.
- Association with arthritis.

Treatment

All ulcerative colitis patients are treated with 5-aminosalicylic acid (5-ASA), or sulfasalazine (a compound of 5-ASA and sulfapyridine). It is broken down into its active component by colonic bacteria and acts as an anti-inflammatory agent.

Some patients receive prednisolone, and they are treated with antibiotics in cases of septicaemia. Azathioprine can induce remission in some cases.

Surgery is curative in ulcerative colitis. Colectomy with an ileorectal, or ileoanal anastomosis with an ileal reservoir, avoids the need for an ileostomy.

A colectomy also removes the risk of cancer in the diseased bowel, in patients with total or sub-total colitis, who have had the disease for more than 10 years.

Prognosis depends on the extent of the disease and it is better in proctitis (disease limited to the rectum) than in severe fulminant disease (which carries a 15–25% mortality).

Comparison of Crohn's disease and ulcerative colitis

It is important to distinguish between a diagnosis of Crohn's and ulcerative colitis as the management of each is different (Fig. 8.6).

Miscellaneous intestinal inflammatory disorders
Acute manifestation of HIV infection

Diarrhoea, weight loss, and malabsorption are common in chronic HIV infection, usually caused by a pathogen, most commonly the coccidian protozoal parasite *Cryptosporidium*. *Microsporidia*, another protozoal parasite, may also cause diarrhoea.

Cytomegalovirus may mimic inflammatory bowel disease and mucocutaneous lesions may be formed at the lower (and upper) end of the GI tract by the herpes simplex virus, particularly in the perianal region.

Mycobacterium tuberculosis infection of the bowel may also occur and *Candida* infections are common.

Comparison of ulcerative colitis and Crohn's disease	
Crohn's disease	**Ulcerative colitis**
Affects anywhere from mouth to anus	Only affects large bowel (but backwash ileitis occurs in 10%)
Deep ulcers and fissures (rose-thorn ulcers) in mucosa	No fissures, horizontal undermining ulcers
Malignant change less common than ulcerative colitis	Malignant change relatively common
10% have fistulae	Fistulae rare
60% have anal involvement	25% have anal involvement
Fibrous shortening and early strictures of intestine	Muscular shortening of colon but strictures rare and late
Skip lesions	No skip lesions
Fat and vitamin malabsorption (if small intestine affected)	No fat or vitamin malabsorption
Granulomas in 50%	No granulomas
Marked lymphoid reaction	Mild lymphoid reaction
Fibrosis	Mild fibrosis
Serositis	Mild serositis (if any)
No raised ANCA	Raised ANCA
Increased incidence in smokers	Decreased incidence in smokers

Fig. 8.6 Comparison of ulcerative colitis and Crohn's disease.

Graft-versus-host disease

Transplanted bone marrow contains many T lymphocytes and, if the host's immune system is deficient (as it usually is), the grafted bone marrow may reject the host. This leads to skin rashes, hair loss (often sparse anyway because of previous treatment), acute diarrhoea, liver disease, and death.

Irritable bowel syndrome

Irritable bowel syndrome (IBS) is a functional bowel disease. There is no structural aetiology, such as inflammation, infection or neoplasia. It is diagnosed on the basis of exclusion of organic diseases and the presence of symptoms.

Irritable bowel syndrome is very common, affecting 10–20% of all adolescents and adults in the West, and it is more prevalent in women. It is comprised of a cluster of symptoms including:
- Abdominal discomfort or pain.
- Changes in bowel habit.
- Bloated feeling.
- Disordered defecation.
- Abdominal tenderness on examination.
- Mucoid stools.
- Urgency to defecate.
- Straining.
- Tenesmus.
- Referred pain to the left lower quadrant.

It is diagnosed by:
- Exclusion of structural or metabolic abnormalities (e.g. ulcers, IBD, lactose intolerance)
- Presence of symptoms: abdominal pain for 12 weeks or more in a 12 month period.
- Presence of two or more accompanying symptoms:
  - Pain relieved by defecation.
  - Onset of pain associated with a change in frequency of the stools.
  - Onset of pain associated with a change in the form of the stools.

Irritable bowel syndrome is generally referred to as constipation predominant or diarrhoea predominant.

Treatment is symptomatic. Loperamide is given for diarrhoea and methylcellulose is given for constipation. Paracetamol or codeine may be given as analgesia.

Malabsorption syndromes

General aspects of the malabsorption syndromes

Malabsorption is the decreased absorption of nutrients and it may be caused by a number of conditions, including biochemical disorders (such as absent or defective digestive enzymes) and disease of the small intestine.

Causes of malabsorption

The causes of decreased nutrient absorption include:

- Reduced surface area of small intestine.
- Infection, leading to damage of the mucosa and bacterial removal of nutrients.
- Defective intraluminal hydrolysis or solubilization (due to lack of enzymes).
- Abnormalities of mucosal epithelial cells (involving loss of digestive enzymes or carriers).
- Drug-induced mechanisms.
- Lymphatic obstruction.
- Rapid passage though the small intestine.
- Failure of nutrients to reach the small intestine (e.g. because of a bypass fistula).
- After surgical resection of gut and/or radiation therapy.

Systemic effects of the malabsorption syndrome

Whatever the cause, the results of malabsorption are essentially the same.

Patients complain of frothy, greasy stools, which are difficult to flush away (steatorrhoea), diarrhoea, weight loss, and abdominal distension.

Anaemia may be due to deficiency of iron, folate, or vitamin B_{12}. Vitamin K deficiency can lead to bleeding disorders, purpura (extravasation of red cells into the skin, characterized by red skin lesions, which do not blanch on pressure) and petechiae (flat, red or purple spots about the size of a pinhead in the skin or mucous membranes).

Endocrine disorders may result from generalized malnutrition and deficiencies of vitamin A and B_1 may lead to peripheral neuropathy.

Deficient absorption of amino acids can result in hypoalbuminaemia and oedema. Dermatitis and hyperkeratosis may also be evident in the skin. The musculoskeletal system may also be affected with osteopenia and tetany.

Fig. 8.7 summarizes the systemic effects of malabsorption.

Specific malabsorption syndromes
Coeliac disease

Coeliac disease is caused by an abnormal reaction to gluten (found in wheat flour), which damages the enterocytes of the small intestine (causing villous atrophy and malabsorption).

It is associated in 90% of cases with human leucocyte antigen DQ2 (HLA-DQ2) and, in a smaller percentage, with HLA-B8 and HLA-DR3. It is also associated with dermatitis herpetiformis, an uncommon but extremely itchy skin disease typically found on the forearms and extensor surfaces.

Injury to the enterocytes appears to be due to an abnormal immune response to gliadin (a component of gluten).

Stem cells are unable to keep up with the rate of loss of enterocytes. This results in villous atrophy and the presence of immature cells, which are unable to absorb nutrients normally on the flattened surface. This, in turn, causes malabsorption and an intolerance of lactose and other sugars because of a secondary disaccharide deficiency resulting from the loss of surface epithelial cells.

The production of gastrointestinal hormones may also be deficient. This has a knock-on effect on pancreatic secretion and bile flow. Malabsorption of fat therefore predominates.

Anaemia, due to iron deficiency is a common secondary complication, as the duodenum and proximal jejunum are affected more than the ileum.

The condition predisposes to T cell lymphomas in the small intestine (an unusual small bowel lymphoma amongst the non-coeliac population, in whom most small bowel lymphomas are B cells).

There is also a higher incidence of other gastrointestinal cancers such as cancer of the stomach and oesophagus. Splenic atrophy may occur and all or any of the other features of malabsorption can be present.

Diagnosis is by jejunal biopsy showing evidence of villous atrophy.

Treatment is a permanent gluten-free diet, and the vast majority of patients show a marked improvement on dietary change. Gluten is present in wheat, barley, oats, and rye and these must all be excluded. It is not, however, present in rice or maize.

Fig. 8.7 Systemic effects of malabsorption.

night blindness
keratitis
(vitamin A)

mouth ulcers
glossitis
stomatitis
(vitamin B, C; folate
and iron)

rash
(essential fatty acids)

abdominal distension,
abdominal pain
borborygmi (carbohydrates
→↑ gut bacteria)

weight loss (general)
anaemia
(iron, folate,
vitamin B_{12})

diarrhoea (H_2O + electrolyte loss)
steatorrhoea (fat)

ascites
(protein)

urinary tract oxalate
stones
(↑ absorption of dietary oxalate)

peripheral
neuropathy
(vitamin B_{12}, E,
thiamine and folate)

rickets (vitamin D, Ca^{2+})
osteomalacia

bruising
(vitamin K and vitamin C)

oedema
(protein)

others: failure to thrive ⎤
short stature   ⎥ children
amenorrhoea   ⎦

Tropical sprue

Tropical sprue describes the malabsorption of two or more substances, following an enteric infection acquired in tropical areas of the world. These include:

- Asia.
- Caribbean islands.
- Puerto Rico.
- South America.

The malabsorption is usually accompanied by malnutrition and diarrhoea. It can be endemic in the tropics.

It is similar to coeliac disease in that villous atrophy is present, but it does not respond to a gluten-free diet.

Treatment is with broad-spectrum antibiotics as it is believed to be caused by bacteria overgrowth of enterotoxigenic organisms such as *Escherichia coli*,

Klebsiella pneumoniae, and *Enterobacter cloacae* in the upper small bowel. It does not appear to lead to intestinal lymphomas. Megaloblastic anaemia caused by folate deficiency is common.

Whipple's disease

This is a rare bacterial infection usually occurring in men over the age of 50 years. It is caused by *Tropheryma whippelii* (a Gram-positive actinomycete)

Diagnosis is by jejunal biopsy, which shows intact villi where the normal cells of the lamina propria have been replaced by macrophages containing PAS-positive glycoprotein granules. Similar cells may be found in lymph nodes, spleen, and liver. Treatment is with the antibiotic tetracycline. Whipple's disease is 10 times more common in men. If it is diagnosed in a woman, tetracycline should not be prescribed if the patient is pregnant, as tetracycline is teratogenic.

Bacterial overgrowth syndrome

The small intestine normally supports a large number of flora but these are kept in check by peristalsis, the acidity of chyme leaving the stomach, and the secretion of immunoglobulins into the intestinal lumen by the mucosal cells.

Where one or more of these factors is reduced, bacterial overgrowth may result in malabsorption.

Jejunal biopsy may show a normal mucosa. Diagnosis is by aspiration of the contents of the jejunum, which show increased numbers of both aerobic and anaerobic organisms.

These organisms may inactivate bile acids in the lumen by dehydroxylation, leading to fat malabsorption. The gut flora may catabolize ingested protein, metabolize sugars, and bind vitamin B_{12}, preventing its absorption.

Treatment is with antibiotics, such as tetracycline, metronidazole, or ciprofloxacin.

Giardiasis

Giardiasis, prevalent in the tropics, is an important cause of traveller's diarrhoea. It is caused by the flagellate protozoan, *Giardia lamblia*, which lives in the duodenum and jejunum, and it is transmitted by the faecal–oral route. It is more common amongst male homosexuals, in the immunosuppressed, and in those with achlorhydria. Cases may occur in Britain among people who have never been abroad.

Asymptomatic carriage may occur. Alternatively, symptoms may develop within 1 or 2 weeks of ingesting cysts.

Giardia lamblia exists as a trophozoite and a cyst; the cyst being the transmissible form. Intestinal damage varies from slight changes in villous architecture to partial villous atrophy with severe malabsorption.

Diagnosis is by examination of stool. Cysts and trophozoites may be found, but their absence does not exclude the diagnosis: in some cases they are only excreted at intervals. The parasite may also be seen in duodenal aspirates and in a jejunal biopsy.

Blood tests may show IgM antibodies to *Giardia* in acute infection and, later, anti-*Giardia* IgG.

Treatment is with metronidazole or quinacrine.

Abetalipoproteinaemia

Abetalipoproteinaemia is a rare autosomal recessive disorder, in which there is a failure to synthesize apo B-100 in the liver and apo B-48 in interstitial cells.

Normally, lipids (principally triglyceride cholesterol and cholesterol esters) are surrounded by a stabilizing coat of phospholipid because they are insoluble. Apoproteins are embedded in the surface of the complex of lipids and phospholipids to form lipoproteins.

In abetalipoproteinaemia, lipoproteins containing B apoproteins (for example, chylomicrons) cannot be made.

Chylomicrons are principally responsible for transporting the digestion products of fat in the diet to the liver and peripheral tissues after dietary fat has been absorbed from the gut.

An absence of chylomicrons leads to accumulation of triglycerides within the absorptive cells of the gut. Lipid vacuolation can be seen in these cells on biopsy.

Acanthocytosis (red blood cells with spiky membrane abnormalities) is seen in the blood. Other complications include atypical retinitis pigmentosa and neurological abnormalities, both linked to the malabsorption of the fat-soluble vitamins A, D, E, and K. Neurological damage can be prevented with vitamin E injections.

The disease is characterized by failure to thrive, diarrhoea, and steatorrhoea in infancy.

Disaccharide deficiency

Normally, disaccharides in the diet are hydrolysed by lactase or sucrase on the luminal surface of mucosal cells. Lactase activity is high at birth, but it declines during childhood and it is low in adults. The decline in lactase activity differs according to race: lactase levels are higher in Caucasians but lower in African, Oriental, and Mediterranean populations.

Disaccharide deficiency leads to diarrhoea, bloating, and flatulence, particularly with a high-milk diet.

Diarrhoea in lactase deficiency is caused by a failure to digest and absorb lactose. Lactose is broken down by bowel bacteria into its constituents, glucose and galactose, and then to lactic acid. This process causes osmotic diarrhoea.

Increased disaccharide residues in the lower small intestine and colon lead to increased gas production and flatulence.

Congenital lactase deficiency is rare. Acquired deficiency due to decreased activity of lactase is common, however, and seen in about 15% of Caucasians and 70–90% of other races.

Congenital disaccharide deficiency becomes apparent early in life because of milk intolerance, which leads to the production of explosive, watery, frothy stools and abdominal distension.

The more common acquired lactase deficiency often becomes apparent during viral and bacterial enteric infection.

Classification of malabsorption syndromes is given in Fig. 8.8.

Obstruction of the bowel

Bowel obstruction may have mechanical or non-mechanical causes (pseudo-obstruction).

The signs and symptoms are similar, regardless of the cause, and depend primarily on the level of the obstruction.

Vomiting is a symptom of high obstruction, but it may be absent (or occur late) in low-level obstruction.

Conversely, distension and colic are early symptoms of obstruction lower in the intestine.

Obstruction causes distension of the gut, with a build-up of gas and intestinal secretions above the level of the obstruction. There is progressive depletion of extracellular fluid and the multiplication of bacteria, especially coliforms, *Streptococcus faecalis*, *Clostridium perfringens*, and *Bacteroides*.

Diagnosis requires a thorough history (as always!) and erect and supine radiography. This shows distended, gas-filled loops of bowel with multiple horizontal fluid levels.

Treatment depends on the cause and level of the obstruction, and whether the bowel is strangulated. Strangulated bowel is an emergency, which requires urgent surgery.

Simple obstruction (not due to strangulation) may be treated conservatively initially. Conservative treatment consists of 'drip and suck': intravenous fluids and continuous aspiration by nasogastric tube.

In general, obstruction high in the gastrointestinal tract presents with vomiting. Obstruction lower down causes distension.

Major causes of bowel obstruction

The major causes of obstruction are:

- Intrinsic lesions (due to malignancy, IBD, congenital strictures, and diverticular disease).
- Luminal occlusions (due to foreign material, faecaliths, polypoid tumours, and meconium in cystic fibrosis).
- External constrictions (due to intussusception, adhesions, hernias, volvulus, and intra-abdominal tumours).

Fig. 8.8 Classification of malabsorption syndromes.

Classification of malabsorption syndromes	
Cause of malabsorption	Mechanism
Defective intraluminal hydrolysis	Lack of enzyme production Dysfunctional enzymes
Primary mucosal cell abnormalities	Loss of enzymes in mucosa Loss of carrier molecules Damage to mucosa via drugs or inflammation
Decreased surface area of intestines	Inflammation Drug induced damage
Infection	Due to enterotoxic microorganisms in the food Due to external injury to the bowel Due to antibiotics
Iatrogenic	Antibiotics, leading to decreased commensals and increased opportunistic infection
Drug induced	Toxicity Increased motility Increased fluid secretion Carrier inhibition Decreased enzyme production No uptake of fats from lacteals
Unexplained	Unknown

- Functional obstructions (due to Hirschsprung's disease, paralytic ileus, and bowel infarction).

Paralytic (adynamic or neurogenic) ileus is atony of the intestine resulting in a lack of peristalsis.

It occurs transiently after almost every laparotomy. Other causes include interruption of the autonomic innervation of the gut, peritonitis (which may cause toxin mediated paralysis of the intrinsic nerve plexuses of the gut), potassium depletion, uraemia, diabetic coma, and drugs (especially anticholinergics).

Meconium ileus occurs in about 10–15% of neonates with cystic fibrosis, a congenital condition characterized by defective mucus secretion. Meconium is unusually sticky, and it may obstruct the lower ileum.

An enema may resolve the obstruction; if it does not, surgery may be required.

Faecaliths are small, hard masses of faeces that can obstruct the bowel. They are particularly found in the appendix, causing inflammation.

Hernias

A hernia is the protrusion of any organ or tissue through its coverings and outside its normal body cavity.

Hernias are common, occurring in about 1% of the population, and they may be congenital or acquired (Fig. 8.9), reducible, irreducible, or strangulated (Fig. 8.10).

Reducible hernias can be pushed back into the compartment from which they came, irreducible ones cannot, and strangulated hernias have had their blood supply cut off by the neck of the sac.

Strangulated hernias present with signs and symptoms of obstruction and, untreated, become gangrenous and necrose.

The most common sites of herniation through the abdominal wall are:

- Inguinal.
- Femoral.
- Umbilical.
- Incisional.
- Ventral.
- Epigastric.

Inguinal hernias may be:

- Direct (protruding through the posterior wall of the inguinal canal).
- Indirect (passing through the inguinal canal).

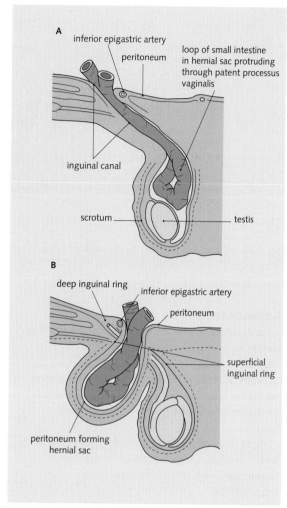

Fig. 8.9 (A) Congenital indirect hernia passing into scrotum through patent processus vaginalis. (B) Acquired direct hernia, passing through a defect in the abdominal wall. (Redrawn with permission from Hall-Craggs ECB. *Anatomy as a Basis for Clinical Medicine.* London: Waverly Europe 1995.)

Direct inguinal hernias are less commonly seen (20% of inguinal hernias) and they lie medial to the inferior epigastric vessels. Indirect hernias are much more common and they can strangulate. The inferior epigastric vessels separate the sites of direct and indirect hernias.

Treatment depends on the type of hernia. Reducible hernias often require no treatment so long as they remain reducible. Strangulated hernias must be treated surgically.

Synthetic meshes are often used to reinforce closure of hernia orifices.

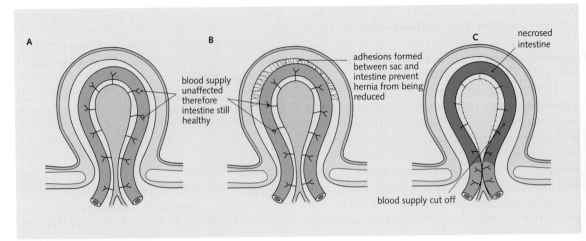

Fig. 8.10 (A) Reducible hernia. (B) Irreducible hernia. (C) Strangulated hernia. Reducible hernias can be pushed back into the compartment from which they came, irreducible ones cannot. Strangulated hernias have had their blood supply cut off.

Adhesions

Adhesions occur where two parts of the body that are normally separate are connected by bands of fibrous tissue.

Some are congenital, but most occur as a result of post-inflammatory scarring (e.g. after peritonitis, endometriosis, or scars that form as a result of surgery).

Adhesions may cause external constriction of the bowel, leading to obstruction or strangulation. Urgent surgery is required to relieve the strangulation.

Examine the patient's abdomen. If there are scars from past abdominal surgery, consider adhesions as a cause of the obstruction.

If the bowel is strangulated, surgery is necessary.

Intussusception

Intussusception occurs when one segment of bowel slides inside the adjacent segment (Fig. 8.11), like a telescope. It is most common in early childhood (95% of all cases), and it occurs mainly at the ileocaecal valve. The ratio of males to females affected is 2:1.

The aetiology is unclear, but it may be related to an adenovirus causing enlargement of lymphatic tissue in the intestinal wall. This protrudes into the lumen and is pushed into the adjacent section by peristalsis.

In some cases a polyp (such as Peutz–Jeghers polyps), Meckel's diverticulum, or carcinoma may project into the lumen and be pushed along in a similar way. Occasionally, a tuberculosis infection of

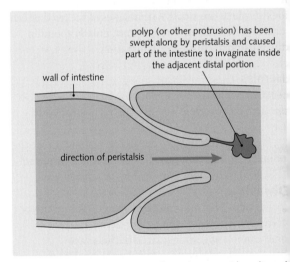

Fig. 8.11 Intussusception. One bowel segment has slipped inside an adjacent one.

the Peyer's patches may cause intussusception in adults.

Patients present aged 5–12 months of age, with periods of screaming, vomiting, blood in the faeces, and drawing up of the legs.

The child is pale and the tumour may be felt as a sausage-shaped mass on palpation of the abdomen.

Peritonitis and gangrene may occur within 24 hours if untreated. A barium enema may resolve the intussusception by forcing the invaginated segment back with hydrostatic pressure. Alternatively, surgery may be required.

Volvulus

Volvulus occurs when a loop of bowel is twisted 180 degrees about its mesenteric axis. This usually occurs in the sigmoid colon, but it may be found in the caecum, small intestine, gall bladder, or stomach.

Volvulus is most common in:
- Developing countries.
- Elderly men.
- The mentally handicapped.

Occasionally, it occurs in infancy when a loop of the small intestine malrotates around adhesions running from the duodenum to the caecum.

Risk factors include chronic constipation, adhesions, and abnormally mobile loops of intestine.

Twisting of the bowel causes obstruction and occlusion of the vessels supplying the affected section. Potentially fatal gangrene and peritonitis may occur if the volvulus is not treated. Symptoms include the sudden onset of colicky pain.

Diagnosis is by plain radiography, which shows a dilated section of bowel, full of gas, and forming a characteristic loop, or inverted U. Treatment depends on the site of the volvulus: surgery is often necessary. Sigmoid volvulus is sometimes resolved by sigmoidoscopy and the passing of a flatus tube.

Colonic diverticulosis

Definitions

- Diverticulum is an outpouching of the wall of the gut. They occur at weak points in the wall, usually due to increased pressure from within the gut or pulling from outside.
- Diverticulosis means that diverticula are present.
- Diverticular disease means that diverticula are causing symptoms, such as abdominal pain or change in bowel habit. However, the pain is due to muscle spasm, not inflammation.

Diverticulitis means that one or more diverticula are inflamed. This is usually caused by an infection and leads to inflammatory abdominal pain and diarrhoea, or constipation.

Diverticulosis

Diverticula may be congenital or acquired, and they occur in any part of the gut.

Congenital diverticula are outpouchings of the full thickness of the bowel wall. They are found most commonly in the duodenum and jejunum.

Congenital diverticula are usually asymptomatic, but they may lead to bacterial overgrowth, steatorrhoea, and vitamin B_{12} malabsorption. They may perforate or haemorrhage.

Acquired colonic diverticula increase in incidence with increasing age, and they are present in about 50% of people aged over 50 years. There is no difference in distribution between the sexes.

They are more common in the left side of the colon than the right, and they are usually found in the sigmoid and descending colon.

They form when the muscle layer of the wall thickens (hypertrophies) and high intraluminal pressures force a pouch of mucosa out through an area of weakness in the muscle layer. Areas of weakness often occur near blood vessels (Fig. 8.12).

Acquired diverticula do not consist of all three layers of the intestinal wall and this differentiates them from congenital ones.

Low-fibre diets are a risk factor. The pouches may become inflamed (diverticulitis) if the neck of the diverticulum becomes obstructed by faeces. Bacterial overgrowth then occurs in the diverticulum, with the risk of abscess formation, perforation (peridiverticulitis), and peritonitis.

Fistulae (abnormal communications between two epithelial surfaces) may also form, usually into the bladder or vagina (causing the patient much distress).

Diagnosis of diverticula is often incidental during other investigations and, as over 90% of cases are asymptomatic, in many cases no treatment is required.

Patients should, however, be advised to increase the amount of fibre and liquids in their diet (fibre has no beneficial effect unless there is sufficient liquid in the diet).

Patients with acute diverticulitis often present in a similar way to those with appendicitis, except that the pain is usually in the left iliac fossa instead of the right. The most common site of diverticula is the sigmoid colon.

Signs include tenderness and guarding on the left side of the abdomen, pyrexia and tachycardia. Radiographs should be taken to exclude air under the diaphragm (an indication of perforation).

In the absence of complications, acute diverticulitis is treated conservatively with a liquid diet and appropriate antibiotic treatment.

Obstruction or peritonitis is treated in the same way as if caused by other pathology.

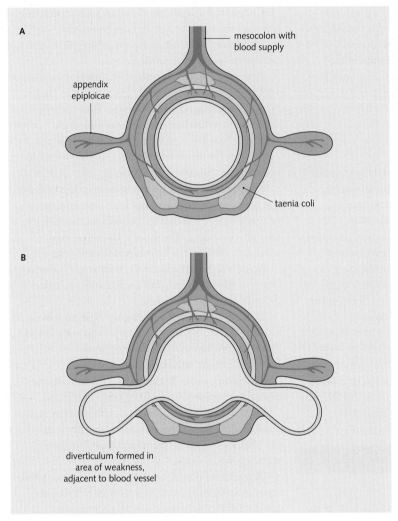

Fig. 8.12 In the diverticulum, high intraluminal pressure has forced pouches of mucosa through weak muscle areas. (Redrawn with permission from Ellis H, Calne R. *Lecture Notes on General Surgery*, 8th edn. Oxford: Blackwell Science, 1993.)

Labels on figure:
- mesocolon with blood supply
- appendix epiploicae
- taenia coli
- diverticulum formed in area of weakness, adjacent to blood vessel

Fistulae may heal of their own accord, but not in the presence of inflammation, and surgery is often indicated.

Vascular disorders

Ischaemic bowel disease

Essentially, the causes of ischaemic bowel disease are the same as ischaemia in other parts of the body.

Common causes include:
- Stenosis.
- Thrombosis.
- Emboli.

Uncommon causes include:
- Atrial thrombi.
- Cardiac failure.
- Septicaemia.

- Trauma.
- Anaphylaxis.
- Tumour infiltration.
- Vasculitis.
- Strangulation.

Ischaemic bowel disease may occur in the small intestine or the colon. Small bowel ischaemia may be chronic or acute. The effect depends on the size of the ischaemic area and the length of time ischaemia has persisted.

It may be classified as mucosal, mural, or transmural, the effects of which are summarized in Fig. 8.13.

The blood supply to the wall is 'from outside in' and mucosal or mural infarction often results from underperfusion. Transmural infarction is usually due to mechanical compromise of the artery.

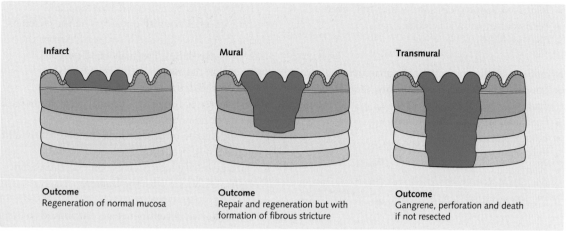

Infarct

Outcome
Regeneration of normal mucosa

Mural

Outcome
Repair and regeneration but with formation of fibrous stricture

Transmural

Outcome
Gangrene, perforation and death if not resected

Fig. 8.13 The effects of acute intestinal infarction.

The splenic flexure and an area of the rectum are particularly prone to ischaemic damage. These are the watershed areas where the arterial supply switches from the superior to the inferior mesenteric artery, and from the inferior mesenteric and hypogastric arteries, respectively (Fig. 8.14).

Reperfusion injury commonly occurs following hypoperfusion and, like reperfusion injury seen in the heart and brain, it is mediated by free radicals, which cause damage to cell membranes.

Damage to the mucosa causes release of proteolytic enzymes, which may cause deeper damage to the wall. However, complete regeneration is more common.

After mural infarction, ulcers form, the mucosa haemorrhages, and granulation tissue forms. This is replaced by fibrotic tissue, which can form a stricture. Transmural ischaemia leads to gangrene, perforation, and, if untreated, death.

Transmural infarction should be suspected in any elderly patient with atherosclerosis or atrial fibrillation with a tender abdomen and absent bowel sounds.

Symptoms in acute small bowel ischaemia include:
- Acute, severe abdominal pain, mainly around the right iliac fossa.
- No abdominal signs, such as distension.
- Shock, due to hypovolaemia.

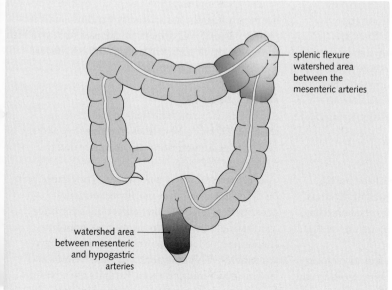

Fig. 8.14 Areas of large bowel particularly prone to ischaemic injury.

splenic flexure watershed area between the mesenteric arteries

watershed area between mesenteric and hypogastric arteries

- Increased haemoglobin and white cell count.
- Persistent metabolic acidosis.
- Gasless abdomen on X-ray.

Symptoms of chronic intestinal ischaemia include:
- Severe, colicky post-prandial pain, in the left iliac fossa.
- Food avoidance and weight loss.
- Bloody diarrhoea.
- Pyrexia.
- Tachycardia.
- Leucocytosis.
- Thumb-printing oedema on X-ray.

Diagnosis relies on abdominal X-ray and endoscopy. A sigmoidoscopy shows a normal rectal mucosa, but it also shows blood and mucus coming from further along the bowel. A full colonoscopy is not performed, due to the risk of perforation.

Histological changes in chronic ischaemic bowel disease include fibrosis, haemorrhage, ulceration, and granulation. On biopsy, the mucosa has a large infiltration of polymorphonuclear cells. Macrophages laden with haemosiderin are uncommon, but thought to be characteristic of ischaemic bowel disease.

The patient is treated with fluid replacement, heparin, and antibiotics. Surgery is absolutely necessary to remove the dead segment of bowel. Revasculization may also be attempted.

The prognosis is poor in acute bowel ischaemia, with a less than 20% survival rate.

Angiodysplasia

Angiodysplasia occurs when vascular anomalies (most commonly arteriovenous malformations) cause bleeding from the large bowel. They are more common in the elderly, and they can be diagnosed by angiography or colonoscopy. The right side of the colon is affected more commonly than the left.

Treatment is by diathermy coagulation or surgical removal.

Haemorrhoids

Haemorrhoids are the enlargement of the normal spongy blood-filled cushions in the wall of the anus. They are the most common cause of rectal bleeding, and patients normally complain of blood on the toilet paper after defecation.

The anal cushions are at the 3, 7, and 11 o'clock positions, when viewed in the lithotomy position and attached by elastic tissue and smooth muscle.

However, gravity, increased anal tone, and straining on defecation all put stress on the cushions, making them protrude and bleed readily from the underlying capillaries. Pregnancy and portal hypertension can also cause haemorrhoids.

Haemorrhoids are classified as:
- First degree (confined to the anal canal, and which bleed but do not prolapse).
- Second degree (which prolapse on defecation, but spontaneously reduce).
- Third degree (which prolapse on defecation, but require reduction with the fingers).

Normally, faecal continence is contributed to by three anal vascular cushions, which drain into the superior rectal veins and then into the inferior mesenteric veins. Internal haemorrhoids can be made worse by anything impairing drainage of the superior rectal veins.

Patients present with bright red bleeding from the rectum, and they are often very anaemic. Mucus discharge and pruritus ani (anal itching) accompanies this. Often internal haemorrhoids are asymptomatic.

Diagnosis involves rectal examination, proctoscopy, and exclusion of any abdominal malignancies, which may also cause bleeding.

Haemorrhoids can be treated by:
- Infra-red coagulation.
- Injection sclerotherapy.
- Banding (rubber band ligation).
- Cryotherapy.
- Haemorrhoidectomy.

The choice of treatment depends on the type of haemorrhoids, the associated symptoms, and the patient history. All patients are advised to have a high fibre diet, drink plenty of water, and use a faecal softening agent, if necessary.

Anal fissures

Anal fissures are midline longitudinal tears in the anal mucosa. About 90% are posterior, and the 10% that occur anteriorly are normally due to parturition.

Most are caused by hard faeces. They cause pain on defecation, and they usually accompany constipation. Bleeding on defecation is common.

Treatment involves application of lidocaine (lignocaine), a local anaesthetic gel, and glyceryl trinitrate (GTN) ointment. Chronic fissures and spasms may require surgery. Patients are advised to increase their dietary fibre and fluid intake.

Neoplastic disease of the bowel

Neoplasms of the bowel, as in the rest of the body, may be benign or malignant. Polyps may be metaplastic and completely benign. They can also be neoplastic and give rise to malignancies. The asymptomatic nature of most polyps means that they are found by chance. The process of cancer progression is shown in Fig. 8.15.

Non-neoplastic polyps

Non-neoplastic polyps make up the vast majority of epithelial polyps found in the large intestine (about 90%), and they increase in frequency with age. They are present in about half the population over the age of 60 years.

Most epithelial polyps are found in the large bowel; they are relatively rare in the small intestine. Mesenchymal polyps may also be found, but these are even more rare than epithelial ones.

Hyperplastic polyps

Hyperplastic (metaplastic) polyps are relatively common in the rectum, especially in the elderly. They are sessile (without a stalk) and they have well formed crypts containing mature goblet or absorptive cells.

They are usually small (less than 5 mm in diameter), and they have no malignant potential.

Hamartomatous polyps

Hamartomas are overgrowths of mature tissue, which, although disordered in arrangement, are benign.

Hamartomatous polyps are usually large and pedunculated (have a stalk). They fall into two main categories: juvenile and Peutz–Jeghers polyps.

Juvenile polyps

Juvenile polyps are usually solitary focal hamartomatous malformations of mucosal tissue.

A hamartoma is a malformation containing two or more mature cell types, which are normally present in the organ in which they arise. They are always benign.

They occur in children and teenagers, but they are most common below the age of 5 years, and about 80% of them occur in the rectum.

They are often large (up to 3 cm in diameter) with long stalks (up to 2 cm in length) but they have no malignant potential.

Juvenile polyposis is an autosomal dominant condition presenting with ten or more colonic polyps. The risk of colonic cancer is increased in this disorder. Children with this must begin a screening programme to help spot cancer in its early stages.

Peutz–Jeghers polyps

Peutz–Jeghers syndrome is a rare autosomal dominant syndrome characterized by multiple polyps scattered throughout the gastrointestinal tract. Abnormal pigmentation also occurs in the skin and oral mucosa. The polyps may bleed and cause anaemia. Although the polyps themselves are not premalignant, being hamartomas, people with Peutz–Jeghers syndrome do have a slightly increased risk of developing certain carcinomas, notably in the gastrointestinal tract and ovary.

Neoplastic epithelial lesions
Adenomas

Adenomas are derived from glandular epithelium, and they are the most important of the epithelial polyps. They are relatively common, especially in the elderly.

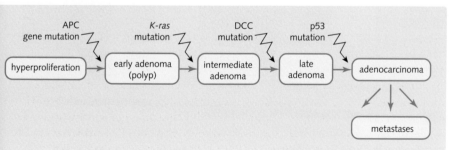

Fig. 8.15 The process of cancer progression, showing the consecutive gene mutations involved.

Of all adenomas, 75% are tubular, 10% villous, and the remainder a mixture of the two (tubulovillous).

Tubular adenomas are smaller than villous adenomas (up to 1 cm in diameter) and they are usually pedunculated. They look a little like a blackberry on a stalk.

Villous adenomas, on the other hand, are usually sessile and larger (up to several centimetres in diameter) and, as the name suggests, have villi lined with dysplastic columnar epithelium protruding from their surface.

Villous adenomas have a greater tendency to malignant change, and they carry the additional risk of electrolyte imbalance and, more rarely, acute renal failure resulting from their secretion of electrolyte-rich mucus.

Familial adenomatous polyposis

People with familial adenomatous polyposis, a rare autosomal dominant disorder, almost always develop cancer of the intestine by the age of 35 years. Familial adenomatous polyposis is characterized by the development of numerous adenomas in the large and, to a lesser extent, the small intestine during the teens and twenties.

The gene involved in familial adenomatous polyposis is called APC and is on the long arm of chromosome 5 (between q21 and q22). Non-steroidal anti-inflammatory drugs (NSAIDs) are thought to be protective.

Colorectal cancer

Colorectal cancer is common in the developed world, and it is the second biggest cause of cancer death in the UK (coming second to lung cancer).

It is closely related to diet. Its incidence is low in Japan but, amongst second generation Japanese living in the United States, the incidence is the same as that of the indigenous American population.

Dietary factors carrying a greater risk of colorectal cancer are:

- Low fibre.
- High carbohydrate.
- High fat.

Fibre increases the bulk of faeces, as long as fluid intake is adequate, and this reduces the time taken for the contents of the intestine to pass through and out of the rectum. In a low-fibre diet, faeces remain in the intestine for longer, altering the normal flora, and this is thought to predispose to cancer.

Inadequate intake of the free radical scavengers, vitamins A, C, and E, also leads to an increased risk of colorectal and some other cancers.

Survival after diagnosis of colorectal cancer depends on the stage. Dukes' classification is most widely used (Fig. 8.16).

Dukes' stages for colorectal carcinoma are:

- Stage A: invaded submucosa and muscle layer of the bowel, but confined to the wall.
- Stage B: breached the muscle layer and bowel wall, but no involvement of lymph nodes.
- Stage C1: spread to immediately draining pericolic lymph nodes.
- Stage C2: spread to higher mesenteric lymph nodes.
- Stage D: distant visceral metastases.

Other neoplasms
Carcinoid tumours

The normal intestine secretes a number of gastrointestinal hormones from endocrine cells.

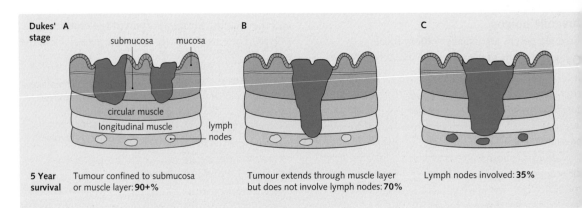

Fig. 8.16 Staging of colorectal cancer by Dukes' classification.

These cells are known as APUD (amine precursor uptake and decarboxylation) cells, and they comprise enterochromaffin and enteroendocrine cells.

Neuroendocrine cells are also found in other organs (e.g. the lung, pancreas, and biliary tract), and tumours may arise in neuroendocrine cells in the gut and elsewhere. These tumours are slow growing, and they are called carcinoid.

Carcinoid tumours are potentially malignant but their malignant potential depends on the site. Larger tumours in the appendix and ileum tend to spread to regional lymph nodes and the liver. Small tumours (less than 2 cm diameter) near the tip of the appendix rarely do so.

Because of the cells in which they arise, tumours produce hormones that may have local or systemic effects:

- 5-HT produced by midgut carcinoid tumours causes diarrhoea and borborygmi as a result of local stimulation of the contractility of the intestine.
- 5-HT may also be produced from metastases in the liver and give rise to the carcinoid syndrome with facial flushing, cyanosis, and pulmonary and tricuspid valve stenosis or incompetence.
- Adrenocorticotrophic hormone (ACTH) may be secreted and can result in Cushing's syndrome.

Palliative treatment is usually chosen. Survival can be anything from 3 years to 30 years, even if metastases are present.

Borborygmi are abdominal gurgles caused by fluid and gas movement in the intestines.

Gastrointestinal lymphoma

Intestinal lymphoma is rare, but is the second most common extranodal origin of lymphoma (after gastric lymphoma). Lymphomas are more common in the small intestine than in the large, and they may be of B cell or T cell lineage.

T cell lymphomas are associated with coeliac disease, B cell lymphomas are not and most occur sporadically.

Alpha-chain disease, most commonly found in the Mediterranean (but also in South America and the Far East), is characterized by a proliferation of plasma cells in the lamina propria of the upper small bowel; a B lymphocyte disorder may lead to lymphoma of the small intestine.

Patients often present with a palpable abdominal mass and obstruction, haemorrhage, or perforation. Those with coeliac disease may fail to respond to gluten withdrawal and have weight loss. Seventy per cent of patients excrete alpha-chains in the urine.

Mesenchymal tumours

These may occur in any part of the alimentary tract, and they include leiomyomas (arising from smooth muscle), lipomas, and Kaposi's sarcoma (a malignant neoplasm of vascular endothelium, commonly associated with acquired immune deficiency syndrome—AIDS).

Neoplasms of the small intestine

Small intestinal tumours are much less common than those in the large intestine. Single isolated polyps suggest malignancy, but they can be benign.

They are caused by:
- Lipoma (benign).
- Leiomyoma (benign).
- Adenoma (often benign).
- Adenocarcinoma (malignant).
- Carcinoid (malignant).
- Metastases, from lung, or melanoma (malignant).

Multiple polyps occur more commonly and they are usually due to:
- Nodular lymphoid hyperplasia.
- Peutz–Jeghers hamartomas.
- Cronkhite–Canada syndrome (adenoma associated with alopecia and nail dystrophy).
- Multifocal adenocarcinoma.

Neoplasms of the appendix

Carcinoid tumours, adenocarcinomas, and lymphomas may all occur in the appendix, but they are rare. Proliferation of the epithelium may also occur causing an increase in secretion of mucus and dilating the lumen of the appendix (mucocele).

The most common cause of a mucocele is mucinous cystadenoma.

A less common cause is mucinous cystadenocarcinoma, from which neoplastic cells may implant into the peritoneum causing pseudomyoxoma peritonei (a distended peritoneal cavity containing semisolid mucin), which may be fatal.

Mucoceles may also be caused by simple epithelial hyperplasia.

Disorders of the peritoneum

Inflammation (peritonitis)

Peritonitis is inflammation of the peritoneum.

It may be limited to a small area, for example, where an abscess has formed, but it is usually generalized, extending to both the visceral and parietal peritoneum. Untreated, it is usually fatal.

Whatever the cause, the onset is usually sudden, with severe pain that is localized at first but becomes generalized, with guarding, tenderness to palpation, and the eventual disappearance of bowel sounds (due to ileus).

The patient will look shocked, with tachycardia, and lie still, sometimes with his or her knees drawn up.

He or she will take very shallow breaths as any movement of the peritoneum (e.g. movement of the diaphragm in inspiration) is extremely painful.

Peritoneal infection

This is caused by organisms that spread from the intestinal lumen or from outside as a result of surgery or penetrating injury (Fig. 8.17). Causes of infection include:

- An ulcer that has eroded through the wall of the gut, producing acute perforation of the bowel.
- Acute salpingitis (inflammation of the fallopian tubes).
- Strangulated bowel.
- Peritoneal dialysis.
- Cholecystitis.
- Diverticulitis.
- Appendicitis.

In short, anything that disrupts the integrity of the intestinal wall and allows organisms out of the lumen into the peritoneal cavity, or disrupts the integrity of the abdominal wall and allows organisms in from the outside world, can cause peritoneal infection.

The organism responsible varies depending on the site of the offending lesion.

Infection from the bowel is most common and organisms include:

- *Bacteroides.*
- *Escherichia coli.*
- *Clostridium perfringens.*
- *Pseudomonas.*
- *Klebsiella.*

The most common organisms introduced from outside the body are *Staphylococcus aureus* and streptococci.

Diagnosis

As always, diagnosis is on the history and clinical findings. In addition, erect radiographs should be taken to look for air under the diaphragm (a sign of perforation) and blood tests performed to exclude pancreatitis.

Exploratory laparotomy may be necessary.

Treatment

The patient will be shocked and resuscitation is essential, with intravenous fluids and correction of electrolyte imbalance.

The cause, once identified, should be removed, and the infection treated with appropriate antibiotics.

As with any patient in pain, adequate analgesia should be given.

Sclerosing peritonitis (retroperitoneal fibromatosis)

This is a rare condition characterized by marked fibrosis behind the peritoneum and an infiltrate of

Fig. 8.17 Summary table of peritoneal infection.

Summary of peritoneal infection		
Mechanism of infection	Event causing infection	Bacteria involved
From inside body	• Appendicitis • Salpingitis • Cholecystitis • Bowel perforation (e.g. ulcer or diverticular)	• Bacterioides • *E. coli* • *Clostridium perfringens* • Pseudomonas • Klebsiella
From outside the body	• Penetrating injury • Peritoneal dialysis • Surgery	• *Staphylococcus aureus* • Streptococci

inflammatory cells (lymphocytes, plasma cells, and neutrophils).

The fibrous tissue may encroach on adjacent structures (most commonly the ureters), producing symptoms that vary according to the structures involved.

Patients often present in middle age with malaise, fever, weight loss, and renal failure.

Blood tests may show a raised erythrocyte sedimentation ratio (ESR; a very non-specific sign) and anaemia. The diagnosis may be made with certainty on an abdominal CT scan. Surgery may be required. The cause is unclear, but it may be autoimmune. It is sometimes associated with the carcinoid syndrome.

Mesenteric cysts

Cysts may form in the mesenteries of the abdomen. They present in children as either a painless abdominal mass, or as acute abdominal pain, caused by rupture, torsion, or obstruction.

They may originate from:
- Walled-off infections following pancreatitis (pseudocysts).
- Diverticula of the developing foregut and hindgut.
- The urogenital ridge (the embryological origin of part of the urinary and genital systems).
- Sequestered lymphatic channels.

They may also be of malignant origin.

Neoplasms

As with all tumours, those of the peritoneum can be divided into primary or secondary, and malignant or benign.

Benign tumours of the peritoneum are very rare.

Tumours may arise from any organ or structure in the abdomen, or seed from elsewhere, and arise from any tissue.

Tumours arising from the mesothelium of the peritoneum are called mesotheliomas and (although more rare) they are similar to mesotheliomas arising in the pleura and pericardium.

Primary mesothelioma

Primary mesothelioma of the peritoneum is very rare but when it does occur it is usually associated with heavy asbestos exposure (80% of cases). Asbestos is also associated with pleural mesotheliomas, and the risk of developing one is increased up to several hundredfold if the person who was exposed also smokes.

Of patients with primary mesothelioma, 50% also have pulmonary fibrosis. Fifty per cent of cases of primary mesothelioma stay confined to the abdominal cavity, but the intestines may become involved in the remainder and lead to intestinal obstruction.

Secondary mesothelioma

The peritoneum is a common site of transcoelomic metastasis, especially from the ovaries and pancreas. Less commonly, seeding may occur from extra-peritoneal tumours.

This results in ascites (an effusion of fluid into the peritoneal cavity), with a fluid rich in protein (an exudate).

The fluid also contains the neoplastic cells that have seeded from the primary, and these are visible on appropriate staining of a sample of fluid aspirated from the peritoneal cavity.

The presence of neoplastic cells is important in distinguishing this from other causes of ascites.

Exudates and transudates are both abnormal collections of fluid outside the vascular system:
- An exudate results from an increase in vascular permeability and is rich in protein (>2 g per 100 mL).
- A transudate is due to increased intravascular pressure or hypoproteinaemia and is low in protein (<2 g per 100 mL).

Treatment of intestinal disorders

Laxatives

Laxatives are the type of drug used to treat constipation. They fall into the categories of:
- Bulking agents (e.g. bran, ispaghula husks, or methylcellulose).
- Osmotic laxatives (e.g. lactulose and magnesium sulphate, or Epsom salts).
- Faecal softeners (e.g. oral liquid paraffin and glycerine suppository).
- Stimulant laxatives (e.g. senna, cascara, or bisacodyl suppository).
- Bowel cleansing solutions (e.g. Picolax).

Bulking agents absorb water, and bulk up and soften faeces. Osmotic laxatives act by retaining water by osmosis and keeping liquid in the stools. Both of these groups distend the gut, stimulating motility and defecation.

Faecal softeners act as lubricants to ease the passage of faeces.

Stimulant laxatives increase intestinal motility, via the propulsive peristaltic reflex. Bowel cleansing solutions are used to prepare the bowel for colonoscopy or a barium meal. They are not treatments for constipation.

Anti-diarrhoeal drugs

Anti-diarrhoeal drugs fall into two major categories, absorbents (or bulk-forming drugs) and opiate agonists (anti-motility drugs).

- Absorbents and bulk-forming drugs act to bulk out fluid faeces (e.g. kaolin, methylcellulose, and ispaghula).
- Anti-motility drugs act by decreasing propulsive activity and increasing segmenting activity in the intestine. This allows more time for absorption of fluids (e.g. morphine, loperamide, codeine phosphate, and co-phenotrope).

Anti-spasmodic drugs

These are used to treat colicky pain and stop intense contractions, which can cause ischaemia. These may give symptomatic relief of IBS by relaxing the muscle of the bowel, although controlled clinical trials show no evidence of them being very effective. Muscle relaxants include:

- Peppermint oil (which is a Ca^{2+} channel antagonist).
- Alverine and mebeverine (which relax smooth muscle by increasing the intracellular cAMP concentration).
- Atropine, propantheline, and dicycloverine (dicyclomine), which are indirect relaxants and act as antagonists of muscarinic receptors.

Motility stimulants

These drugs act to stimulate motility in a region of the gut where motility is impaired. Direct motility stimulants are dopamine receptor antagonists (e.g. metoclopramide). They are used to:

- Stimulate peristalsis.
- Increase lower oesophageal sphincter (LOS) tone.
- Stimulate gastric emptying.

- List the embryological origin, site, and frequency of Meckel's diverticulum.
- How does Hirschsprung's disease arise? How does it differ from acquired megacolon?
- What are atresia and stenosis of the small and large intestines?
- What are the main categories of diarrhoea, and how are they defined?
- What might cause infectious enterocolitis?
- What causes Chagas' disease, and how does the illness present?
- Compare and contrast Crohn's disease and ulcerative colitis.
- What is irritable bowel syndrome? How is it diagnosed and treated?
- What causes malabsorption?
- Briefly describe the mechanisms causing coeliac disease.
- What is abetalipoproteinaemia? What effect does this disease have on absorption in the small intestine?
- What are the major causes of bowel obstruction?
- What is a hernia, and what types are found in the inguinal region?
- What is intussusception? How does it occur?
- What is a volvulus? What are the risk factors associated with it?
- What is the difference between diverticular disease and diverticulitis?
- What causes diverticulosis? How might this be prevented?
- Summarize the causes, classification, complications, and management of bowel ischaemia.
- How do haemorrhoids form? How are they classified?
- What are the main kinds of hamartomatous polyps?
- What is familial adenomatous polyposis? Draw a diagram to show how the gene mutations change a premalignant neoplasm into colorectal adenocarcinoma.
- What are the dietary factors contributing to colorectal cancer? What is Dukes' staging of colorectal cancer?
- What are carcinoid tumours?
- How does peritonitis occur? How does the patient present with this?
- How can the peritoneum become infected?
- Briefly describe the neoplasms found in the peritoneum.
- What is the treatment for peritonitis?
- What laxatives are available to treat constipation? What are their mechanisms of action?
- How do anti-spasmodic drugs work?
- What drugs are available to treat diarrhoea? How do they work?

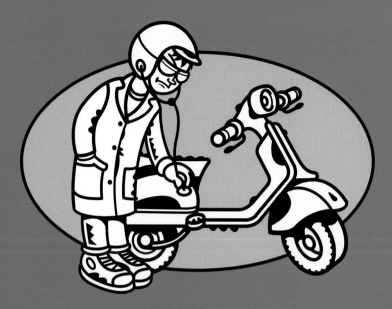

CLINICAL ASSESSMENT

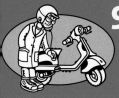

9. Common Presentations of Gastrointestinal Disease

Belching

Belching describes the passing of gas from the stomach up the oesophagus and through the mouth. This is common, particularly after drinking fizzy drinks and in anxious individuals who involuntarily swallow air.

It is almost always benign, especially if there are no other symptoms, but it may occur in obstruction. Air in the gastrointestinal tract cannot get beyond the obstruction and it comes back up to be expelled through the mouth.

It is more likely to be pathological if other symptoms such as abdominal pain, vomiting, or weight loss are present (Fig. 9.1).

Dysphagia

Dysphagia means having difficulty in swallowing. This is a symptom of a number of conditions, principally obstruction, stricture, neurological lesions, or uncoordinated peristalsis as in achalasia (Fig. 9.2).

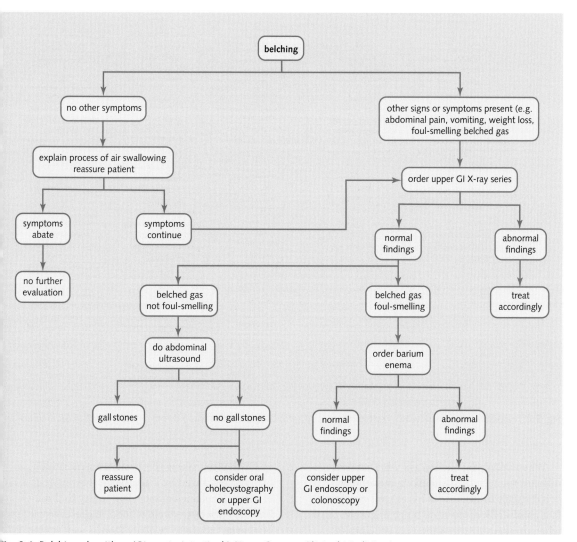

Fig. 9.1 Belching algorithm. (GI, gastrointestinal.) (From Greene, *Clinical Medicine.*)

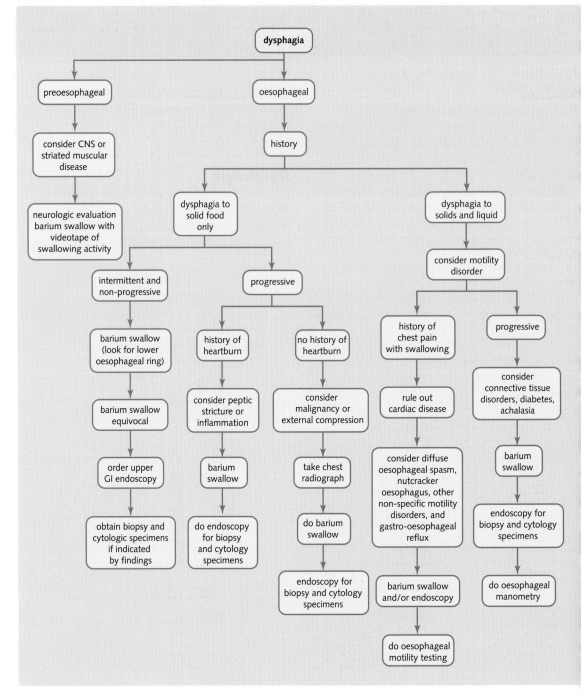

Fig. 9.2 Dysphagia algorithm. (CNS, central nervous system; GI, gastrointestinal.) (From Greene, *Clinical Medicine.*)

When taking the history, ask whether it is difficult to make the swallowing movement. Is it difficult to swallow fluids as well as solids? Is it painful? Does the neck bulge or gurgle when drinking? Does swallowing precipitate coughing?

Difficulty making the swallowing movement is likely to be caused by a neurological lesion (e.g. a cerebrovascular accident). The ability to drink liquids, but not to swallow food, suggests a stricture. However, failure to swallow food as well as fluid is seen in achalasia.

Constant, painful dysphagia with weight loss may be caused by a malignant stricture. Bulging or gurgling is a symptom of a pharyngeal pouch (Killian's dehiscence).

Heartburn, indigestion, and peptic symptoms

Heartburn is common, especially in developed countries. It is pain behind the sternum (retrosternal) that may radiate up towards the throat. It is worse on bending and lying flat. It can also be worse after drinking alcohol or eating something acidic or spicy (Fig. 9.3).

It is important to distinguish this from the retrosternal pain of a myocardial infarct (typically described as a central crushing pain, as if someone were tightening a band around the chest).

Indigestion has different meanings to different people, and it is commonly used to mean any discomfort experienced after eating or drinking. It is important to establish exactly what the patient means by the word (Fig. 9.4).

Nausea and vomiting

Nausea is a feeling that one is about to vomit. It is often accompanied by hypersalivation, which protects the mouth against the acid contents of the stomach. Differential diagnoses are given in Fig. 9.5.

Some patterns of vomiting are almost diagnostic, for example, the projectile vomiting seen in pyloric stenosis in babies (Fig. 9.6).

The content of the vomit (especially blood or bile), the frequency and amount all give important information. The presence of bile suggests that the lesion is below the ampulla of Vater.

Abdominal distension

Abdominal distension may be caused by one of the five Fs (flatus, fluid, fetus, fat, or faeces).

Obstruction low in the gastrointestinal tract typically leads to distension. Obstruction higher up causes vomiting.

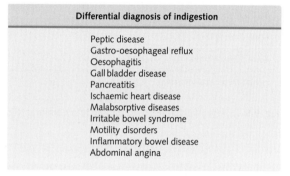

Differential diagnosis of indigestion
Peptic disease
Gastro-oesophageal reflux
Oesophagitis
Gall bladder disease
Pancreatitis
Ischaemic heart disease
Malabsorptive diseases
Irritable bowel syndrome
Motility disorders
Inflammatory bowel disease
Abdominal angina

Fig. 9.4 Differential diagnoses of indigestion. (From Greene, *Clinical Medicine.*)

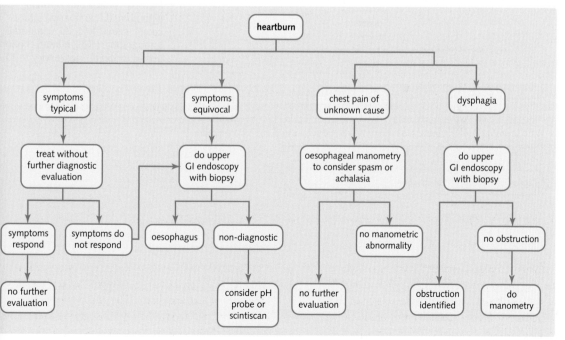

Fig. 9.3 Heartburn algorithm. (GI, gastrointestinal.) (From Greene, *Clinical Medicine.*)

Differential diagnosis of nausea and vomiting			
		Predominant symptoms	
Associated abdominal pain	**Associated neurological signs**	**Acute**	**Recurrent or chronic**
Viral gastroenteritis	Increased intracranial pressure	Digitalis toxicity	Psychogenic vomiting
Acute gastritis	Midline cerebellar haemorrhage	Ketoacidosis	Metabolic disturbances
Food poisoning	Vestibular disturbances	Opiate use	Gastric retention
Peptic ulcer disease	Migraine headaches	Cancer chemotherapeutic agents	Bile reflux after gastric surgery
Acute pancreatitis		Early pregnancy	Pregnancy
Small bowel obstruction		Inferior myocardial infarction	
Acute appendicitis		Drug withdrawal	
Acute cholecystitis		Binge drinking	
Acute cholangitis		Hepatitis	
Acute pyelonephritis			
Inferior myocardial infarction			

Fig. 9.5 Differential diagnoses of nausea and vomiting. (From Greene, *Clinical Medicine.*)

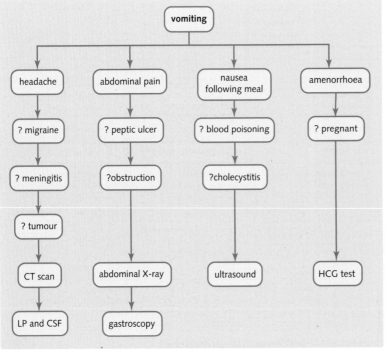

Fig. 9.6 Nausea and vomiting algorithm. (LP, lumbar puncture; C[S] cerebrospinal fluid; CT, computed tomography; HCG, human chorion[ic] gonadotrophin—pregnancy test.)

Distension may have intraluminal, intramural, or intraperitoneal causes (Fig. 9.7).

As with other disorders, the rate of onset (i.e. the rate at which the abdomen distended) is important. A neoplasm, for example, will not produce distension as quickly as gas.

Benign causes are also less likely to cause other symptoms. Aetiologies are given in Fig. 9.8.

Abdominal pain

Because of the embryological development of the gut, pain in a structure that develops from the foregut may be referred to the epigastric region, midgut structures to the umbilical area, and hindgut structures to the suprapubic area.

There are many possible causes of abdominal pain (Fig. 9.9), and it may be acute or chronic (Figs 9.10 and 9.11). Accompanying symptoms will give clues as to the mechanisms behind the pain.

Gastrointestinal bleeding

In general, bright red blood signifies fresh blood and dark, black blood is from an old bleed. Bright red blood from the anus is most likely to have come from low down in the gastrointestinal tract, such as the rectum or anus. Dark blood in the stools (melaena) will indicate bleeding from higher up in the gut.

Profuse bleeding from the upper gastrointestinal tract will result in haematemesis (blood in the vomit), and this needs to be diagnosed and treated quickly, as acute bleeding, particularly from oesophageal varices, can be fatal (Fig. 9.12).

By far the most common cause of rectal bleeding is piles (haemorrhoids). Patients usually say they notice blood on the toilet paper.

Jaundice

Jaundice is characterized by a yellow skin and sclera (observed in a good light), and it is caused when plasma bilirubin levels exceed 45 μmol/L.

The mechanisms by which levels may become elevated are described in Chapter 6.

It is classified as prehepatic, hepatic, or posthepatic jaundice. Jaundice may also be described as intrahepatic and extrahepatic (Fig. 9.13).

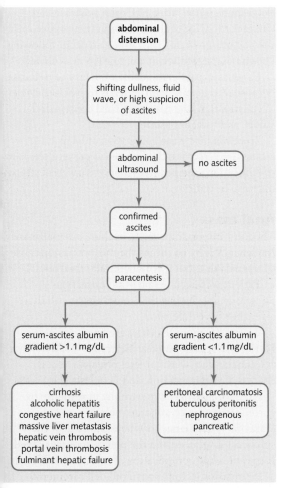

Fig. 9.7 Abdominal distension algorithm. (From Greene, *Clinical Medicine.*)

Aetiologies of abdominal distension
Gaseous causes
Functional gas/bloat syndrome
Gastric outlet obstruction
Small bowel obstruction
Ileus
Intestinal pseudo-obstruction
Pneumatosis cystoides intestinalis
Perforated viscus
Solid causes
Organomegaly
Liver
Spleen
Kidney
Tumour mass
Constipation with faecal retention
Pregnancy
Obesity
Fluid causes
Ascites
Perforated viscus
Abdominal haemorrhage
Cysts
Abscesses
Pancreatic pseudocysts
Gastric outlet obstruction
Small bowel obstruction
Ileus
Intestinal pseudo-obstruction
Bladder outlet obstruction

Fig. 9.8 Causes of abdominal distension. (From Greene, *Clinical Medicine.*)

Principal mechanisms of abdominal pain	
Obstruction	**Metabolic disturbance**
Gastric outlet	Diabetic ketoacidosis
Small bowel	Porphyria
Large bowel	Lead poisoning
Biliary tract	
Urinary tract	**Nerve injury**
	Herpes zoster
Peritoneal irritation	Root compression
Infection	**Muscle wall disease**
Chemical irritation (blood, bile, gastric acid)	Trauma
Systemic inflammatory process	Myositis
Spread from a local inflammatory process	Haematoma
Vascular insufficiency	**Referred pain**
	Pneumonia (lower lobes)
Embolization	Inferior myocardial infarction
Atherosclerotic narrowing	Pulmonary infarction
Hypotension	
Aortic aneurysm dissection	**Psychological stress**
Mucosal injury	Depression
	Situational stress
Peptic ulcer disease	Intrapsychic conflict
Gastric cancer	
Altered motility	
Gastroenteritis	
Inflammatory bowel disease	
Irritable colon	
Diverticular disease	

Fig. 9.9 Mechanisms of abdominal pain. (From Greene, *Clinical Medicine.*)

Diarrhoea and constipation

Severe diarrhoea causes electrolyte disturbances, and it is a significant cause of mortality in children worldwide.

It may be classified as acute or chronic. Acute cases are usually due to dietary indiscretion or infections. Chronic diarrhoea often has more serious causes (Fig. 9.14). Fig. 9.15 shows an algorithm for the management of acute diarrhoea.

Constipation is a subjective complaint. Some people believe they must open their bowels at least once a day to remain healthy but in fact anything from once every three days to three times a day is well within the normal range.

In the absence of other symptoms, a high-fibre diet may improve things, as long as sufficient fluid is taken with the fibre.

However, constipation may also be due to obstruction (Fig. 9.16).

Flatulence

Flatulence often causes great embarrassment, but some degree of flatulence is perfectly normal (about 10–20 releases a day). The sources of intestinal gas are described in Chapter 7.

Excessive gas may cause painful abdominal distension (resulting in a taut, drum-like abdomen), and it may be due to an abnormal increase in gas from any of the normal sources.

Causes include the incomplete breakdown of food because of an enzyme deficiency, leading to malabsorption. In the absence of other symptoms, simple exclusion of certain foods may relieve the symptoms (Fig. 9.17).

Anorectal pain

Anorectal pain may be caused by spasm of the sphincter, fissures, haemorrhoids, or abscesses (Fig. 9.18).

Fissures are cracks in the anal canal, and they are intensely painful on defecation (much more so than might be expected from their size). They may be caused by trauma from passing a constipated stool.

Fissures and other acquired anal abnormalities are a common complication of Crohn's disease (see Chapter 8). Most of them occur in the midline on the posterior margin. They may also occur following childbirth, particularly if a perineal tear occurred.

Patients are understandably reluctant to defecate because of the pain, and this leads to a vicious cycle of constipation, the passing of hard constipated stools, and further fissuring.

Treatment is by the application of local anaesthetic cream to the fissure (to prevent the pain of defecation) and laxatives if necessary. Anal stretch may also be indicated.

Anal mass

The most important thing to exclude is a malignancy. Malignancy is by no means the most common cause of an anal mass, but it is a potentially fatal one.

Patients often complain of tenesmus (an uncomfortable feeling that something is still there after they have defecated).

The most common causes are haemorrhoids (varices), hypertrophied anal papillae, condylomata acuminata (viral warts), rectal prolapse, rectal abscess, faecal impaction, and neoplasia (Fig. 9.19).

Anal papillae may hypertrophy in response to chronic irritation or inflammation.

Rectal prolapse occurs where the tone of the sphincter is reduced and the pelvic floor weakened. It may be a late complication of multiple childbirth.

Neoplasms include squamous cell carcinomas, malignant melanoma, Bowen's disease, Paget's disease and basal cell carcinoma.

A rectocele (the protrusion of the rectum through the weakened posterior wall of the vagina) may also occur. The patient may say she can feel 'something drop', especially when straining.

It is essential to perform a rectal examination and proctoscopy at the first opportunity to investigate an anal mass.

Faecal incontinence
This may be of faeces or flatus.

The internal sphincter is an involuntary one, relaxing reflexly in response to distension by intestinal contents.

The external sphincter is under voluntary control, allowing us to defer defecation until a convenient moment.

Structural changes such as a loss of the angle of the rectum and anus (which contributes to faecal continence), neuromuscular and neurological lesions may all lead to incontinence (Fig. 9.20).

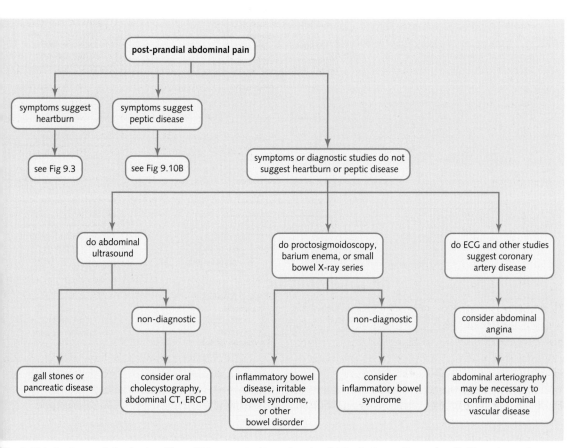

Fig. 9.10A Post-prandial pain algorithm. (CT, computed tomography; ECG, electrocardiography; ERCP, endoscopic retrograde cholangiopancreatography.) (From Greene, *Clinical Medicine*.)

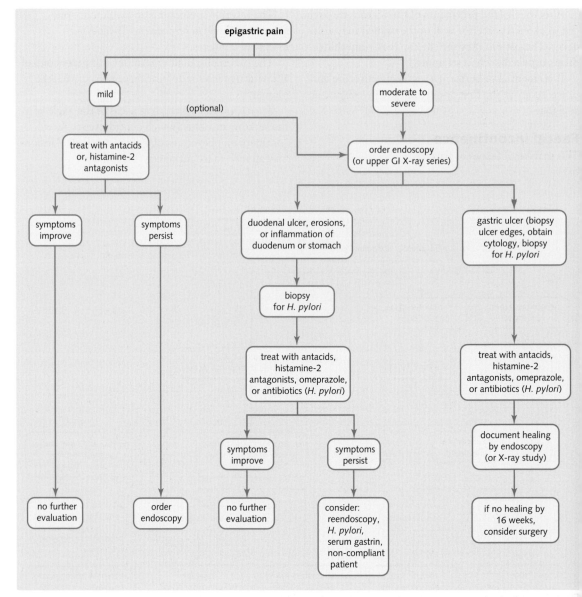

Fig. 9.10B Algorithm for the evaluation of epigastric pain. (GI, gastrointestinal.) (From Greene, *Clinical Medicine.*)

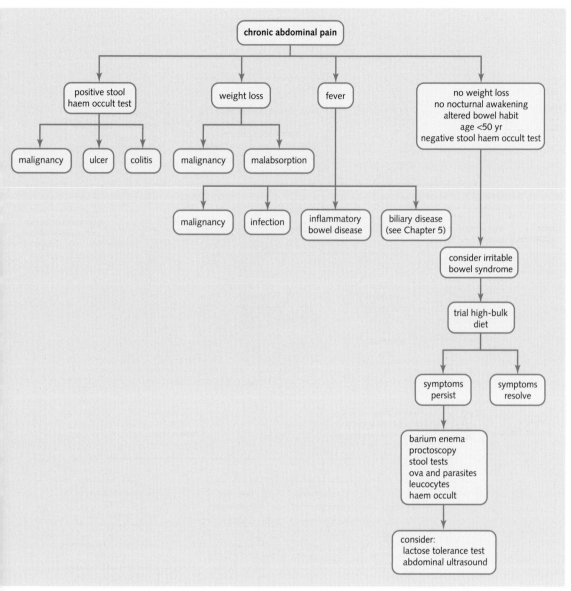

Fig. 9.11 Chronic abdominal pain algorithm. (From Greene, *Clinical Medicine.*)

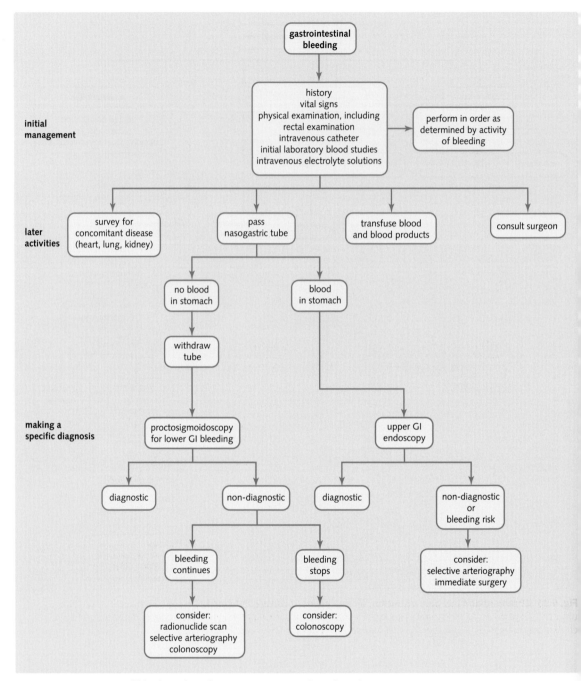

Fig. 9.12 Gastrointestinal bleeding algorithm. (From Greene, *Clinical Medicine.*)

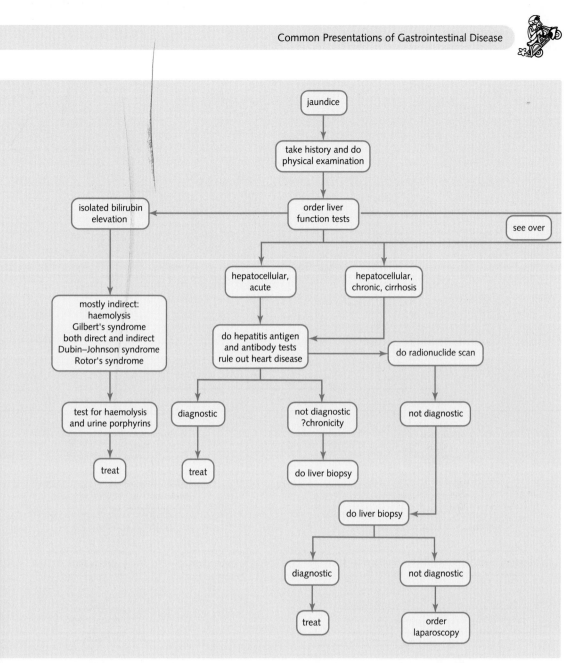

Fig. 9.13 Jaundice algorithm. (CT, computed tomography; MRI, magnetic resonance imaging; US, abdominal ultrasonography; ERCP, endoscopic retrograde cholangiopancreatography; PTC, percutaneous transhepatic cholangiography; GGT, γ-glutamyl transpeptidase.) (From Greene, *Clinical Medicine.*)

189

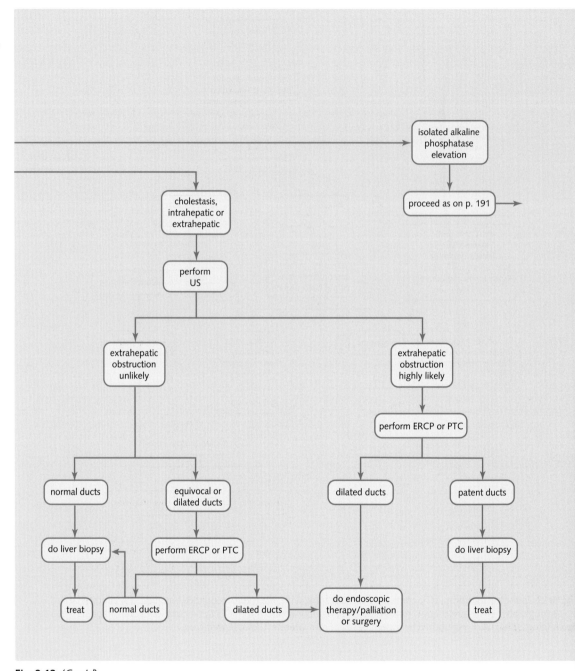

Fig. 9.13 (*Contd*)

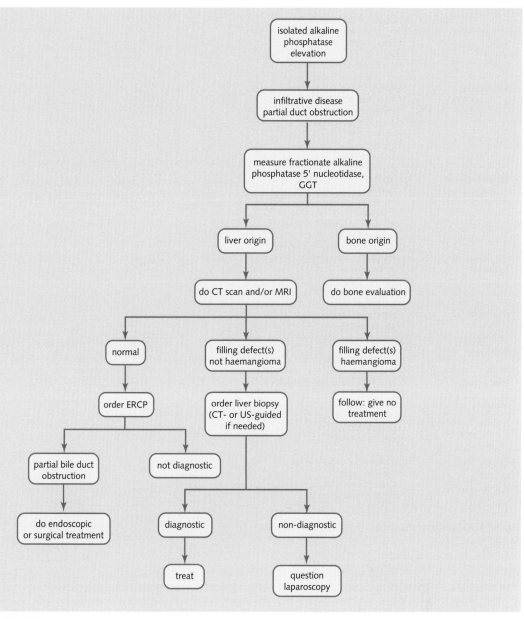

Fig. 9.13 (*Contd*)

191

Common aetiologies of diarrhoea	
Viral	Norwalk agent Rotavirus Enteric adenovirus
Bacterial toxin	*Staphylococcus* *Clostridium perfringens* *Clostridium difficile* *Clostridium botulinum* *Bacillus cereus* Toxigenic *Escherichia coli* *Vibrio cholerae*
Bacterial invasion	Shigella Invasive *E. coli* *Salmonella* Gonorrhoea *Yersinia enterocolitica* *Vibrio parahaemolyticus* *Campylobacter fetus* and *jejuni*
Parasites	*Giardia lamblia* *Cryptosporidium* *Entamoeba histolytica*
After infection	Lactase deficiency Bacterial overgrowth
Drugs	Laxatives Antacids with magnesium
Food toxins	Ciguatoxin, scombroid, pufferfish
Metabolic	Hyperthyroidism Adrenal insufficiency Hyperparathyroidism Diabetes mellitus
Chronic illness	Inflammatory bowel disease Ischaemic colitis Malabsorption Irritable bowel syndrome

Fig. 9.14 Aetiology of diarrhoea. (From Greene, *Clinical Medicine.*)

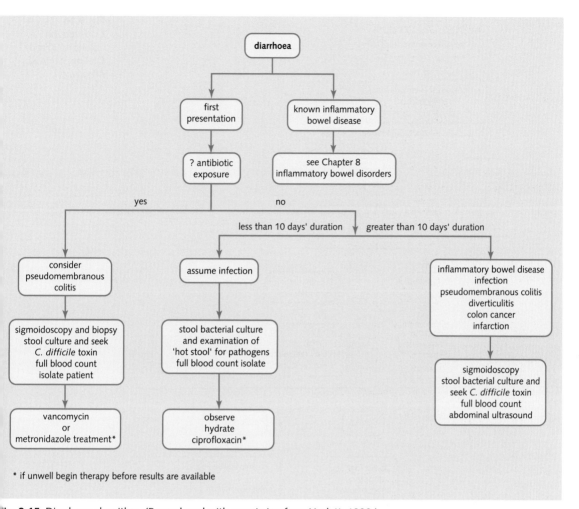

Fig. 9.15 Diarrhoea algorithm. (Reproduced with permission from Haslett, 1999.)

193

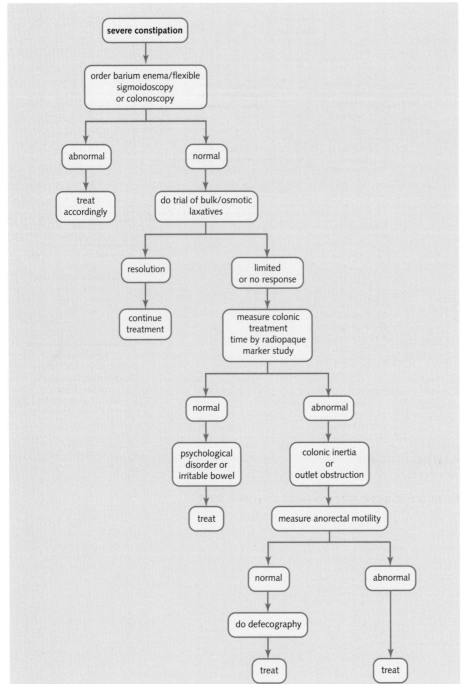

Fig. 9.16
Constipation algorithm. (From Greene, *Clinical Medicine*.)

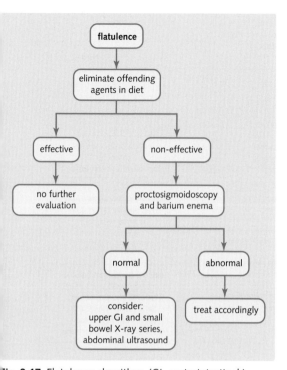

Fig. 9.17 Flatulence algorithm. (GI, gastrointestinal.) (From Greene, *Clinical Medicine.*)

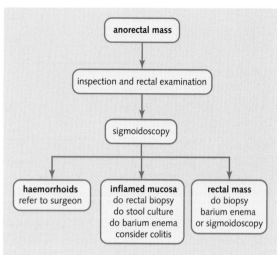

Fig. 9.19 Anal mass algorithm.

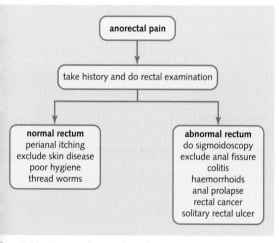

Fig. 9.18 Anorectal pain algorithm.

195

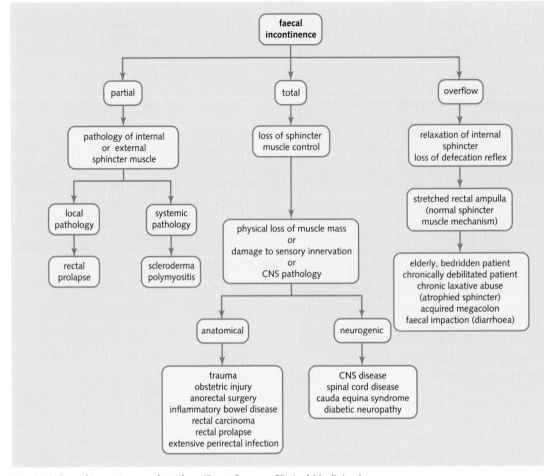

Fig. 9.20 Faecal incontinence algorithm. (From Greene, *Clinical Medicine*.)

- What is dysphagia?
- What might cause dysphagia?
- What are the differential diagnoses of indigestion?
- Why do we salivate prior to vomiting?
- What can be used to investigate abdominal pain if the symptoms are not suggestive of heartburn or peptic disease?
- What sign in abdominal distension might make you suspect ascites?
- List the causes of chronic abdominal pain.
- What is haematemesis? What is it a sign of?
- How is jaundice classified?
- What are the different mechanisms leading to faecal incontinence? Give an example of the aetiology for each mechanism.

Taking a history

Things to remember when taking a history

Most diagnoses are made on the history alone. Investigations should confirm the diagnosis arrived at on the history.

Remember that at this stage (when you meet to take the history) the patient has far more information about his or her condition than you do.

Introduce yourself, be polite, listen carefully, and look interested (even if you have been up all night!). Give the patient the time and the opportunity to tell you what you need to know, and put him or her at his or her ease. Many symptoms are embarrassing.

Maintain eye contact (even if the patient doesn't) and watch carefully for clues. How ill does the patient look? Is he or she agitated or distressed? Is he or she in pain; can you notice any tremors? Has he or she lost a lot of weight (cachexia)?

Look around the bedside for clues, such as inhalers, oxygen, a walking stick or frame, cards from family and friends, sputum pots, reading material and glasses, special food preparations, etc.

The structure of a history

When recording a history, use the headings below. You are less likely to leave things out if your history is structured. It is also easier for others to find the information they need quickly when looking at your notes.

When writing in the patient's notes, make sure you include everything, date the entry, and sign your name legibly. Remember to state your position (e.g. medical student). It is good practice to include a bleep number, if you have one.

Description of the patient

This should be a brief description giving details of the patient's age, sex, ethnic origins, and occupation. It should allow others who have not met the patient to picture him or her in their mind's eye.

Presenting complaint (PC)

Write one or two lines summarizing the symptoms felt by the patient, not your diagnosis. For example,

write 'abdominal pain' or 'chest pain', not 'appendicitis' or 'myocardial infarction'!

History of presenting complaint (HPC)

A complete description of the problem that brought the patient to see you including:

- How and when the symptoms started.
- The speed of onset: was it rapid, or slow and insidious?
- The pattern of symptoms, their duration and frequency. Are they continuous or intermittent? How often do they appear?
- If the symptoms include pain, you should spend at least half a page describing it!
- What was the patient doing when it started?
- What does it feel like: a sharp, stabbing pain? Crushing, like a tight band around the chest? Is the pain colicky?
- Are there any relieving factors that make it better? What does the patient do when it comes on? Does the patient lie absolutely still (as in peritonitis) or roll around? If he or she rolls around, it is probably visceral pain (the contractions of a hollow organ such as the uterus, or intestinal spasm).
- Are there any precipitating factors? Does anything make it worse, e.g. does exercise bring on chest pain or does eating cause abdominal pain?
- If the pain is abdominal, or retrosternal, ask about its relationship to food.
- Has the patient had it before? Is this exactly the same or a little bit different?
- What happened last time? Did he or she have any treatment (and did it work?) or investigations, or did it go away by itself?
- Why has the patient come to the doctor this time?
- Find out the extent of any deficit. Is there any loss of function, anything he or she can't do, or any movement he or she can't make?
- Is there anything else the patient thinks might be relevant, however trivial?

When asking about pain, remember the pneumonic: SOCRATES.

Site.

Onset.

Character: sharp, dull, shooting, crushing, stabbing, etc.

Radiation.

Associated factors: nausea, vomiting, diarrhoea, migraine, etc.

Timing: duration, episodes.

Exacerbating and relieving factors: lying down, sitting up, drinking coffee, etc.

Severity.

Past medical history (PMH)

Has the patient had any medical contact in the past? This question often needs persistence. It is amazing how many people forget operations, spells in hospital, or visits to the GP!

Always ask for symptoms of past complaints. The diagnosis might be wrong, or misremembered, but patients nearly always remember how they felt.

Ask what previous investigations have been carried out.

Drug history

Ask about all drugs, including contraceptive pills and over-the-counter medicines, as well as medicines that have been prescribed.

NSAIDs (non-steroidal anti-inflammatory drugs) are commonly taken as over-the-counter medicines, and they can cause ulcers.

Does the patient have any allergies? It is difficult to defend a compensation claim where a patient has been given a drug to which he or she is known to be allergic!

Lots of people say they are allergic to drugs when what they have actually had is a normal side effect, e.g. diarrhoea after taking penicillin. It is important to establish whether they really are allergic, as you may be denying them the best treatment, but do not give them anything they say they are allergic to unless you are absolutely sure they are not!

Ask about alcohol, smoking, and illicit drug use. Industrial toxins are important in claims for compensation.

The government has set targets for reducing smoking in the *Health of the Nation* document and GPs are now under an obligation to give advice on healthier life-styles when seeing new patients.

Remember to ask if the patient actually took the prescribed medication, if non-compliance is suspected. However, this requires some tact and rapport with the patient.

Family history

Ask about the causes of death of close relatives, especially parents and siblings. Practice drawing quick sketches of family trees. Make a note on the family tree of any diseases (such as cancer or heart disease) that relatives may have had, to help you notice trends.

Social history

The purpose of this assessment is to see the patient as a whole and gain some idea of how the illness affects this particular patient, what support he or she has, and whether he or she can reduce any health risks.

It should include information about the patient's:

- Marital status.
- Children and other dependants.
- Occupational history. This is especially relevant regarding exposure to toxins, musculoskeletal disorders, and psychiatry.
- Accommodation. Put yourself in the patient's position. Will he or she be able to cope at home?
- Diet. Is it adequate? High cholesterol? Vegetarian?
- Exercise. Does he or she take any? Is it appropriate?

Is there any risk behaviour? This overlaps with alcohol, smoking, and drug abuse, but also ask about sexual practices here, if appropriate.

Systems enquiry

Briefly go through all the systems of the body and ask specifically whether the patient has experienced any symptoms relating to them.

Going through the systems logically will help ensure nothing is forgotten.

Summary

The history should end with a brief summary, describing the patient again and recapping the most important features. For example:

- Reginald Smith, a 69-year-old retired bank manager, presenting with dysphagia, which started about 3 months ago and has become progressively worse. The patient had a hernia operation 3 years ago, but there is nothing else of note in his past medical history. He has smoked 30 cigarettes a day since his early 20s. His father died of cancer of the stomach at the age of 50.

General inspection

The main purpose of a general inspection is to determine how ill the patient is (Fig. 10.1).

Bear this in mind as you introduce yourself and take a history. If the patient is very ill, do not waste valuable time asking questions that can wait until later.

Look at the patient's facial expression. Is he or she comfortable; in obvious distress; looking furtive, receptive, or hostile?

Assess the patient's body posture and mobility, and his or her weight and size.

Is he or she appropriately dressed? Very bright and clashing clothes may be a sign of manic depression. An unusual object to which the patient seems to attach a particular significance may indicate schizophrenia (e.g. the patient might believe the piece of string hanging over one ear is a transmitter through which he or she receives messages).

Many diseases and conditions do not have a direct effect on the gut. However, always remember that the patient may be receiving medication for a pre-existing condition, and this may affect the dose of drug you are intending to give for his or her gut condition (e.g. he or she may already be receiving enzyme-inducing drugs for another condition). Current medication might even be producing his or her gut symptoms (e.g. diarrhoea caused by antibiotic therapy).

Finally, treatment for a pregnant or breastfeeding woman needs to be chosen carefully.

Hands and limbs

A surprising amount of information can be gleaned from a careful inspection of a patient's hands (Fig. 10.2).

General inspection of the patient		
Test performed	Sign observed	Diagnostic inference
Inspection of skin colour	Pallor	Anaemia, shock, myxoedema
Inspection	Yellow skin (and sclera)	Jaundice
	Pink nodules and/or areas of baldness on scalp (alopecia neoplastica)	Metastases from internal carcinoma, usually from gastrointestinal tract, breast, kidney, ovary or bronchus
	Dark pigmented flexures, especially armpits and under breasts (acanthosis nigricans)	Obesity, endocrine disease, genetic, adenocarcinoma of gastrointestinal tract, or other internal malignancy
	Vellus hair over face and body (hypertrichosis lanuginosa)	Anorexia, neoplasm
	Patient sitting forward on edge of bed using accessory muscles of respiration (respiratory distress)	Airways obstruction, anaemia, heart failure, pulmonary embolism, obesity
	Abdominal distension	Fluid, fat, faeces, fetus, flatus
	Large masses	Neoplasm, cysts, congenital abnormalities
	Telangiectasia (abnormal dilatation of blood vessels)	Cirrhosis, outdoor occupation
	Severe muscle wasting and loss of body fat (cachexia)	Severe illness
Inspection and questioning	Itchy tissue-paper skin (ichthyosis)	Lymphoma, drugs, malabsorption, malnutrition
	Generalized itching	Jaundice, systemic malignancy
	Painful tender veins in different sites at different times (thrombophlebitis migrans)	Carcinoma of pancreas

Fig. 10.1 General inspection of the patient.

Examination of the hands		
Test performed	**Sign observed**	**Diagnostic inference**
Inspection of ends of fingers	Clubbing (an exaggerated longitudinal curvature, loss of the angle between the nail and nail bed and bogginess)	The causes of clubbing may be divided into gastrointestinal, thoracic and cardiac. Gastrointestinal causes include: inflammatory bowel disease (especially Crohn's disease), cirrhosis, gastrointestinal lymphoma and malabsorption (e.g. coeliac disease)
Arms straight with wrists fully extended	Hands flap (liver flap or asterixis)	CO_2 retention, cirrhosis, portosystemic encephalopathy
Inspection of palms of hands	Palmar erythema (redness around the edges of the palms)	Cirrhosis, pregnancy or polycythaemia
Inspection of nails	Leuconychia (white nails)	Hypoalbuminaemia
	Koilonychia (spoon shaped)	Iron deficiency, syphilis
	Terry's lines (white nails with normal pink tips)	Cirrhosis
	Mees' lines (paired white parallel bands across the nails)	Hypoalbuminaemia
	Beau's lines (horizontal grooves across the nail)	Chemotherapy, previous severe illness
Inspection	Purpura (purple lesions which do not blanch on pressure)	Clotting disorder, vasculitis, drugs, infections, amyloidosis
Inspection of position of fingers	Dupuytren's contracture (fibrosis and contracture of the palmar fascia)	Ageing, liver disease, trauma (if unilateral) or epilepsy
Inspection	Lentigines (small, circumscribed, brown macules)	Peutz–Jeghers syndrome
Feel and inspection of skin of palm	Excessive sweating	Alcoholism, anxiety
Pinch a fold of skin up on back of hand	Skin fold takes a relatively long time to disappear	Dehydration
Inspection	Dark warty palms (tripe palms)	Adenocarcinoma of gastrointestinal tract, other internal malignancy
	Calcified nodules	CREST syndrome
	Tendon xanthoma	Familial hypercholesterolaemia
Inspection of palm	Simian crease	Down syndrome

Fig. 10.2 Examination of the hands.

A proper history should always be taken before a detailed physical examination (unless of course the patient is obviously very ill).

You should have shaken hands at the beginning. This may give you your diagnosis. If the patient takes your hand but cannot release it, you can fairly confidently say he or she has myotonic dystrophy, an uncommon but chronic condition often cropping up in clinical oral examinations!

Physical examination of the patient should start with an inspection of the hands. This is relatively non-invasive and allows the patient to get used to your touch. It also gives you a lot of information.

Skin lesions are described in the 'General inspection' section, above.

When examining a patient, be methodical. Examine the hands and then work your way up the arm (Fig. 10.3) to the head and neck.

Head and neck

Head
Face, scalp, and eyes

Always warn a patient that you are about to look in his or her eyes. You need to get pretty close to have a

Examination of the limbs		
Test performed	Sign observed	Diagnostic inference
Palpation	Pulses	Information about cardiovascular system
Inspection	Central dilated arteriole with small red vessels radiating out from it, like a spider (spider naevus)	If more than five or six: pregnancy, cirrhosis, or other chronic liver disease
	Scratches	Pruritus
	Muscle wasting	Damage to innervation of muscles, malnutrition, chronic illness
	Thinning of skin	Steroid use

Fig. 10.3 Examination of the limbs.

proper look and this can be misinterpreted! Examination of the head and face is covered in Fig. 10.4.

Mouth

Use a pen torch to inspect the inside of the mouth (Fig. 10.5). If necessary, gently depress the tongue with a wooden tongue depressor. Wear gloves if you need to feel anything in the mouth, and ask the patient to remove any false teeth.

Stomatitis simply means ulceration of the mucosal surface of the mouth—it can occur in the mouth or at the edges, where the upper and lower lips meet.

Neck

Inspect both the front and back of the neck.

Then stand behind the patient and palpate for enlarged nodes in the back, front, and sides of the neck (Fig. 10.6). Always palpate for the supraclavicular lymph nodes carefully, as this is a common site for gastrointestinal metastases.

Thoracic examination

Most signs and symptoms in the thorax signal cardiovascular or respiratory disease.

This section is intended as a quick guide to the signs, symptoms, and diagnostic inferences that have particular relevance to gastrointestinal disease. A book on respiratory or cardiovascular medicine should be consulted for a fuller description of the examination of the thorax.

Observation

Undress the patient to the waist.

Be sensitive to the patient, especially if female. Do not ask him or her to remove his or her underwear unless and until necessary and then only for as long as necessary.

Position the patient, so that they are lying at 45° (half sitting up position).

Have a chaperone present when examining a female, if you are male.

Stand at the end of the bed and observe the chest for a few seconds before moving nearer to the patient again and having a closer look.

From the end of the bed, assess the rate of breathing (about 12 breaths per minute is normal) and look for any signs of respiratory distress (these may not have been obvious with clothes on).

Check for any scars, signs of asymmetry, or abnormality of the chest wall such as a funnel chest (pectus excavatum) or a pigeon chest (pectus carinatum). Check also for a curved spine scoliosis (combined lateral and rotational curvature), lordosis (abnormally extended spine), kyphosis (abnormally flexed spine), or tilt (lateral deformity) (Fig. 10.7).

Palpation

Feel for the trachea by pressing two fingers gently into the sternal notch. The trachea should be central. Explain to patients that you are about to do this, as it is uncomfortable.

Feel for the apex beat with the flat of your hand, i.e. the lowest and most lateral place at

Examination of the head and face		
Test performed	**Sign observed**	**Diagnostic inference**
Inspection of colour of sclera in a good light	Yellow	Jaundice
Inspection of colour of conjunctiva of lower lid	Pale	Anaemia
Inspection	Red eye from subconjunctival haemorrhage	Bleeding disorder from liver disease or other cause, diabetes, vomiting
	Inflamed connective tissue beneath conjunctiva (episcleritis)	Reiter's syndrome (may follow dysentery)
	Red eye from conjunctivitis	Stevens–Johnson syndrome
	Chronic red eye	Cirrhosis, renal failure, hereditary haemorrhagic telangiectasia (Rendu–Osler–Weber syndrome), iron deficiency anaemia, ataxia telangiectasia
	Acute swelling of eyelids	Adverse reaction to penicillin, bee sting or other allergen, infection
	Firm, chronic swelling of eyelids	Lymphoma, sarcoidosis
	Yellow swelling in periorbital area (xanthelasma)	Hypercholesterolaemia, age
	Erythematous, swollen eyelids	Dermatomyositis
	Malar flush	Mitral stenosis
	White ring around edge of iris (arcus)	Hypercholesterolaemia, ageing
	Protruding eye with sclera visible above iris	Graves' disease
	Constricted pupils	Ageing, drugs (opiates, glaucoma treatment), damage to sympathetic innervation (e.g. Horner's syndrome if unilateral)
	Swollen, purple nose and ears (lupus pernio), prominent scars, orange–brown papules, nodules and plaques	Sarcoidosis
	Patches of hair loss on scalp (alopecia neoplastica)	Metastases from internal carcinoma (usually from gastrointestinal tract, kidney, ovary, bronchus, or breast)
	Flushing	Carcinoid syndrome
	Periorbital oedema, erythema of face and neck	Dermatomyositis
Inspection of cornea	Brown rings (Kayser–Fleischer rings) at periphery	Wilson's disease
Pupil reaction	Pupils constrict to accommodation but not to light (Argyll–Robertson pupil)	Syphilis

Fig. 10.4 Examination of the head and face.

which you can feel the heart beat. It is normally in the 5th intercostal space in the midclavicular line.

Place your thumbs together and spread your fingers out around the patient's side. Ask the patient to take deep breaths in and out, and see how far your thumbs move apart and whether each thumb moves an equal distance. You are checking for the amount and symmetry of chest expansion.

Palpate the thorax and ask the patient to say 'ninety-nine'. This is called tactile vocal fremitus, and it demonstrates a clear or consolidated lung. The vibrations of the voice feel distant and muffled in a normal lung, but feel clear and loud in a consolidated lung.

Examination of the mouth		
Test performed	Sign observed	Diagnostic inference
Inspection	Puckered mouth	Scleroderma
	Swollen gums	Pregnancy, acute leukaemia, puberty, phenytoin, infection
	Fissuring at edges of mouth (angular cheilosis or stomatitis)	Iron-deficiency anaemia, malabsorption, candidal or other infection
	Vesicles on lips and in perioral area	Herpes simplex infection
	Blue spots on mucosa	Hereditary haemorrhagic telangiectasia (Osler–Weber–Rendu syndrome)
	Small pigmented areas on lips and on mucosa (lentigines)	Peutz–Jeghers syndrome
	Bleeding and necrosis of gums	Acute leukaemia
	Bleeding gums	Vitamin C deficiency
	Beefy, raw, red tongue	Pernicious anaemia, malabsorption, pellagra
	Dry discoloured tongue	Gastrointestinal or other infection
	Ulcer	Carcinoma, lymphoma, trauma, infection (tuberculosis, herpes, Vincent's angina, diphtheria, measles), Stevens–Johnson syndrome, Behçet's syndrome, drugs, pemphigus, bullous pemphigoid
	Swellings	Cysts, stones in salivary glands, infection
	High arched palate	Marfan's syndrome
	Black tongue	Antibiotic treatment
	Blue tongue and lips	Cyanosis
Inspection and touch with spatula	White patches that cannot be brushed off (leucoplakia)	Trauma, infection (including HIV)
	White patches that can be brushed off	Candidal infection (thrush)
Smell	Halitosis	Infection, poor hygiene, hepatic coma, uraemia, diabetic coma

Fig. 10.5 Examination of the mouth.

Percussion

It takes practice to develop a good technique for percussion. Put the middle finger of one hand flat against the patient's skin and hit this finger with the middle finger of your other hand. The movement should come from the wrist.

The clavicle can be percussed without putting your own middle finger over it. Simply tap the bone gently with the middle finger of one hand.

Solid organs are dull to percussion (i.e. sound dull when percussed); organs containing air (e.g. healthy lungs) are resonant.

Percuss in the mid-axillary line and on the back, comparing left and right sides.

Auscultation

Remember to put the stethoscope in your ears the right way around (pointing towards the front) and ensure it is switched to the side you are using (the bell or diaphragm). The bell is better for listening to low sounds.

Politely ask the patient not to talk to you while you are listening with the stethoscope!

Medical notes often say 'vesicular breath sounds'. This simply means normal!

Normal breath sounds are louder on inspiration, tailing off in expiration, and they are caused by the movement of air in the larger airways rather than in the alveoli. Compare breath sounds on both sides.

203

Examination of the neck		
Test performed	**Sign observed**	**Diagnostic inference**
Inspection of JVP (jugular venous pressure)	JVP raised (vertical height of column of blood in internal jugular vein exceeds 3 cm, measured from the sternal angle with the patient lying at 45°)	Superior mediastinal obstruction, e.g. carcinoma of bronchus (if JVP non-pulsatile), right heart failure, fluid overload, tricuspid incompetence, cardiac tamponade (if JVP pulsatile)
Palpation	Swellings	Infection, carcinoma, bronchial cyst, thyroglossal or other cyst, goitre (iodine deficiency or thyroid disorder)
	Enlarged lymph nodes (lymphadenopathy)	Infection, carcinoma
	Enlarged supraclavicular lymph node on the left (Virchow's node)	Carcinoma of stomach
Palpation of trachea	Deviation, not central	Superior mediastinal mass, collapse of one lung, fibrosis
Palpation of carotid pulse	Character of pulse	Information about cardiovascular system

Fig. 10.6 Examination of the neck.

Crackles sound like the noise you hear if you rub strands of hair together in front of your ears. They may be fine or coarse (caused by bubbling of air through fluid).

Stridor is increased noise on inspiration, due to partial blockage of the upper airways. Wheezes are louder on expiration, although they may be heard on inspiration if airway narrowing is severe.

Remember to auscultate the apical region of the lungs, by placing the bell of the stethoscope just posterior to the clavicles and lateral to the base of the neck.

Check for vocal resonance by auscultating the lungs and asking the patient to say 'ninety-nine'. Sounds are muffled and distant over normal lung tissue, but louder and clearer over consolidated lung (because solid material transmits sound better than air). Tactile vocal fremitus also demonstrates this.

Listen to the heart sounds in the designated sites, for the aortic, pulmonary, tricuspid, and mitral (apex) sounds. Listen to the apex of the heart with the bell of the stethoscope (Fig. 10.8).

To remember that the stethoscope bell is better for listening to low sounds, think of 'bellow'.

Abdominal examination

Observation

The abdomen should be examined from the nipples to the knees, but not all at once. Respect the patient's dignity and only uncover as much as you need to at any one time.

Ask the patient to remove his or her clothes and lie flat on the bed or the couch, with his or her head on one pillow and arms by his or her sides.

Cover the patient with a folded sheet or blanket (you can usually find one at the end of the bed or examining couch). It is easy to move this up or down, exposing or revealing different parts, as you complete your examination.

Briefly expose the patient from the nipples to the pubic bone. Stand at the end of the bed to look at the abdomen as a whole and check for:

- Asymmetry.
- Distension.
- Dilated veins.
- Caput medusae (described below).
- Purpura.
- Spider naevi.
- Bruising.
- Visible peristalsis and/or pulsation.
- Masses.
- Scars.
- Striae (Fig. 10.9).

Then have a closer look at individual areas, checking more closely for all of the above. Skin lesions are

Examination of the thorax		
Test performed	**Sign observed**	**Diagnostic inference**
Inspection	Enlarged breasts in the male (gynaecomastia)	Liver disease, prepuberty, drugs (spironolactone, steroids, digoxin, phenothiazines)
	Loss of body hair	Cirrhosis
Inspection of skin	Figs 10.1, 10.2 and 10.3	
Inspection of sputum pot	Blood (haemoptysis)	Infection, carcinoma or other tumour of lung, tuberculosis, clotting disorder, pulmonary infarction, trauma, vasculitis, foreign body, mitral stenosis
	Green or yellow sputum	Infection, asthma
	Frothy pink sputum	Pulmonary oedema
	Offensive smelling sputum	Anaerobic infection
	Clear, white or grey (mucoid) sputum	Chronic bronchitis
Assessment of expansion	Diminished movement on one side	Pathology on that side
Percussion	Hyperresonance	Emphysema, asthma, pneumothorax
	Dull	Obesity, consolidation, fibrosis, collapse
	Duller in upper lobe	Old tuberculosis
	Stony dull	Pleural effusion
Auscultation	Wheezing	Airflow obstruction, asthma, bronchitis, left ventricular failure
	Quiet breath sounds	Obesity, hyperinflation
	Absent breath sounds	Pneumothorax, collapse
	Fine crackles	Fibrosing alveolitis, congestion caused by heart failure
	No breath sounds, but bowel sounds heard in chest	Diaphragmatic hernia
	Coarse crackles	Excess secretions (bronchiectasis)

Fig. 10.7 Examination of the thorax.

described above. Ask the patient to breathe in deeply two or three times and look for any abdominal masses that may come into view.

Palpation

Make sure you have warm hands, and tell the patient that you are about to feel his or her abdomen.

Before you do so, ask whether the abdomen is tender anywhere. If it is, then start your palpation as far away from the tender area as possible.

Ask the patient to tell you if he or she feels anything. This is better than asking him or her to let you know if it hurts. Most people will understandably tense their abdominal muscles if they think you are about to cause them pain.

Never take your eyes off the patient's face while you are palpating. You are looking for any signs of pain or discomfort. Do not hurt the patient!

Gently palpate all four quadrants and then go around again, palpating more deeply. Patients with tender abdomens are naturally apprehensive about having them palpated. When you have been around the quadrants once without hurting them, however, they will often relax their abdominal muscles enough to let you palpate more deeply and feel deeper structures (which is what you need to do).

You should be looking for:

- Enlarged organs (organomegaly).
- Tenderness.
- Guarding (tensing of the abdominal muscles).

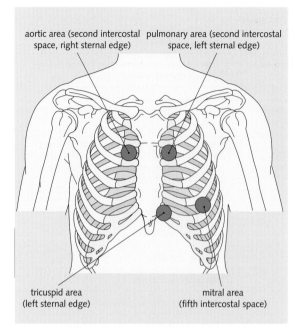

aortic area (second intercostal space, right sternal edge)　pulmonary area (second intercostal space, left sternal edge)

tricuspid area (left sternal edge)　mitral area (fifth intercostal space)

Fig. 10.8 The sites for auscultation of the heart sounds on the anterior wall of the thorax. This shows where best to hear the valves, not their physical location.

- Rovsing's sign (more pain in the right iliac fossa than in the left iliac fossa, when palpated).
- Obvious masses.

To examine the liver, start at the right iliac fossa and move your hand up, using the long, flat edge of your index finger to feel for the liver edge. The normal position of the liver is shown in Fig. 10.10.

Its edge can usually be felt just below the edge of the costal margin. You need to palpate quite deeply to feel it. Ask the patient to take deep breaths in and out; the edge should be felt moving against your fingers with respiration (Fig. 10.11).

To examine the spleen, start in the right iliac fossa and move up diagonally to the left costal margin. A grossly enlarged spleen can extend into the right iliac fossa! A normal spleen cannot be felt.

Most books say the spleen has a palpable notch but many clinicians say they have never been able to feel it!

If you can feel an upper margin, you are not feeling the spleen (you cannot get 'above' the spleen).

The kidneys should be 'balloted', using two hands. This is the procedure of bouncing the kidney between the hand at the renal angle and the hand positioned anteriorly to this. It is easier to do, once demonstrated!

Percussion

The liver and spleen are dull to percussion. You can trace their margins (and confirm organomegaly) by percussing in the directions you palpated when examining them both (Fig. 10.12). Always percuss for the upper border of the liver as well as the lower one. The liver may be pushed down by a hyperinflated chest or other respiratory pathology. Hepatomegaly may be wrongly diagnosed if the upper border has not been located.

Auscultation

You should listen for bowel sounds (there should be some and they should not be too loud) and bruits (evidence of disturbed blood flow).

Listen for at least 1 minute over the ileocaecal valve before declaring that there are absent bowel sounds (Fig. 10.13).

You can also use the stethoscope to confirm the edges of an enlarged liver. Put your stethoscope over the liver and gently scratch the surrounding area with the soft part of the end of your finger (not your nail). The sound will be loud when you are scratching over the liver, but soft as soon as you go over the liver margin.

You can use the same technique to confirm the edges of an enlarged spleen.

 When describing any lump in the body, comment on the site, size, shape, surface, smoothness, and surrounding (e.g. tethered or not)—six Ss!

Rectal and genital examination

Rectal examination

Always wear gloves and make sure your examining finger is well lubricated (Fig. 10.14).

It is absolutely essential to explain that you are going to perform a rectal or genital examination, and why you need to do this.

Make sure you have a chaperone of the same sex as the patient when performing any intimate examination.

Many patients find rectal examinations distressing and embarrassing. It is important to establish a rapport with them first and be sensitive to their feelings.

Inspection of the abdomen		
Test performed	Sign observed	Diagnostic inference
Inspection	Nodule near umbilicus (Sister Joseph's nodule)	Metastasis of gastrointestinal or ovarian carcinoma through the ligamentum teres
	Inflamed indurated lesion (carcinoma erysipelatoides)	Lymphatic extension of carcinoma to the skin
	Pink nodules on anterior trunk	Cutaneous metastases (usually from gastrointestinal tract, kidney, ovary, breast or bronchus)
	Central dilated arteriole with small red vessels radiating out from it, like a spider (spider naevi)	If more than five or six, pregnancy, cirrhosis, or other chronic liver disease
	Distension	Fat, fetus, fluid, faeces, flatus, obstruction
	Firm pressure in the left lower area of distension leaves indentations	Distension caused by faeces (e.g. Hirschsprung's disease or acquired megacolon)
	Visible pulsation	Aortic aneurysm
	Visible peristalsis from left to right	Pyloric stenosis
	Visible peristalsis from right to left	Obstruction in the transverse colon
	Visible peristalsis in the middle (like a ladder)	Obstruction in the small bowel
	Patient lying rigid, taking very shallow breaths	Peritonitis
	Distended stomach but thin limbs	Cushing's syndrome, steroids
	Discoloration around umbilicus (Cullen's sign)	Acute pancreatitis, carcinoma of the pancreas
	Discoloration in the flanks (Grey Turner's sign)	Acute pancreatitis
	Dilated veins (not confined to umbilical region)	Obstruction of inferior vena cava
	Purple striae	Cushing's syndrome, steroids
	White striae	Obesity, previous pregnancy
	Veins radiating out from umbilicus (caput medusae)	Portal hypertension

Fig. 10.9 Inspection of the abdomen.

To perform a rectal examination, ask the patient to lie on his or her left side with his or her knees drawn up. Inspect the anus for redness, bleeding, external haemorrhoids, skin lesions, or fistulae. Before you begin, ask the patient if there is any tenderness and to tell you if they feel any pain during the examination.

Gently insert a well-lubricated index finger into the anal canal and rectum. Note the tone of the anal sphincter.

Gently sweep your finger around the walls to check for any masses or abnormalities.

You should be able to feel the prostate in the male and cervix in the female through the anterior wall of the rectum. The prostate has a shallow central groove.

Withdraw your finger: there should be faecal matter on it but no blood or mucus. Take your glove off cuff first, pulling the glove off inside out, and dispose of it in a clinical waste bag (these are usually yellow).

Genital examination

You should be looking for any signs of infection, gross abnormality, and hernias.

It is best to look for hernias with the patient standing and you kneeling down so that you are at the same level as the area you are examining. Many

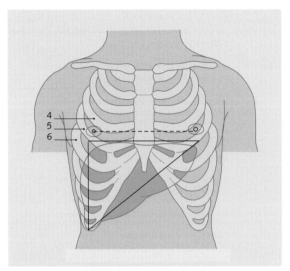

Fig. 10.10 The position of the normal liver in relation to the nipple line and to the 4th, 5th and 6th ribs.

hernias disappear if the patient lies down. Hernias are common. About 1 in 100 people will have a hernia at some time in their life. About 70% of hernias are inguinal, 20% are femoral, and 10% are umbilical.

Palpate over the external and internal rings (above and medial to the pubic tubercle) to detect an inguinal hernia and ask the patient to cough. You may feel a lump when he or she does.

Repeat this procedure below and lateral to the pubic tubercle (to check for a femoral hernia), and above and below the umbilicus (for an umbilical hernia).

Perform the same procedure at other points of weakness (e.g. over scars and at the edges of the rectus muscles).

Try to reduce any swelling (gently push it back into the abdominal cavity).

Palpation of the abdomen		
Test performed	**Sign observed**	**Diagnostic inference**
Palpation	Enlarged liver (hepatomegaly)	Malignancy, infection (especially glandular fever and malaria), hepatitis, sickle-cell disease, porphyria, haemolytic anaemia, connective-tissue disease, portal hypertension, lymphoma, leukaemia, glycogen storage disorders, myelofibrosis
	Pulsatile liver	Tricuspid incompetence
Palpation of right iliac fossa	The right iliac fossa is more painful than the left (Rovsing's sign)	Acute appendicitis
Press on abdomen	Pain occurs when you press in and also when you remove your hand (rebound tenderness)	Peritonitis
Place two fingers over right upper quadrant, ask patient to breathe in	Pain on inspiration (Murphy's sign)	Inflamed gall bladder
Palpation	Sausage-shaped mass	Pyloric stenosis, intussusception
	Mass	Carcinoma, obstruction, hernia, faeces

Fig. 10.11 Palpation of the abdomen.

Percussion of the abdomen		
Test performed	**Sign observed**	**Diagnostic inference**
Percuss the abdomen from flank to flank, ask patient to roll onto one side and percuss from flank to flank again	Flanks are dull to percussion, midline is resonant with patient lying on his or her back, upper flank is resonant but lower flank is dull to percussion with patient lying on his or her side (shifting dullness)	Ascites
Percussion	Hepatosplenomegaly	Portal hypertension, amyloidosis, leukaemia, sickle-cell anaemia, thalassaemia, glandular fever
	Splenomegaly	Lymphoma, leukaemia, portal hypertension, haemolytic anaemia, rheumatoid arthritis, infection

Fig. 10.12 Percussion of the abdomen.

The femoral pulse and lymph nodes in the groin should be palpated. In the male, inspect the penis and scrotum, carefully palpating the testes, epididymis, and spermatic cords. Note any scrotal swelling.

Vaginal examination is not routine and it is only performed when indicated.

Finishing the examination

An examination should also ideally include checking the feet and legs for pitting oedema. This can give clues about respiratory, cardiac, or hepatic function.

Urinalysis should also be performed.

Auscultation of the abdomen		
Test performed	Sign elicited	Diagnostic inference
Auscultation	Absent bowel sounds	Paralytic ileus
	Loud bowel sounds (tinkling)	Intestinal obstruction
	Bruit	Disturbed flow (e.g. atherosclerosis)

Fig. 10.13 Auscultation of the abdomen.

Rectal examination		
Test performed	Sign elicited	Diagnostic inference
Rectal examination and inspection of glove afterwards	Bloody mucus	Chronic inflammatory bowel disease, ulcerating tumour
	Watery mucus	Villous adenoma
	Pale faecal material	Obstructive jaundice
	Bright red blood and slime	Intussusception, colitis
Rectal examination	Nodular prostate	Carcinoma, calcification
	Tender prostate	Prostatitis
	Enlarged, smooth prostate	Age-related benign prostatic hyperplasia
	Narrow empty rectum and a gush of faeces and flatus on withdrawing finger	Hirschsprung's disease

Fig. 10.14 Rectal examination.

- How can pain be described?
- What information can inspection of the patient give before any examination is performed?
- What is clubbing? What can it tell you about your patient?
- What is asterixis (liver flap)? What causes this?
- How do you test for dehydration?
- What signs of hypercholesterolaemia are displayed on the face?
- Write a list of the different signs and their causes found when inspecting the tongue.
- What causes a raised JVP?
- What disease might you suspect on finding enlarged supraclavicular lymph nodes on the left?
- How is percussion of the thorax performed?
- What can you find on percussion of the thorax? What causes these findings?
- Briefly describe how to auscultate the thorax.
- Where are the heart sounds auscultated?
- For what signs do you inspect the abdomen?
- How do you palpate the abdomen?
- How do you palpate the liver and spleen?
- What causes hepatomegaly?
- How do the liver and spleen sound when percussed?
- Briefly describe how to perform a rectal examination.
- What is the best method to follow when examining for hernias?

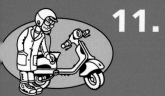
Investigation of gastrointestinal function

Oesophageal manometry

Oesophageal manometry measures pressure changes in different parts of the oesophagus, and it is used to investigate suspected motility disorders.

A fluid-filled continuously perfused catheter is passed through the nose into the oesophagus (in much the same way as a nasogastric tube). Contraction of the oesophagus causes a pressure change that is transmitted up the fluid column and recorded as a trace.

In normal individuals, a pressure wave should pass down the oesophagus to the lower oesophageal sphincter, which then relaxes to allow the oesophageal contents to pass into the stomach. Abnormal traces are seen in motility disorders.

Investigation of gastric function

Refluxed acid may overwhelm the normal protective lining of the oesophagus, leading to ulceration. Suspected reflux may be investigated by measuring the pH in the lower oesophagus over the course of 24 hours with a pH-sensitive probe.

A normal trace shows the pH above 4 for most of the time—if the pH is below 4 for more than 4% of the time, significant reflux is said to have occurred.

Disorders of gastric acid secretion may be investigated using the pentagastrin test. The patient fasts overnight and the resting juice in the stomach is aspirated using a nasogastric tube. Pentagastrin, a synthetic analogue of gastrin, is then given (6 mg/kg body weight) to stimulate acid secretion, and gastric contents are again aspirated for 1 hour and analysed.

A large volume of resting juice suggests gastric stasis, a high acid secretion suggests Zollinger–Ellison syndrome, and a failure to stimulate acid secretion with pentagastrin indicates achlorhydria.

Plasma levels of gastrin (a hormone which stimulates gastric acid secretion and growth of the gastric mucosa) may also be measured.

The levels of gastrin will be high in Zollinger–Ellison syndrome as G cells in the pancreas, duodenum or, more rarely, the stomach, secrete large amounts of gastrin in this disorder and cause hyperacidity, leading to ulceration.

Levels will also be high if the patient is taking drugs that inhibit gastric acid secretion and such drugs should be stopped before gastrin levels are measured.

Liver function tests

The functions of the liver are described in Chapter 4. 'Liver function tests' are usually defined as the measurement of serum levels of:

- Albumin.
- Bilirubin.
- Aminotransferases (AST and ALT).
- Alkaline phosphatase.
- γ-glutamyltransferase.
- Proteins.

The prothrombin time is a measurement of the clotting ability of the plasma: prothrombin is made in the liver and is a vitamin K-dependent clotting factor with a short half-life. A prolonged prothrombin time gives an indication of the amount of prothrombin synthesized by the liver and, therefore, of the liver's synthesizing capacity.

However, prothrombin time is also increased in vitamin K deficiency. If there is any doubt about the cause, vitamin K should be given to the patient and prothrombin time measured again after 18 hours. By then it should have returned to normal if the cause was vitamin K deficiency.

Deficiency of vitamin K may occur in biliary obstruction because it is a fat soluble vitamin and bile salts are needed for its absorption.

Serum albumin is a good indicator of chronic liver disease. It is another protein synthesized by the liver and its levels will fall in chronic disease. Its half-life is longer than that of prothrombin, however, and levels may be normal in acute disease.

Biochemical tests

Bilirubin levels increase in liver disease. Aminotransferases (transaminases) are present in hepatocytes and leak into the plasma in liver cell damage.

Alanine aminotransferase (ALT) is present in the cytoplasm of hepatocytes, and its level increases in hepatocellular injury.

Asparatate aminotransferase (AST) is a mitochondrial enzyme present in:

- The liver.
- The cardiac muscle.
- The kidneys.
- The brain tissue.

It is less specific than alanine aminotransferase and its level increases in:

- Hepatic necrosis.
- Myocardial infarction.
- Congestive cardiac failure.
- Muscle injury.

Other enzymes of the liver

An isoenzyme of alkaline phosphatase is present in the canalicular and sinusoidal membranes of the liver. Other isoenzymes are present in bone, intestine, and placenta.

Levels rise following damage to any of these structures but electrophoresis can be used to determine the particular isoenzyme (and therefore its source).

Hepatic alkaline phosphatase is raised in infiltration of the liver, cirrhosis, and cholestasis (from both intrahepatic and extrahepatic causes). The highest levels are seen in hepatic metastases and primary biliary cirrhosis.

Gamma-glutamyltransferase (γ-GT) is present in the mitochondria of many tissues, including the liver, and raised levels are seen following the administration of phenytoin (an antiepileptic drug and enzyme inducer) and the ingestion of even a moderate amount of alcohol.

If γ-GT is raised but alkaline phosphatase levels are normal, the cause of the damage is probably alcohol.

If both γ-GT and alkaline phosphatase are high, the cause may be cholestasis or intrahepatic malignancy.

If the alkaline phosphatase is raised, but the γ-GT is normal, then one should suspect bone disease (e.g. Paget's disease).

Immunological tests

Immunoglobulins are raised in liver disease. Normally, sinusoidal and Kupffer's cells phagocytose antigens absorbed from the gut, and antibodies are made in the lymph nodes and spleen.

In chronic liver disease, phagocytosis is reduced and lymphoid and plasma cells that infiltrate the portal tracts produce immunoglobulins. IgM is raised in primary biliary cirrhosis and IgG raised in autoimmune chronic active hepatitis.

Additional tests

- α_1-antitrypsin. Deficiency of α_1-antitrypsin can produce cirrhosis.
- α-fetoprotein. This is raised in patients with hepatocellular carcinoma and in pregnant women. Less elevated levels are found in hepatitis, teratoma, and chronic liver disease.

Patterns of abnormality are important in diagnosis.

- Raised levels of AST and ALT reflect hepatocellular damage.
- Raised alkaline phosphatase and γ-GT indicate cholestasis or intrahepatic abscess and malignancy.

Endoscopic examinations

Endoscopy is a relatively non-invasive procedure that gives very valuable information about a number of gastrointestinal tract disorders. It is worth going to a hospital's endoscopy suite to see the procedure in action. The results are shown on a television screen, and it is possible to gain a very clear view.

Gastroscopy (oesophagogastroduodenoscopy)

Patients are normally told gastroscopy involves 'swallowing a small camera', which understandably makes them very apprehensive. It is better to say: '. . . a thin tube, no thicker than your little finger'. Some patients are given mild sedation (which can cause slight amnesia), but many manage with just an oral local anaesthetic spray.

The patient is laid on their left side and the endoscope is passed down their oesophagus.

Patients must fast overnight beforehand and the endoscopy is performed as a day case procedure. Gastroscopy is commonly used to investigate upper gastrointestinal disorders. Forceps for taking biopsies can be passed through the biopsy channel of the endoscope.

Always perform a digital rectal examination before proctosigmoidoscopy or colonoscopy. The patient may have a large tumour in the anal canal or rectum, and damage may be caused if a scope is inserted without checking first.

Endoscopic ultrasound

Endoscopic ultrasound (EUS) is a procedure in which an ultrasound image is obtained while performing an endoscopy. The ultrasound transducer is incorporated into the end of the endoscope to produce images alongside the camera image (Fig. 11.1).

Endoscopic retrograde cholangiopancreatography

Endoscopic retrograde cholangiopancreatography (ERCP) involves injection of contrast material into the biliary and pancreatic systems, via endoscopy, followed by radiological screening (Fig. 11.2).

Two different contrasts are used: low iodine for the common bile duct (so as not to obscure gall stones) and a higher iodine contrast for the pancreatic duct.

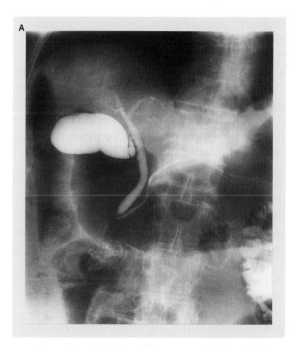

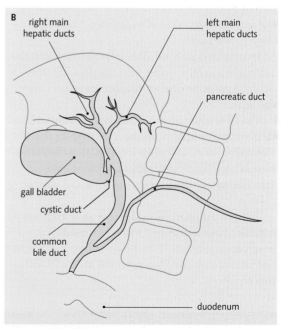

Fig. 11.2 Endoscopic retrograde cholangiopancreatography (ERCP) image, showing a normal biliary and pancreatic duct system (A) and explanatory diagram (B). ([A] Reproduced with permission from Haslett, 1999.)

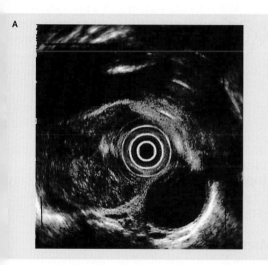

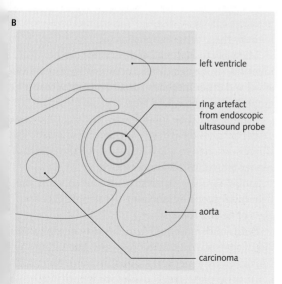

Fig. 11.1 Endoscopic ultrasound image of oesophageal carcinoma (A) and the explanatory diagram (B). [A] Reproduced with permission from Haslett, 1999.)

Diathermy instruments and grasping forceps can be passed through the endoscope and used to remove stones in the common bile duct after the ampulla of Vater has been incised (sphincterotomy). Obstructions in the biliary tree can also be relieved using a stent.

ERCP may introduce infection leading to cholangitis and prophylactic antibiotics are usually given. Pancreatitis may also occur.

Colonoscopy, sigmoidoscopy, and proctoscopy

These procedures give information about the lower gastrointestinal tract.

Proctoscopy is commonly performed in outpatients and involves the use of a proctoscope: a rigid tube with a detachable, disposable end that is used for one patient only and then removed and thrown away. Before the proctoscope is used, an obturator is inserted into its lumen to avoid the discomfort of inserting a hollow tube into the patient's anal canal and the end of the instrument is well lubricated.

The patient is then asked to lie on his or her left side with knees drawn up to the chest; the proctoscope is gently inserted; the obturator is removed; and air is pumped in through the proctoscope to inflate the rectum. It is kinder to explain to the patient that any associated noise is caused by the air being pumped in, otherwise he or she may think it is caused by flatulence and become very embarrassed!

Proctoscopy gives valuable information about the anal canal and rectum but, because the instrument is rigid, it cannot be used to visualize structures above the flexure.

The fibre sigmoidoscope and colonoscope are both flexible instruments, with the former being shorter. The colonoscope will allow inspection of the entire large bowel, but the sigmoidoscope only gives information on the anal canal, rectum and sigmoid colon.

The procedure in sigmoidoscopy and colonoscopy is similar to proctoscopy. However, bowel preparation is required for 2 days before colonoscopy and patients are given analgesia and sedated for the procedure.

Routine investigations

A number of simple tests are available to confirm (or disprove) diagnoses arrived at from the history of a patient in outpatients or casualty.

A probable diagnosis should have been decided, and appropriate questions asked to support or exclude it while taking the history (unless of course the patient is unconscious and no history is available). The tests ordered should be relevant to the possible diagnoses. Unnecessary or inappropriate tests waste finite resources, and they are time-consuming.

The results described below are particularly relevant to gastrointestinal disease: other texts in the *Crash Course* series should be consulted for other systems.

The pattern of deviation from normal levels is more important than individual rises or falls: do not rely too heavily on a single abnormal result. If all the tests were conducted on a healthy person, the chances are that at least one of them would be abnormal!

Haematological and clinical chemistry tests

The results of the more common tests are described in Figs 11.3 and 11.4.

Microbiology

Microbiology is the study of microorganisms and their effects on humans. Bacteria, viruses, fungi, and parasites can cause disease. Various methods exist to identify these different organisms.

Many bacteria, fungi, and parasites can be identified using light microscopy, but viruses are too small and other methods (described below) must be employed for their detection.

Samples must be solidified by freezing (in urgent cases) or treated with wax or transparent plastic and thinly sectioned to allow light to shine through and render individual structures visible.

Liquid samples may also be examined under the light microscope by smearing the sample over the glass plate and fixing it.

Both solid and liquid samples may be stained to aid diagnosis with the microscope. The Gram stain (designed by a medical student in the 19th century) is particularly useful for identifying bacteria.

Cell culture is useful in deciding which antibiotic is most effective against particular bacteria. Samples

General haematological tests		
Normal ranges	Raised	Lowered
Leucocyte count 4–11 $\times 10^9$	Infection—see below for details	Chemotherapy, steroids
Erythrocyte count men: 4.5–6.5 $\times 10^{12}$ women: 3.9–5.6 $\times 10^{12}$		
PCV (packed corpuscular volume) men: 0.4–0.54 L/L women: 0.37–0.54 L/L	Polycythaemia	
MCV (mean corpuscular volume) 76–96 fL	Excessive alcohol consumption, vitamin B_{12} and folate deficiency, liver disease	Iron deficiency anaemia, thalassaemia
MCH (mean corpuscular haemoglobin) 27–32 pg		
Neutrophils 2.0–7.5 $\times 10^9$/L 40–75% of total white cell count	Bacterial infections, trauma, surgery, haemorrhage, inflammation, infarction, drugs (e.g. steroids), disseminated malignancy, polymyalgia, myeloproliferative disorders, polyarteritis nodosa	Vitamin B_{12} deficiency, folate deficiency, bone marrow failure, tuberculosis, brucellosis, typhoid, kala-azar, septicaemia, hypersplenism, certain autoimmune diseases, drugs (e.g. sulphonamides, carbimazole)
Lymphocytes 1.3–3.5 $\times 10^9$/L 20–40% of total white cell count	Viral infection, toxoplasmosis, brucellosis, whooping cough, chronic lymphoid leukaemia	HIV infection, marrow infiltration, drugs (steroids), systemic lupus erythematosus, legionnaire's disease, uraemia, chemotherapy, radiotherapy
Eosinophils 0.04–0.44 $\times 10^9$/L 1–6% of total white cell count	Atopic conditions, parasitic infections, malignancy, polyarteritis nodosa	
Basophils 0–0.1 $\times 10^9$/L 0–1% of total white cell count	Ulcerative colitis, viral infection, malignancy, polycythaemia rubra, cell-mediated lympholysis, haemolysis, myxoedema	
Monocytes 0.2–0.8 $\times 10^9$/L 2–10% of total white cell count	Acute and chronic infection, malignancy	
Platelet count 150–400 $\times 10^9$/L	Inflammatory disease, colitis, Crohn's disease	Lymphoma, viral infection, drugs, marrow failure, idiopathic thrombocytopenic purpura, disseminated intravascular coagulation, hypersplenism
Reticulocyte count 25–100 $\times 10^9$/L	Anaemia, haemorrhage	
ESR (erythrocyte sedimentation rate, mm/h) rises with age, upper limit is: men: age ÷ 2 women: (age + 10) ÷ 2	Anaemia, malignancy, infection, sarcoidosis, lymphoma, CT disease, abdominal aneurysm	Heart failure, polycythaemia
Prothrombin time 10–14 s (often expressed as INR, by definition 1 is normal)	Liver disease, warfarin	
Activated partial thromboplastin time 35–45 s	Haemophilia, Christmas disease	

Fig. 11.3 General haematological tests.

are smeared on an agar plate, small areas of which have been impregnated with different antibiotics, and then incubated. Small patches of agar on which no bacteria have grown can be seen around those antibiotics that are most effective against the bacteria in question.

Histology and cytology

Histology is the study of tissue samples taken on biopsy or following surgical removal, usually to confirm whether tissue is malignant or not.

The sample may be examined using light microscopy or electron microscopy.

Blood tests		
Normal range	Raised	Lowered
Alanine aminotransferase 5–35 IU/L	Liver disease (hepatocellular damage), shock	
Albumin 35–50 g/L	Dehydration	Malabsorption, malnutrition, malignancy, liver disease
Alkaline phosphatase 30–300 IU/L	Liver disease (cholestasis)	
α-fetoprotein <10 kU/L	Hepatocellular carcinoma, hepatitis, chronic liver disease, teratoma	
α-amylase 0–180 somogyi U/L	Acute pancreatitis	
Aspartate transaminase 5–35 IU/L	Liver disease (hepatocellular damage), myocardial infarction, skeletal muscle damage	
Bilirubin 3–17 µmol/L	Jaundice	
Calcium Ion, 1.00–1.25 mmol/L Total, 2.12–2.65 mmol/L	Malignancy, sarcoidosis, tuberculosis, hyperparathyroidism	Malabsorption, acute pancreatitis, massive blood transfusion, hypoparathyroidism
Caeruloplasmin 200–350 mg/L		Wilson's disease
Copper 11.0–22.0 µmol/L		Wilson's disease
Cholesterol 3.9–7.8 mmol/L	Hyperlipidaemia	
Creatinine kinase 25–195 IU/L men 25–170 IU/L women	Myocardial infarction	
Ferritin 12–200 µg/L	Haemochromatosis	
Folate 2.1 µg/L		Malabsorption, alcoholism, drugs, malignancy, haemolysis
γ-GT 0–0.50 µkat/L	Alcoholic liver disease, biliary obstruction	
Iron 14–32 µmol/L men, 11–29 µmol/L women		Iron deficiency anaemia
LDH 70–250 IU/L	Hepatocellular damage, myocardial infarction	
Magnesium 0.75–1.05 mmol/L		Diarrhoea, alcohol, total parenteral nutrition
Potassium 3.5–5.0 mmol/L	Trauma (including surgery), catabolic states, renal failure, transfusion of stored blood, haemolysis	Pernicious anaemia treated with B_{12}, diarrhoea, laxative abuse, vomiting, villous adenoma
Total protein 60–80 g/L		Malabsorption, Ménétrièr's disease, nephrotic syndrome, malnutrition
Sodium 135–145 mmoL/L	Dehydration	Vomiting, diarrhoea, fistulae, ileus, intestinal obstruction, cystic fibrosis
Triglyceride 0.55–1.9 mmol/L	Hyperlipidaemia	
Urea 2.5–6.7 mmol/L	Dehydration	
Urate 210–480 µmol/L men 150–390 µmol/L women	Lymphoma, gout, leukaemia, haemolysis, drugs, alcohol	Coeliac disease, Wilson's disease, pernicious anaemia
Vitamin B_{12} 0.13–0.68 nmoL/L		Malabsorption, pernicious anaemia, gastrectomy

Fig. 11.4 Blood tests. (γ-GT, γ-glutamyltransferase; LDH, lactate dehydrogenase.)

Cytology is the study of cell samples taken by smears (for example of the cervix) or fine needle aspiration of cystic or other lesions.

The cells are stained and examined under a microscope to detect the presence of abnormal and inflammatory cells.

Breath tests

A hydrogen breath test can be performed after giving the patient a lactulose solution to drink. This can detect an overgrowth of bacteria, if there is more than 20 parts per million of hydrogen gas in less than 2 hours.

A urea breath test can be performed to confirm the presence of *Helicobacter pylori* in the stomach. It uses ^{14}C-urea or ^{13}C-urea isotopes. The *H. pylori* urease enzyme converts the urea to ammonia and CO_2, which is collected in a breath sample. It is a good non-invasive investigation.

Imaging of the gastrointestinal system

Plain radiography and contrast technique

Substances absorb X-rays to different extents, depending on their atomic number. Those that absorb most appear white, those that absorb least appear black.

Borders are only seen at the interfaces between different densities (e.g. the interface between the wall of the stomach and the gastric air bubble), but may be enhanced by the introduction of contrast media, for example, barium.

When commenting on any X-ray, always follow the same order. Do not come straight out with a diagnosis!

1. Check the film has been taken properly and the information recorded on it:
   - Look at the name and the date. Is it the correct patient and the X-ray you want to examine? Many patients have lots of different X-rays with their notes, and it is easy to pick up the wrong envelope of films!
   - Is it an AP (anteroposterior) or PA (posteroanterior) film?
   - Check the alignment of the spine (or the clavicles on a chest X-ray). Was the patient straight when it was taken? If not, organs may be displaced and look abnormal even if they are not.

2. Check the outlines of all the structures you would expect to see on a normal X-ray. Are they all visible? Can you see anything you would not normally expect? Is any area more (or less) opaque than normal?
3. Describe the gross pathology that might have caused these abnormalities (e.g. stricture in the oesophagus, rose-thorn ulcers in the ileum).
4. Suggest the most probable diagnosis, and some differential diagnoses.

The use of X-rays should be avoided in pregnancy whenever possible. In men and women of reproducing age, a lead guard must be placed over the genital organs, to prevent X-ray damage to the gonads.

Abdominal films may be taken with the patient supine (best for seeing the distribution of gas) or erect (better for spotting air under the diaphragm and for seeing fluid levels).

The intestines are lower down in erect X-rays than in the supine position. Before X-rays became available doctors had only seen intestines in supine bodies at dissections and operations and a number of unfortunate people had completely unnecessary operations to hitch up their guts when erect abdominal X-rays were first taken!

Look at the pattern of gas (central in ascites, displaced to the left lower quadrant in splenomegaly). Extraluminal gas in the liver or biliary system suggests a gas-forming infection or the passing of a stone. In the colonic wall it suggests infective colitis.

Air under the diaphragm may be caused by:
- Perforation of the bowel.
- A section of intestine lying between the liver and the diaphragm.
- A gas-forming infection.
- A pleuro-peritoneal fistula (tuberculosis, trauma, or carcinoma), following surgery or laparoscopy.
- Giving birth.
- Air being forced up the vagina and through the fallopian tubes (in female water skiers).

Look for opaque areas of calcification, commonly caused by stones (although only 10% of gall stones are radio-opaque), pancreatitis, or atherosclerosis.

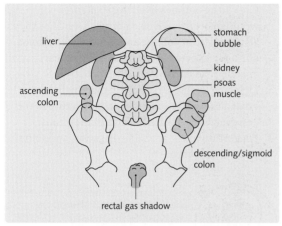

Fig. 11.5 Structures normally visible on plain abdominal X-ray. (© RA Hope & JM Longmore, TJ Hodgetts & PS Ramrakha, 1993. Reprinted from *Oxford Handbook of Clinical Medicine* edited by RA Hope & JM Longmore, TJ Hodgetts & PS Ramrakha, 3rd edn, 1993, by permission of Oxford University Press.)

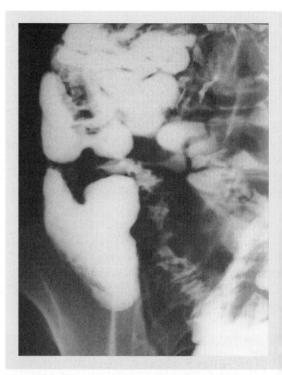

Fig. 11.6 A small bowel barium study in Crohn's disease demonstrates narrowing and distortion of the terminal ileum. (Courtesy of Dr A Grundy.)

A loop of intestinal gas (sentinel loop) can be caused by local peritoneal inflammation resulting in a localized ileus.

Fig. 11.5 shows the structures normally visible on plain abdominal X-ray.

Contrast radiographs

These may be single or double contrast (e.g. air and barium). Double-contrast films give a better picture of surface mucosa.

Barium may be administered orally and different parts of the gastrointestinal tract can be visualized using this technique depending on the delay before taking the X-ray.

A barium enema is often used to visualize the lower gastrointestinal tract (Fig. 11.6).

Angiography

Angiography is another form of contrast imaging used to visualize blood vessels.

It may show the site of gastrointestinal bleeding (although endoscopy is often the investigation of choice) and the blood supply to specific organs such as the liver (showing architectural abnormalities).

Computerized tomography

Computerized tomography (CT) scanners have been in use since 1972, and they produce computerized images of the body in a series of slices, based on the amount of X-rays absorbed by different tissues at different angles (Fig. 11.7).

They are more effective for imaging soft tissues (including tumours) than radiography, and the level of radiation is generally lower.

CT scans may be plain or contrast—contrast is often used to delineate the bowel.

Magnetic resonance imaging

Magnetic resonance imaging (MRI) scanners are large electrical coils that align the nuclei of hydrogen atoms in the body so that they lie parallel to each other (normally they lie in random directions).

The nuclei are then temporarily knocked out of alignment by radio pulses, and they emit radio signals as they fall back into alignment.

These signals are analysed to produce sliced images of the body, similar to CT scans.

Most scanners will be set so that fatty tissue, containing a high density of hydrogen atoms, produces a bright image. Conversely, bone tissue produces dark images. However, techniques used may vary according to the requirements of the scan.

MRI scans are often preferred in pregnancy as they do not use radiation, but they can interfere with pacemakers, hearing aids, and other electrical devices.

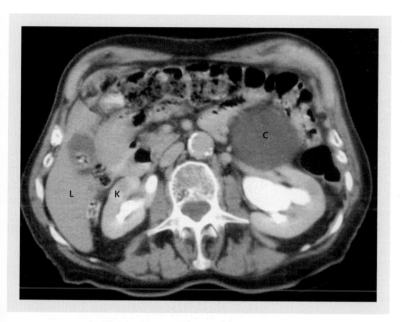

Fig. 11.7 Computerized tomography (CT) scan of a kidney cyst. The cyst (C) is displacing the pelvicalyceal system (compare with right kidney [K]). (L, liver.) (Courtesy of Dr A Grundy.)

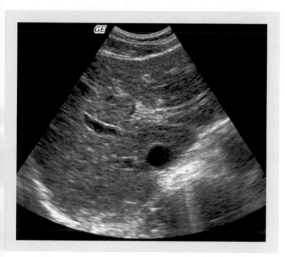

Fig. 11.8 Ultrasound of cirrhosis of the liver, showing the classical coarse, grainy appearance. (Courtesy of Dr J Pilcher.)

Radioisotope scanning

Radioisotope scanning is used to study the uptake of isotopes by various organs.

Different isotopes are taken up by different organs and structures. Hot lesions take up more isotope than the surrounding tissue, cold ones take up less.

Technetium (^{99m}Tc) colloid is used to scan the liver and ^{99m}Tc HIDA (hepatic iminodiacetic acid) for the biliary tree, as it is taken up by the liver, cleared to the gall bladder and excreted in bile. Liver lesions greater than 2 cm in diameter show up as cold spots in scanning with ^{99m}Tc colloid.

Ultrasonography

Ultrasonography has been used since the 1970s, and it is often the investigation of choice for abdominal masses (Fig. 11.8).

Ultrasonographic machines emit very high frequency sound waves, which pass readily through fluids, but are reflected back from acoustic interfaces such as soft tissue, bone or gas—the reflected echoes are analysed to produce images.

Ultrasonographic scans are non-invasive and safe in pregnancy.

- How can suspected reflux be investigated?
- What is measured in liver function tests? For each test, list the causes of abnormal serum levels.
- What is prothrombin time?
- Briefly describe the different types of endoscopic examination.
- What is an ERCP used to investigate?
- What are the causes of a lowered neutrophil count?
- Why is cell culture useful to clinicians?
- What should one look for on an X-ray before making a diagnosis?
- Briefly explain the principle of MRI and state which tissues show up as bright and dark images.
- What does extraluminal gas in the liver or biliary system suggest?

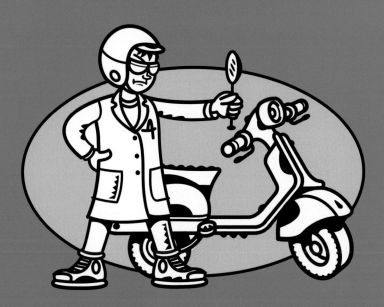

SELF-ASSESSMENT

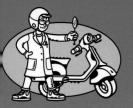

Multiple-choice Questions

Indicate whether each answer is true or false.

1. Ketone bodies (acetoacetate and β-hydroxybutyrate):

(a) Are used in health as fuels for tissues such as the heart.
(b) Are not found in the fasting state.
(c) May be metabolized to acetone.
(d) Are formed from acetyl CoA.
(e) Are not useful fuels for the brain.

2. The anti-diarrhoeal agents morphine and loperamide:

(a) Are opiate receptor antagonists.
(b) Would be suitable to treat cholera-induced diarrhoea.
(c) Induce a pattern of segmenting contractions in the colon.
(d) Reduce fluid secretion in the intestine.
(e) Can cause constipation.

3. Concerning the enteric nervous system:

(a) It is part of the autonomic nervous system.
(b) It contains neurons that use NO as a neurotransmitter.
(c) Ranitidine alters its activity directly.
(d) It only affects the small intestine.
(e) Some of its neurons use substance P as a neurotransmitter.

4. Irritable bowel syndrome is characterized by:

(a) Pain in the right hypochondrium.
(b) Proctitis.
(c) Pain relieved by defecation.
(d) Bloating.
(e) Odynophagia.

5. Concerning the lower oesophageal sphincter (LOS):

(a) It is formed by the cricopharyngeus muscle.
(b) It is unaffected by achalasia.
(c) Relaxation only occurs during swallowing.
(d) Noradrenaline produces relaxation of the LOS during swallowing.
(e) Prokinetic agents such as cisapride can increase its tone.

6. The bacterium *Helicobacter pylori*:

(a) Forms a part of the normal gut flora.
(b) Is detectable only by biopsy.
(c) Has a urease enzyme.
(d) Increases gastric acid secretion by stimulation of gastric antral D cells.
(e) Is frequently eradicated using ranitidine.

7. Endocrine regulation of gut function includes:

(a) Secretin stimulates contraction of the gall bladder.
(b) Gastrin release can be modulated via nerves.
(c) PZ-CCK results in the pancreatic secretion becoming enzyme rich.

(d) GIP slows gastric emptying.
(e) CCK stimulates gastric emptying.

8. The oxyntic cell:

(a) Can be found in the gastric antrum.
(b) Has H_1 receptors on the cell surface.
(c) Is stimulated by acetylcholine via the generation of cAMP.
(d) Will have its secretion abolished by vagotomy.
(e) Is the target cell for omeprazole.

9. Immunoglobulin A:

(a) Is secreted as a dimer.
(b) Is secreted without an accessory chain.
(c) Has its most important site of action at mucosal surfaces.
(d) Is synthesized by the M cells of Peyer's patches.
(e) Can bind toxins such as cholera toxin.

10. The sphincter of Oddi:

(a) Is contracted by CCK.
(b) Regulates the flow of bile into the duodenum.
(c) Relaxes in response to gastrin.
(d) Contracts in the interdigestive period.
(e) Diverts bile from the cystic duct into the common hepatic ducts during digestion.

11. In the small intestine:

(a) Protein can be absorbed by a process coupled to sodium.
(b) The glycocalyx of the microvilli does not contain enzymes.
(c) Water is absorbed by pumping K^+ ions into the intercellular spaces.
(d) Peristaltic reflexes are mediated exclusively by acetylcholine.
(e) Intrinsic factor is required for the absorption of vitamin B_{12}.

12. Concerning normal intestinal flora:

(a) They usually cause disease.
(b) In the large bowel they are predominantly aerobes.
(c) They prevent some pathogens from colonizing the colon.
(d) *Bacteroides* are the predominant obligate anaerobe.
(e) They may produce metabolites of benefit to the host.

13. Concerning infections of the gut:

(a) *Vibrio cholerae* produces secretory diarrhoea through the action of the toxin on cAMP levels in the epithelial cells.
(b) *Clostridium perfringens* causes enterocolitis through preformed toxins in food.

223

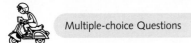

(c) *Clostridium difficile* causes necrotizing enterocolitis.
(d) Rotavirus can cause vomiting and diarrhoea in children.
(e) The secretory diarrhoea produced by *Vibrio cholerae* is due to the active secretion of K^+ into the lumen.

14. Hirschsprung's disease:

(a) Is due to an absence of ganglion cells in the Auerbach's and Meissner's plexuses.
(b) Is a common cause of chronic constipation in the newborn.
(c) Is diagnosed by barium enema alone.
(d) Is more common in males.
(e) Causes perforation of the bowel.

15. During the embryonic development of the pancreas:

(a) The pancreas develops from the endoderm.
(b) There are two embryonic pancreatic buds.
(c) Annular pancreas is a congenital disorder that can cause obstruction of the duodenum.
(d) The hindgut gives rise to the pancreas, liver, and gall bladder.
(e) There is always an accessory pancreatic duct formed.

16. Concerning congenital disorders of the oesophagus:

(a) Atresia affects 1 in 20 births.
(b) Atresia is caused by a failure of the oesophageal endoderm to grow quickly enough when the embryo elongates.
(c) In 50% of cases, atresia and fistula occur together.
(d) The infant is at risk of aspiration pneumonia in tracheoesophageal fistula.
(e) There are no surgical treatments available.

17. Clubbing is caused by:

(a) Crohn's disease.
(b) Hepatitis A infection.
(c) Gastrointestinal lymphoma.
(d) Coeliac disease.
(e) Cirrhosis.

18. Haemochromatosis is characterized by:

(a) Yellow discolouration of the skin.
(b) Diabetes mellitus resulting from insufficient insulin production.
(c) Liver enlargement.
(d) A genetic defect on chromosome 6.
(e) Saturation of the iron-binding protein lactoferrin.

19. Reye's syndrome:

(a) Is characterized by brain and liver damage.
(b) Can occur after a genitourinary infection.
(c) Has been linked to aspirin.
(d) Is characterized by seizures and deepening coma.
(e) Has a mortality of approximately 20%.

20. Barrett's oesophagus:

(a) Is a premalignant condition.
(b) Results from prolonged acid reflux.

(c) Involves the change from its normal epithelium to stratified squamous epithelium.
(d) Can become adenocarcinoma.
(e) Occurs in 20% of symptomatic cases of reflux.

21. Causes of sqamous cell carcinoma of the oesophagus include:

(a) Achalasia.
(b) Genetic predisposition.
(c) Nitrites/nitrous amides in foodstuffs.
(d) Smoking.
(e) Plummer–Vinson syndrome.

22. Causes of cirrhosis include:

(a) Autoimmune liver disease.
(b) Budd–Chiari syndrome.
(c) Gall stones.
(d) Haemochromatosis.
(e) Coeliac disease.

23. Hepatitis B:

(a) Is transmitted through the faecal–oral route.
(b) Can be vaccinated against.
(c) Is secreted in the breast milk.
(d) Can cause hepatocellular carcinoma.
(e) Is endemic in Australia.

24. Cullen's sign (discolouration around the umbilicus) may be seen in:

(a) Cushing's syndrome.
(b) Acute pancreatitis.
(c) Hirschsprung's disease.
(d) Carcinoma of the pancreas.
(e) Peritonitis.

25. Mouth ulcers are seen in:

(a) Crohn's disease.
(b) Herpes.
(c) Uraemia.
(d) Diphtheria.
(e) Lymphoma.

26. Diarrhoea:

(a) Can be defined as an increase in the volume, decrease in viscosity, and increase in the frequency of stools.
(b) Can be caused by decreased motility.
(c) Can be caused by defects in intraluminal digestion and absorption.
(d) Occurs in IBD.
(e) Occurs due to excessive use of motility stimulants.

27. Bile:

(a) Contains only water, bile acids, and cholesterol.
(b) Contains unconjugated bile acids.
(c) Contains conjugated bilirubin.
(d) Is required for the uptake of protein in the small intestine.
(e) Is required to help emulsify fats in the stomach.

28. Irritable bowel syndrome:

a) Is a functional disorder.
b) Requires surgery.
c) Is more common in women.
d) Is diagnosed by exclusion of organic causes alone.
e) Is relieved by metaclopramide.

29. The causes of acute pancreatitis include:

a) Hyperthermia.
b) Azathioprine.
c) Alcohol.
d) NSAIDs.
e) Gall stones.

30. In the liver:

a) Phagocytosis is one of the roles of the hepatocytes.
b) The spaces of Disse are located in between the Kupffer cells.
c) Ito cells secrete collagen.
d) The sinusoids have an incomplete lining of endothelial cells.
e) Bile canaliculi are sealed by zonulae occludentes.

31. Peritonitis presents with:

a) Shock.
b) Bradycardia.
c) The patient lying still with his or her knees drawn up.
d) The patient breathing deeply.
e) Dullness in the flanks on percussion of the abdomen.

32. Oesophageal varices:

a) Occur in the lower oesophagus.
b) Are not visible on endoscopy.
c) May bleed resulting in haematemesis.
d) May be caused by portal hypertension.
e) May be treated by sclerotherapy.

33. The following statements are true:

a) Percussion of the thorax sounds hyperresonant in emphysema.
b) Frothy pink sputum may infer a pulmonary infection.
c) The lungs are the only area of the body that sounds resonant on percussion.
d) Rovsing's sign indicates acute pancreatitis.
e) Absent bowel signs are caused by paralytic ileus.

34. The following statements are true:

a) A nodular prostate on rectal examination infers carcinoma of the prostate.
b) On inspection, white striae on the abdomen are indicative of Cushing's syndrome.
c) On palpation of the abdomen, rebound tenderness is indicative of peritonitis.
d) On palpation of the abdomen, a sausage-shaped mass is indicative of a hernia.
e) Splenomegaly can be palpated in the right iliac fossa.

35. The following statements are true:

a) A raised prothrombin time indicates liver disease.

(b) A lowered neutrophil count (neutropenia) may be caused by sulphonamides.
(c) A raised platelet count is seen in idiopathic thrombocytopenic purpura (ITP).
(d) A lowered albumin may be caused by malabsorption.
(e) A raised basophil count may be caused by ulcerative colitis.

36. Concerning the stomach:

(a) The blood supply is from the coeliac artery.
(b) The left gastric artery anastomoses with the right gastric artery.
(c) The fundus lies above the cardiac orifice.
(d) Like the liver, the stomach is only partly covered by peritoneum.
(e) Innervation of the stomach is by both sympathetic and parasympathetic nerves.

37. Concerning the mixing and digestion of food in the stomach:

(a) Muscular contraction in the gastric antrum is important in food mixing.
(b) Fatty chyme in the duodenum speeds up gastric emptying.
(c) Some salivary digestion continues to occur in the stomach.
(d) Stomach acid secretion is important because it breaks down protein chains as well as protecting against pathogenic bacteria.
(e) Pepsin is secreted from chief cells on the tips of gastric villi.

38. Gastrin secretion:

(a) Can start before food has even entered the mouth.
(b) Is stimulated by distension in the stomach.
(c) Is eliminated after a vagotomy.
(d) Is inhibited by high levels of amino acids in the chyme.
(e) Is the cause of ulcers in Barrett's oesophagus.

39. Concerning gastric tone and motility:

(a) Upon entry of food into the stomach, relaxation of the stomach wall occurs via adrenergic fibres.
(b) The muscularis externa is thicker in the antral region of the stomach.
(c) Cholinergic stimulation from the vagus decreases gastric motility.
(d) A group of 'pacemaker' cells on the distal body of the stomach can initiate peristaltic contractions.
(e) The peristaltic contractions occur at a rate of 10 per minute.

40. Concerning protection of the gastric mucosa:

(a) Mucus is secreted by enterochromaffin cells in the body of the stomach.
(b) Prostaglandins inhibit mucus production.
(c) Hyperparathyroidism causes excess acid secretion.
(d) Having Zollinger–Ellison syndrome is protective against ulcer formation.
(e) Bicarbonate ions help maintain the protective mucus layer.

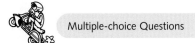

41. Concerning ulceration:

(a) Peptic ulcers only occur in the duodenal cap and the stomach.
(b) Peptic ulcers are more common in people with blood group A.
(c) Duodenal ulcers occur more commonly than gastric ulcers.
(d) 70% of duodenal ulcers are associated with *H. pylori* infection.
(e) Curling's ulcer is caused by extreme hyperacidity at the gastric mucosa.

42. Regarding acid reducing drugs:

(a) H_2 histamine receptor antagonists are the most powerful acid inhibitory and ulcer healing drugs.
(b) Sucralfate is a mucosal strengthener.
(c) Ranitidine and omeprazole act at the same site on the oxyntic cell.
(d) Vancomycin is used in the triple therapy regimes for *H. pylori* eradication.
(e) Misoprostol is a synthetic bicarbonate analogue, which can prevent NSAID-associated ulcers.

43. Concerning motility in the small intestine:

(a) Segmentation brings about rapid propulsion of intestinal contents towards the anus.
(b) Segmentation involves contraction and relaxation of both circular and longitudinal muscles.
(c) The MMC begins in the stomach.
(d) During the MMC, the pyloric sphincter contracts and closes tightly.
(e) The MMC is only present during the fasting state.

44. Concerning motility in the large intestine:

(a) Storage is facilitated in the colon by adrenergic nerve fibres.
(b) Contraction of the taeniae coli causes segmental contractions.
(c) Mass movement is responsible for colonic evacuation.
(d) The gastro-colic reflex is a neuronal and hormonal reflex.
(e) Parasympathetic stimulation increases contraction of the proximal colon.

45. Dietary fibre:

(a) Can increase the bulk of stools by 5 g for every gram of fibre.
(b) Can increase the excretion of nitrogenous waste.
(c) Binds and holds anions, thus facilitating their excretion.
(d) Includes carbohydrates with β-glycosidic linkages.
(e) Has no link with cancer of the colon.

46. The following statements are true:

(a) The puborectalis muscle encircles the rectum at the junction with the anal canal.
(b) Parasympathetic innervation to the rectum is derived from S1, S2, and S3 nerves.
(c) The anal columns are muscular ridges found on the outer surface of the anal canal.

(d) The anal columns only contain the terminal branches of the superior rectal vein.
(e) The pectinate line is the junction between the endodermal and ectodermal parts of the anal canal.

47. The following statements are true:

(a) Paralytic ileus may be caused by potassium depletion.
(b) Faecaliths are small hard masses of faeces found particularly in the sigmoid colon.
(c) Hernias occur in 10% of the population.
(d) Adhesions may cause internal constriction of the bowel.
(e) Intussusception occurs mainly at the ileocaecal valve.

48. The following statements are true:

(a) The muscular layers of the upper third of the oesophagus are made up of striated muscle.
(b) Asking a patient to stick out their tongue is a good test of function of the glossopharyngeal nerve.
(c) The gastroduodenal vein returns blood from the antrum of the stomach and the duodenum to the hepatic portal vein.
(d) NSAIDs inhibit cyclooxygenase (COX), which is required for prostaglandin production.
(e) Glisson's capsule is a capsule of connective tissue giving definite shape to the pancreas.

49. The following statements are true:

(a) The porta hepatis only contains the hepatic artery (proper), the portal vein, and the lymphatic vessels.
(b) The daily output of bile is less than 700 mL per day.
(c) The head of the pancreas is supplied by the splenic artery.
(d) The innervation to the gall bladder is from the coeliac and hepatic plexuses, the vagus nerve, and the right phrenic nerve.
(e) The liver receives 10% of the cardiac output.

50. The following statements are true:

(a) The pancreas does not produce phospholipase-A_2.
(b) Vitamin D is mainly absorbed in the jejunum.
(c) Starch contains α-1,3 and α-1,5 linkages.
(d) Small peptides are absorbed more rapidly than amino acids.
(e) Chloride is only absorbed in the colon.

51. Regarding the GI tract:

(a) The tract develops from the endodermal germ layer.
(b) Most bacteria are able to survive in the stomach.
(c) The cardiac orifice of the stomach lies behind the 7th costal cartilage about 2–4 cm to the left of the median plane.
(d) The caecum is part of the small intestine.
(e) The gall bladder is essential for life.

52. In the diet:

(a) Carbohydrates with β-glycosidic linkages cannot be absorbed.
(b) Fat should compromise about 40% of the total food intake.
(c) We need about 0.75 g/kg/day of protein.

d) Excess protein has no harmful effects.
e) Vitamins A, B, E, and K are fat soluble.

53. In the oropharynx:

a) The vestibule lies posterior to the teeth.
b) The blood supply to the oral cavity proper is principally from the internal carotid artery.
c) The intrinsic muscles of the tongue have no point of attachment outside it.
d) The external muscles of the tongue are genioglossus, hyoglossus, styloglossus, and palatoglossus.
e) Styloglossus is innervated by the accessory nerve (XI) via the pharyngeal branch of the vagus.

54. In the oropharynx:

a) All of the muscles of the soft palate are supplied by pharyngeal motor fibres carried to the pharyngeal plexus by the vagus nerve (X).
b) The pharynx extends from the base of the skull to the level of C7.
c) The gingiva and hard palate are covered by stratified squamous epithelium.
d) The muscles of mastication develop from the first branchial arch.
e) The medial pterygoid muscle has superior and inferior heads.

55. Regarding the salivary glands:

a) The parotid gland produces serous saliva.
b) The parotid gland is innervated by both the parasympathetic and the sympathetic nervous system.
c) The submandibular gland produces mixed secretions.
d) Salivary excretions are modified as they pass through the salivary ducts.
e) The opening of the parotid gland lies opposite the second lower molar tooth.

56. The oesophagus:

a) Passes through the diaphragm, just to the left of the median plane.
b) Is supplied by the inferior thyroid artery, branches of the thoracic aorta, and branches of the left gastric artery.
c) Develops from the tracheobronchial diverticulum, which appears in week 7 of gestation.
d) Has a venous drainage that forms a portosystemic anastomosis.
e) Has a striated muscle lower sphincter.

57. Regarding the intake of food:

a) The ability to burn off excess calories in the form of heat increases with age.
b) CCK is a satiety hormone.
c) Carbohydrates are primarily metabolized during the day and fats are metabolized at night.
d) Lesions of the ventromedial hypothalamus cause hyperphagia.
e) Lesions of the lateral hypothalamus cause aphagia.

58. Regarding salivation:

a) The components of saliva vary according to the rate and site of production.

b) Saliva has an acid pH.
c) The normal rate of secretion is 1–2 L in 24 hours.
d) During surgery, salivation may cause death via aspiration.
e) Denervation of the salivary glands results in a dry mouth.

59. Regarding swallowing:

(a) The swallowing reflex is triggered by afferent impulses in the trigeminal, facial, and hypoglossal nerves.
(b) It is controlled by centres in the medulla.
(c) Peristaltic tertiary waves propel food towards the stomach.
(d) Food cannot pass down the oesophagus in the absence of peristalsis.
(e) The swallowing reflex inhibits respiration.

60. Regarding vomiting:

(a) Salivation is inhibited prior to vomiting.
(b) Antiemetic drugs should be prescribed as soon as possible.
(c) It is a common side effect of drugs.
(d) The presence or absence of bile is helpful in determining the cause.
(e) The vomiting centre is located in the lateral reticular formation of the medulla.

61. Regarding the stomach:

(a) The fundus lies beneath the pyloric sphincter.
(b) The greater omentum is formed by a reflection of the greater curvature.
(c) The stomach is supplied by branches of the superior mesenteric artery.
(d) It develops from a fusiform dilatation of the foregut that appears at about week 4 of development.
(e) It has an outer oblique muscle layer.

62. In the stomach:

(a) The fundic (gastric) glands are the most numerous.
(b) The appearance of the parietal (oxyntic) glands changes with the presence of food in the stomach.
(c) Chief cells secrete pepsin.
(d) HCl and intrinsic factor are secreted by parietal cells.
(e) Venous drainage is to the hepatic portal system.

63. In the stomach:

(a) A thick, mucopolysaccharide gel protects the stomach wall from enzymatic digestion.
(b) Gastric lipase activity is of great significance in the digestion of lipids.
(c) An acidic resting juice is secreted between meals.
(d) The cephalic phase of secretion is unaffected by ligation of the vagal innervation of the stomach.
(e) H_2 receptor agonists reduce acid secretion.

64. The liver:

(a) Weighs approximately 2.5 kg.
(b) Has a bare area related to the superior vena cava.
(c) Is innervated by both vagi and the coeliac plexus.

(d) Has a substantial capacity to regenerate after injury.
(e) Forms ketone bodies in poorly controlled diabetes.

65. Regarding the metabolism of drugs:

(a) Phase I metabolism by the liver almost always produces less reactive products than the parent drug.
(b) Oxidative phase I reactions are carried out by the mixed function oxygenase system of the smooth endoplasmic reticulum.
(c) Phase II reactions include conjugation with glucuronic acid.
(d) Phenobarbitone and phenylbutazone are enzyme inducing drugs.
(e) In paracetamol overdose, there is depletion of glutathione and saturation of liver enzymes.

66. Regarding bile:

(a) The majority of bile acids in the body are synthesized *de novo* every day.
(b) The critical micelle concentration is the maximum concentration of bile acids found in health.
(c) The principal bile pigment is bilirubin.
(d) An aqueous isotonic solution of the epithelial cells lining the bile ducts accounts for about 80% of the total volume of bile.
(e) Low levels of bile acids in the portal blood stimulate the secretion of bile acids.

67. The gall bladder:

(a) Concentrates and stores bile.
(b) Only contracts during the gastric and intestinal phases of gastric secretion.
(c) Is more likely to contain pigment stones than cholesterol stones.
(d) Is often removed in childhood due to the presence of stones.
(e) Has a capacity of about 150 mL.

68. The pancreas:

(a) Has a poor blood supply.
(b) Is innervated by the splanchnic and vagus nerves.
(c) Produces insulin from month 3 after conception.
(d) Only contains endocrine cell types α and β.
(e) Has islet cells which are most abundant in the body.

69. The exocrine pancreas:

(a) Secretes about ten times its own weight in fluid every day.
(b) Secretes a fluid richer in bicarbonate when the rate of secretion is higher.
(c) Secretes most of its enzymes in an active form.
(d) Has an increased rate of secretion following sympathetic stimulation.
(e) Has an increased rate of secretion in response to insulin.

70. The small intestine:

(a) On X-ray in the adult is difficult to distinguish from the large intestine.

(b) Develops entirely from the embryological foregut.
(c) Herniates outside the abdominal cavity at about week 6 from conception.
(d) Rotates about the inferior mesenteric artery during its development.
(e) Is supplied by branches of the coeliac and superior mesenteric arteries.

71. The mucosa of the small intestine:

(a) Contains tall columnar enterocytes.
(b) Contains mucus-secreting goblet cells.
(c) Contains protein-secreting Paneth cells in the most superficial parts of the glands.
(d) Loses about 17 million enterocytes a day.
(e) May become flattened, leading to malabsorption.

72. Regarding flora of the GI tract:

(a) *Bacteroides fragilis* is commonly found in the mouth.
(b) Bacteria of the *Neisseria* species are often found in the small intestine.
(c) Anaerobes cannot survive in the mouth.
(d) Anaerobes in the intestines produce vitamin K.
(e) *E. coli* makes up about 90% of the bacteria in the bowel.

73. Regarding haematological tests:

(a) The MCV (mean corpuscular volume) is raised in chronic alcohol abuse.
(b) The MCV is lowered in thalassaemia.
(c) Lymphocytes make up about 75% of the total white cell count.
(d) Eosinophils are raised in atopic conditions.
(e) Prothrombin time is decreased in liver disease.

74. In the large intestine:

(a) Mass movements occur about every 15 minutes in the fed state.
(b) Intestinal contents move more quickly through the colon than through the small intestine.
(c) Gastric distension inhibits peristalsis.
(d) In Hirschsprung's disease the internal anal sphincter is hypotonic.
(e) The anal canal can sense the difference between air, liquid, and solid.

75. The following statements are correct:

(a) Progressive dysphagia may be due to malignancy.
(b) Jaundice is usually apparent once plasma bilirubin levels exceed 17 μmol/L.
(c) Diarrhoea is rarely life-threatening.
(d) Flatulence occurring more than five times a day should always be investigated.
(e) Anal masses may present with tenesmus.

76. Regarding signs and symptoms:

(a) Areas of baldness on the scalp may be due to malignancy.
(b) Dark, warty palms are never a cause for concern.
(c) Itchy tissue-paper skin may be present in malabsorption.

(d) Palmar erythema is almost always due to malignancy.
(e) Telangiectasia (abnormal visible dilatation of the blood vessels) is caused by cirrhosis.

77. The following statements are correct:

(a) Contraction of an empty stomach stimulates appetite.
(b) Clubbing may occur in inflammatory bowel disease.
(c) Small pigmented macules may be seen in the mouth in Peutz–Jeghers syndrome.
(d) A high arched palate is common in Down syndrome.
(e) White patches that cannot be brushed off are known as leucoplakia.

78. On inspection of the abdomen:

(a) Sister Joseph's nodule is a sign of carcinoma.
(b) Up to 10 spider naevi are considered normal.
(c) Visible peristalsis from right to left indicates pyloric stenosis.
(d) Grey Turner's sign is discolouration around the umbilicus.
(e) White striae may be seen in pregnancy.

79. Regarding hernias:

(a) Inguinal hernias are almost always direct.
(b) Strangulated hernias are a surgical emergency.
(c) Indirect inguinal hernias lie medial to the inferior epigastric vessels.
(d) Surgical repair of hernias may lead to adhesions.
(e) Reducible hernias should be treated surgically.

80. Regarding liver function tests:

(a) Alanine aminotransferase is present in canaliculi and sinusoidal membranes.
(b) Bilirubin levels normally increase in liver disease.
(c) The pattern of changes is more important than a single rise or fall.
(d) Prothrombin time is increased in vitamin K deficiency.
(e) High levels of both γ-GT and alkaline phosphatase indicate cholestasis.

81. In the small intestine:

(a) The ligament of Treitz is found between the jejunum and the ileum.
(b) Secretory diarrhoea occurs when enterocytes secrete more fluid than they absorb.
(c) Most of the immunoglobulins produced are IgG.
(d) Chyme is propelled forward at about 50 cm per hour.
(e) Peristaltic rushes are normally experienced about three times a day.

82. In the mouth:

(a) Simple cleft palate is more common in the male.
(b) Cleft palate does not affect breastfeeding.
(c) Aphthous ulcers may occur in the mouth in association with inflammatory bowel disease or coeliac disease.
(d) Infection with herpes simplex II is more common than herpes simplex I.
(e) Leucoplakia is a premalignant condition.

83. Regarding the oesophagus:

(a) Oesophageal atresia and fistula rarely occur together.
(b) Diagnosis of oesophageal varices is by biopsy.
(c) Basal cell hyperplasia is seen in reflux oesophagitis.
(d) Killian's dehiscence is more common in middle-aged women.
(e) Chagas' disease may lead to denervation of the oesophagus and dysphagia.

84. The following statements are correct:

(a) Diaphragmatic hernia occurs in about 1/10 000 live births.
(b) Pyloric stenosis is more common among males.
(c) Acute and chronic gastritis may be caused by *Helicobacter pylori* infection.
(d) Body stores of vitamin B_{12} are sufficient for 2 or 3 years.
(e) Vitamin B_{12} is absorbed from the duodenum in the presence of intrinsic factor.

85. The following statements are correct:

(a) A portosystemic anastomosis exists between the epigastric and paraumbilical veins.
(b) Oesophageal varices are a benign condition.
(c) Councilman bodies are seen in the liver in acute viral hepatitis.
(d) Yellow fever causes mid-zonal necrosis.
(e) Cirrhosis is a common cause of portal hypertension.

86. The following statements are correct:

(a) Primary haemochromatosis is characterized by the absorption of too much copper.
(b) Kayser–Fleisher rings are seen in Wilson's disease.
(c) Alpha$_1$-antitrypsin causes lung disease.
(d) Microvesicular steatosis occurs in the liver in Reye's syndrome.
(e) Rubella infection in pregnancy may cause hepatitis in the infant.

87. Regarding viruses:

(a) Diagnosis of hepatitis A is by detection of virus-specific IgM.
(b) Infection with hepatitis A leads to carrier status in 90% of cases.
(c) Hepatitis B is spread by the faecal–oral route.
(d) Hepatitis C has an incubation period of 6–8 weeks.
(e) Hepatitis D is a defective RNA virus.

88. The following statements concern the effects of toxins on the liver:

(a) Zone 1 of the liver is most susceptible to alcoholic liver damage.
(b) Mallory bodies are seen in hepatocytes following alcoholic damage.
(c) Cirrhosis is reversible.
(d) Irreversible steatosis may result from alcohol ingestion.
(e) Unpredictable drug reactions will occur in any individual if the dose is sufficient.

89. The following statements regarding the liver are correct:

(a) Severe ischaemic damage is common.

229

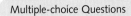

(b) Zone 1 is closest to the central vein.
(c) The Budd–Chiari syndrome is caused by thrombosis of the hepatic artery.
(d) 5-year survival in chronic Budd–Chiari syndrome is about 70%.
(e) Passive congestion results in a 'nutmeg liver'.

90. Regarding pregnancy:

(a) Pregnancy-induced hypertension is more common among primigravidas.
(b) Pregnancy-induced hypertension is a benign condition.
(c) Acute fatty liver is common in early pregnancy.
(d) Intrahepatic cholestasis may lead to stillbirth.
(e) Intrahepatic cholestasis is often benign.

91. The following statements regarding the biliary tract are correct:

(a) Primary biliary cirrhosis is more common in males.
(b) Congenital hepatic fibrosis is inherited as an autosomal-dominant condition.
(c) Caroli's disease is inherited as an autosomal-recessive condition.
(d) Primary biliary cirrhosis is an autoimmune disorder.
(e) 70% of cases of primary sclerosing cholangitis are associated with ulcerative colitis.

92. Regarding the pancreas:

(a) Ectopic pancreatic tissue may be found in the distal end of the oesophagus.
(b) Ranson's criteria are used to stage chronic pancreatitis.
(c) Speckled calcification of the pancreas may occur in chronic pancreatitis.
(d) Pseudocysts are usually multiple.
(e) Diabetic smokers have an increased risk of developing carcinoma of the pancreas.

93. The following statements about congenital abnormalities are correct:

(a) Meckel's diverticulum occurs about 2 inches (5 cm) from the ileocaecal valve.
(b) A Meckel's diverticulum may contain ectopic gastric tissue.
(c) Hirschsprung's disease usually presents with projectile vomiting.
(d) Faeces can be felt in the distal rectum in Hirschsprung's disease.
(e) The incidence of Hirschsprung's disease is higher in children with Down syndrome.

94. Regarding infections and enterocolitis:

(a) Diarrhoea means the passage of more than two stools a day.
(b) Infectious enterocolitis accounts for 50% of deaths before the age of 5 years in developing countries.
(c) Rotavirus infection is common in adults.
(d) *S. aureus* enterocolitis is caused by ingestion of a preformed toxin.
(e) Necrotizing enterocolitis is uncommon before the age of 3 years.

95. Regarding inflammatory bowel disease:

(a) Crohn's disease may occur anywhere from the mouth to the anus.
(b) Crohn's disease is four times more common in males.
(c) Ulcerative colitis is characterized by skip lesions.
(d) Ulcerative colitis is more common amongst smokers.
(e) Cryptosporidium is a common cause of diarrhoea in people with HIV infection.

96. Regarding malabsorption syndromes:

(a) Malabsorption from different causes presents with different signs and symptoms.
(b) Tropical sprue is common in Africa.
(c) Whipple's disease is more common in women.
(d) Treatment of coeliac disease is with tetracycline.
(e) The absence of cysts and trophozoites in stools excludes a diagnosis of giardiasis.

97. Obstruction:

(a) Due to non-mechanical causes is called pseudo-obstruction.
(b) High in the GI tract presents with distension.
(c) May be due to a strangulated hernia.
(d) Should always be treated surgically.
(e) Due to volvulus is more common in developed countries than in developing ones.

98. Regarding colonic diverticula:

(a) Diverticulosis means that diverticula are causing symptoms.
(b) Congenital diverticula are outpouchings of the full thickness of the bowel wall.
(c) Congenital diverticula are usually symptomatic.
(d) Acquired diverticula are more common on the left side of the colon.
(e) Patients with diverticulitis should be advised to decrease the amount of fibre in their diet.

99. Regarding neoplasms of the bowel:

(a) Adenomas may cause electrolyte imbalances.
(b) Colorectal cancer is the second biggest cause of cancer death in the UK.
(c) Diet has no effect on the risk of developing colorectal cancer.
(d) Dukes' classification is used to assess the stage of carcinoid tumours.
(e) B cell lymphomas are associated with coeliac disease.

100. Peritonitis:

(a) Is usually limited to a small area.
(b) Is often due to *E. coli*.
(c) Should be treated by resuscitation and removal of the cause.
(d) May lead to air under the diaphragm being visible o- an erect X-ray.
(e) May be due to retroperitoneal fibromatosis.

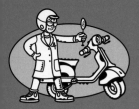
1. List the signals for the release of gastrin. What are its actions?

2. List the main functions of hepatocytes.

3. Describe the main congenital abnormalities of the oesophagus.

4. Describe the nerve supply to the tongue.

5. Why is iron deficiency relatively common among women of reproductive age?

6. Describe how the composition of saliva varies with the rate of flow.

7. What are lipoproteins?

8. How should one perform a rectal examination on an adult male?

9. What signs, symptoms, and results of investigations would lead you to suspect posthepatic jaundice? What are the principal causes of this type of jaundice?

10. Write brief notes on hepatitis B.

11. What are the effects of a carcinoid tumour of the small intestine?

12. What are the main causes and consequence of acute pancreatitis?

13. What are the main effects of gall stones?

14. What is Hirschsprung's disease?

15. List the systemic effects of malabsorption.

16. Mrs. M.H., a 34-year-old woman, has come to see her GP complaining of abdominal pain and feeling breathless a lot of the time. On questioning she admits that the pain is relieved by defecation and that she has been having diarrhoea on and off, and the pain, for about 5 months. Her abdomen is tender on palpation.

   (a) What would you initially consider to be the diagnosis?
   (b) What investigations might you carry out to confirm the diagnosis?
   (c) What treatment is available for the problem?

17. A 7-year-old boy comes into A&E with vomiting, lethargy, and increasing disorientation. The little boy starts to have seizures. On questioning, his mother describes how he has recently been recovering from 'flu'. After extensive investigations, a liver biopsy shows accumulations of triglycerides (steatosis).

   (a) What might be the diagnosis?
   (b) How does this disease progress?

18. A 21-year-old man comes into his GP clinic presenting with a flu-like illness and anorexia. He has recently come back from 12 months of travelling in South-East Asia, where he had a tattoo put on his arm.

   (a) What does the GP test for?
   (b) Who else might be at risk?

19. A 55-year-old man presents with epigastric pain, vomiting, tiredness, and weight loss. On examination, he has abdominal tenderness and a palpable epigastric mass. Blood tests confirm that he has anaemia. The GP sends him for an endoscopy.

   (a) What is the most likely diagnosis?
   (b) What other questions would his doctor ask?

20. An obese 39-year-old lady arrives at her GP complaining of increasing pain on inspiration and abdominal tenderness in the right upper quadrant. On examination, the GP notices that her sclera have a yellow tinge. She tells the GP that she has been passing pale stools.

   (a) What is the problem with this lady?
   (b) What treatment is available?

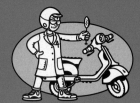

Essay Questions

1. What is malrotation of the gut? How may it arise and what are its effects?

2. Describe the patterns of damage seen in the liver. What causes these patterns of damage?

3. What are the main causes of obstruction of the bowel?

4. What is bile? How is it produced and released into the duodenum?

5. Describe the aetiology, pathogenesis, and pathology of circulatory disorders of the liver. What complications may arise? How do they develop, and how are they treated?

6. Give an account of neoplasms of the GI tract.

7. Do X-ray investigations still have a place in the diagnosis of GI disorders?

8. Discuss the causes and symptoms of jaundice.

9. What are the main causes of epigastric pain? Briefly, discuss how it may be evaluated.

10. What diagnostic inferences may be made from an inspection of the abdomen?

11. Describe the phases of gastric secretion.

12. What makes up the gut flora? Give examples of species found in each region of the bowel, and describe the functions of the gut flora.

13. What are peptic ulcers? How are they treated, and how can they be prevented?

14. Describe motility in the large intestine.

15. Describe the process of gastric emptying.

16. What are the main hormones controlling the GI tract? What are their functions, and when are they secreted?

17. How are pancreatic secretions controlled?

18. What is irritable bowel disease? How is it diagnosed and treated?

19. Give a brief account of the hepatitis viruses. What are the epidemiology, complications, and possible treatments of each virus?

20. Compare and contrast Crohn's disease and ulcerative colitis.

MCQ Answers

1. (a) False—They are used in disease states (e.g. diabetes) as a source of fuel.
   (b) False—They are found in prolonged starvation.
   (c) False—They are metabolized to acetyl-CoA.
   (d) True—Ketogenesis occurs in the liver.
   (e) False—The brain, heart, and muscle can all oxidize and use ketone bodes as fuel.

2. (a) False—They are opiate receptor agonists.
   (b) False—Cholera requires antibiotic and fluid replacement therapy to correct electrolyte imbalance. Anti-diarrhoeal drugs treat the symptoms, not the infection.
   (c) True—They also decrease propulsive activity in the intestine.
   (d) False—They allow more time for fluid absorption.
   (e) True—Too big a dose can cause constipation.

3. (a) True—It includes Auerbach's and Meissner's plexuses.
   (b) True—These are non-adrenergic non-cholinergic (NANC) neurons.
   (c) False—Ranitidine acts as an H_2 receptor antagonist on oxyntic cells.
   (d) False—It is present throughout the entire bowel.
   (e) True—Substance P is an excitatory neurotransmitter and a cotransmitter of acetylcholine.

4. (a) False—Pain is referred to the lower left quadrant.
   (b) False—Proctitis is inflammation of the rectum, and it is not a symptom of IBS.
   (c) True—This is a diagnostic symptom.
   (d) True—This is a common symptom accompanied by abdominal discomfort or pain.
   (e) False—This is retrosternal pain on ingestion; often a symptom of oesophagitis.

5. (a) False—The upper oesophageal sphincter is formed by the cricopharyngeus muscle.
   (b) False—Achalasia causes spasm of the LOS.
   (c) False—The LOS relaxes when a peristaltic wave meets it and just prior to vomiting.
   (d) False—Relaxation of the LOS is produced by NANC fibres. Therefore NO and VIP cause relaxation of the LOS.
   (e) True—Cisapride acts to upregulate the release of acetylcholine, leading to vagal excitation and increased LOS tone.

6. (a) False—It is a pathogenic organism that can cause peptic ulcers.
   (b) False—A urea breath test is diagnostic for H. pylori.
   (c) True—This is used to convert urea to ammonia.

   (d) False—H. pylori is pro-inflammatory due to its urease enzyme and ammonia production.
   (e) False—Eradication requires triple therapy (two antibiotics and a proton pump inhibitor).

7. (a) False—CCK stimulates gall bladder contraction.
   (b) True—Gastrin releasing peptide, via acetylcholine from intramural neurons, upregulates gastrin secretion.
   (c) True—It acts on pancreatic acinar cells to upregulate enzyme secretion.
   (d) True—GIP is released by the duodenum in response to the presence of chyme.
   (e) False—CCK inhibits gastric emptying.

8. (a) True—However, oxyntic cells are mainly found in the gastric glands of the fundus.
   (b) False—They have H_2 receptors.
   (c) True—Histamine, gastrin, and caffeine (via c AMP) also stimulate the oxyntic cells.
   (d) True—This removes acetylcholine stimulation.
   (e) True—Omeprazole is a proton pump inhibitor.

9. (a) True—IgA plays a major role in mucosal defence.
   (b) False—The accessory chain is the secretory component that protects IgA from digestion by proteolytic enzymes.
   (c) True—IgA is also found on the surfaces of B cells as a monomer.
   (d) False—IgA is synthesized by plasma (B) cells.
   (e) True—IgA is very effective against mucosal toxins.

10. (a) False—CCK relaxes the sphincter of Oddi.
    (b) True—It also regulates the flow of pancreatic juice into the duodenum.
    (c) False—Gastrin increases gastrin motility and inhibits gastric emptying.
    (d) True—Bile and pancreatic juice are only released during a meal.
    (e) False—This occurs in the interdigestive period.

11. (a) True—There are a number of different amino acid carriers, some are Na^+-dependent and some are Na^+-independent.
    (b) True—The glycocalyx of the microvilli contains enzymes for digestion and transport.
    (c) False—Na^+ ions are pumped into the intracellular space in exchange for K^+ ions.
    (d) False—It is also mediated by substance P.
    (e) True—The ileal epithelial cells have receptors for the intrinsic factor–vitamin B_{12} dimer.

12. (a) False—They do not cause disease normally and often have important functions.

(b) False—Anaerobes are found in the large bowel.
(c) True—Commensal bacteria compete with pathogenic bacteria for space and nutrients.
(d) True—The large bowel contains about 400 different bacterial species altogether!
(e) True—*Bacteroides fragilis* produces vitamin K.

13. (a) True—The increase in cAMP causes an increase in secretion of Na^+, Cl^- and water.
(b) True—The toxins are also heat stable.
(c) False—It causes pseudomembranous colitis.
(d) True—It can also cause fever and abdominal pain.
(e) False—It is due to increased cAMP and increased secretion of Na^+, Cl^- and H_2O.

14. (a) True—This is due to failure of neuroblasts to migrate in weeks 5–12 of gestation.
(b) True—It may also result in obstruction.
(c) False—It is diagnosed by biopsy and barium enema.
(d) True—It is four times more likely to occur in males.
(e) False—It causes obstruction and constipation.

15. (a) True—It develops from the endodermal lining of the duodenum in weeks 4–6.
(b) True—There is a dorsal and ventral pancreatic bud.
(c) True—It is caused by incomplete migration of the ventral bud, or migration in the opposite direction.
(d) False—The foregut gives rise to these organs.
(e) False—Sometimes an accessory pancreatic duct forms.

16. (a) False—Atresia affects 1 in 200 births.
(b) True—This occurs in week 5 of gestation.
(c) False—In 90% of cases, oesophageal atresia and fistula occur together.
(d) True—A fistula is an abnormal connection between trachea and oesophagus, thus leading to aspiration pneumonia.
(e) False—Treatment of atresia and fistula is by surgery.

17. (a) True—It is more often seen in Crohn's disease than ulcerative colitis.
(b) False—It is not caused by viral hepatitis.
(c) True—Clubbing is seen in malignancies of other organs too.
(d) True—Malabsorption causes clubbing.
(e) True—Cirrhosis is a major GI cause of clubbing.

18. (a) False—It is characterized by a bronze discolouration (yellow discolouration is seen in jaundice).
(b) True—The pancreas does not function properly due to iron accumulation in its cells.
(c) True—Iron accumulation causes liver enlargement.
(d) True—The defect is in the HLA-A3 gene on chromosome 6.
(e) False—There is saturation of the iron binding protein transferrin.

19. (a) True—Acute encephalopathy and microvesicular steatosis of the liver are characteristic.
(b) False—It occurs after an upper respiratory tract infection.

(c) True—Other potential precipitating factors include influenza and varicella infections.
(d) True—Disturbed cardiac rhythm, cessation of breathing, and hepatic failure eventually occur.
(e) False—Overall mortality is about 50%, due mainly to cerebral oedema.

20. (a) True—Barrett's oesophagus results from prolonged reflux of gastric acid into the oesophagus.
(b) True—This occurs when the lower oesophageal sphincter is incompetent.
(c) False—The normal squamous epithelium changes to columnar epithelium.
(d) True—Adenocarcinoma is 30–40 times more likely to occur in Barrett's oesophagus than in normal oesophagus.
(e) True—It is most commonly seen in middle-aged men.

21. (a) True—It is also caused by Plummer–Vinson syndrome and chronic oesophagitis.
(b) True—Coeliac disease also predisposes to squamous cell carcinoma.
(c) True—Fungal contamination of foodstuffs can also cause it.
(d) True—Alcohol intake is a risk factor too.
(e) True—This is an oesophageal disorder caused by an oesophageal web, iron deficiency anaemia, and eventual oesophageal cancer.

22. (a) True—This is caused by autoantibodies, which destroy the hepatic tissue.
(b) True—Budd–Chiari syndrome is a rare condition caused by portal vein thrombosis.
(c) True—Biliary cholestasis can also cause cirrhosis.
(d) True—Haemochromatosis involves iron overload of the liver.
(e) False—Coeliac disease is a malabsorption disorder and can predispose to T cell lymphoma not cirrhosis.

23. (a) False—It is transmitted through blood products, body fluids, sexual contact, breast milk, and vertical transmission.
(b) True—The vaccine may also protect against hepatitis D infection.
(c) True—It can also be passed from mother to child through vertical transmission during pregnancy.
(d) True—Other complications of hepatitis B infection include cirrhosis and chronic hepatitis.
(e) False—It is endemic in South-East Asia, China and tropical Africa.

24. (a) False—A sign of Cushing's syndrome is purple striae on the abdomen.
(b) True—It is often seen with Grey Turner's sign (discolouration in the flanks).
(c) False—Hirschsprung's disease often presents with distension in the left lower quadrant.
(d) True—60% of all pancreatic carcinoma occurs in the head of the pancreas.

(e) False—Peritonitis presents with rebound tenderness on palpation of the lower abdomen and the patient lies very still and takes shallow breaths.

25. (a) True—Crohn's can affect any part of the GI tract from mouth to anus.
    (b) True—Ulcers are usually caused by HSV-1.
    (c) False—Uraemia may present with halitosis.
    (d) True—Tuberculosis infections may cause mouth ulcers too.
    (e) True—Lymphoma and carcinoma can both cause mouth ulcers.

26. (a) True—It may be due to a number of factors including increased secretion or infection.
    (b) True—Gastrointestinal stasis facilitates bacterial overgrowth and, therefore, it can cause diarrhoea.
    (c) True—Failure to absorb, excess secretion, or failure of ion transport may cause diarrhoea.
    (d) True—Diarrhoea is mainly a symptom of ulcerative colitis.
    (e) False—Diarrhoea may be caused by excess use of purgative laxatives.

27. (a) False—Bile contains water, electrolytes, bile pigments, bile salts, cholesterol, and phospholipids.
    (b) False—Bile contains conjugated bile acids.
    (c) True—Bilirubin is conjugated to make it soluble.
    (d) False—Bile is required to facilitate fat uptake.
    (e) False—Bile emulsifies fat in the small intestine.

28. (a) True—There is no structural aetiology, such as infection, inflammation, or neoplasm.
    (b) False—Treatment for IBS is symptomatic.
    (c) True—IBS affects 10–20% of all adolescents and adults in the West.
    (d) False—It is diagnosed by exclusion of organic causes and the presence of symptoms.
    (e) False—Metaclopramide is a motility stimulant and IBS is usually treated with loperamide, methylcellulose and analgesia.

29. (a) False—Hypothermia may cause acute pancreatitis.
    (b) True—This can cause acinar cell injury leading to leakage of enzymes.
    (c) True—Alcohol acts like drugs in causing cell injury, enzyme release and tissue necrosis.
    (d) False—NSAIDs can cause peptic ulcers.
    (e) True—Gall stones cause duct obstruction leading to release of intracellular enzymes.

30. (a) False—Kupffer cells are phagocytic, not hepatocytes.
    (b) False—The space of Disse is located between the hepatocytes and sinusoidal epithelial cells.
    (c) True—This provides a supportive mesh.
    (d) True—The endothelial cells are interspersed with Kupffer cells.

(e) True—Zonulae occludentes prevent leakage of bile into the intercellular spaces.

31. (a) True—Peritonitis is very painful, and this acute inflammation often presents with shock.
    (b) False—The patient will have tachycardia.
    (c) True—Movement of the abdomen causes extreme pain.
    (d) False—The patient will be taking shallow breaths, as inspiration causes pain.
    (e) False—Dullness in the flanks on percussion of the abdomen is only present if there is ascites.

32. (a) True—They only occur at a site of portal systemic anastomosis.
    (b) False—Endoscopy is diagnostic for varices.
    (c) True—Varices may also lead to massive haemorrhage and rapid death.
    (d) True—Cirrhosis also causes varices and portal hypertension.
    (e) True—Banding and vasoconstrictor drugs are also treatments for varices.

33. (a) True—Hyperresonance is also found in asthma and pneumothorax.
    (b) False—Frothy pink sputum infers pulmonary oedema.
    (c) False—The abdomen can sound resonant due to flatus.
    (d) False—Rovsing's sign indicates acute appendicitis.
    (e) True—However, loud bowel sounds (tinkling) indicate intestinal obstruction.

34. (a) True—The prostate should feel smooth with a midline groove.
    (b) False—Cushing's syndrome presents with purple striae on the abdomen.
    (c) True—Rebound tenderness describes the sharp pain on release of the hand as you palpate.
    (d) False—A sausage-shaped mass is due to pyloric stenosis or to intussusception.
    (e) True—The spleen enlarges inferiorly and diagonally.

35. (a) True—It may infer an abnormality in the production of clotting factors, which occurs in the liver.
    (b) True—Carbimazole is another drug that causes neutropenia.
    (c) False—ITP presents with a lowered platelet count.
    (d) True—It may also be due to malignancy, liver disease, or malnutrition.
    (e) True—It is also seen in viral infections, malignancy, and haemolysis.

36. (a) True—This is via the 3 branches of the coeliac artery: the left gastric, splenic, and common hepatic.
    (b) True—The left gastric artery also has a branch that supplies the lower oesophagus.
    (c) True—The fundus is superior to the plane of the cardiac orifice.

(d) False—The anterior and posterior surfaces of the stomach are covered by the peritoneum and meet at the greater and lesser curvatures.

(e) True—Sympathetic—coeliac plexus; parasympathetic—vagus (X).

37. (a) True—This occurs in the distal body and antrum of the stomach.
(b) False—Fatty acids in the duodenum cause slowing of gastric emptying and increase contractibility.
(c) True—It occurs at the centre of the bolus of food.
(d) True—Acid enables activation of pepsin from pepsinogen and provides a hostile environment for pathogenic bacteria.
(e) False—Pepsinogen is secreted from chief cells in the deepest part of the gastric glands.

38. (a) True—This is mediated by the vagus nerve in the cephalic phase.
(b) True—This occurs via local enteric and central vago-vagal reflexes.
(c) False—Gastrin is stimulated by the presence of amino acids and fatty acids; by distension of the stomach; blood-borne calcium and adrenaline.
(d) False—Amino acids in the chyme stimulate gastrin release.
(e) False—In Zollinger–Ellison syndrome, patients have a gastrin-secreting pancreatic adenoma. This can cause ulcers.

39. (a) False—Reflex receptive relaxation is brought about by vagal inhibitory fibres.
(b) True—This is the site where mixing of stomach contents occurs.
(c) False—Cholinergic stimulation from the vagus increases motility and secretion.
(d) True—The peristaltic contractions sweep down towards the antrum.
(e) False—The contractions occur at a rate of three per minute, each lasting 2–20 seconds.

40. (a) False—Mucus is secreted by neck and surface mucus cells in the body and fundus of the stomach.
(b) False—Prostaglandins stimulate mucus production.
(c) True—Hyperparathyroidism increases levels of calcium in the body, which stimulates acid production.
(d) False—In Zollinger–Ellison syndrome, a gastrin-secreting adenoma results in hyperacidity and can cause ulcer formation.
(e) True—Bicarbonate ions raise the pH around the mucus layer and therefore make pepsin less active, thus preventing pepsin degradation of the mucus.

41. (a) False—Peptic ulcers may occur in the distal oesophagus, a Meckel's diverticulum, and where a gastroenterostomy has been performed.
(b) False—Peptic ulcers are more common in people with blood group O.

(c) True—Duodenal ulcers are 2–3 times more common than gastric ulcers.
(d) False—About 95% of duodenal ulcers are associated with H. pylori infection.
(e) False—Curling's ulcer occurs after burns.

42. (a) False—Proton pump inhibitors are the most powerful acid inhibitory and ulcer healing drugs.
(b) True—Sucralfate forms a polymerized, sticky gel in acid conditions that adheres to the base of ulcers and protects them from gastric acid.
(c) False—Ranitidine is a H_2 receptor antagonist and omeprazole is a proton pump inhibitor. Both reduce acid secretion.
(d) False—The triple therapy regimen for H. pylori eradication consists of amoxycillin, metronidazole, and omeprazole or clarithromycin, tinidazole, and omeprazole.
(e) False—Misoprostol is a synthetic prostaglandin analogue, which can help prevent NSAID-associated ulcers.

43. (a) False—Peristalsis brings about rapid propulsion. Segmentation mixes the digested food and exposes it to the absorptive surfaces.
(b) False—Segmentation only involves contraction and relaxation of the circular muscles.
(c) True—The MMC begins in the stomach and moves towards the terminal ileum.
(d) False—During the MMC, the pyloric sphincter is open wide.
(e) True—The MMC stops immediately on ingestion of food and motility switches to the fed-state pattern.

44. (a) False—Storage is facilitated by NANC fibres, via NO and VIP release.
(b) True—The taeniae coli are three bands of longitudinal muscle, which gather the colon into haustra.
(c) True—Mass movement describes the intense contractions that occur only a few times a day.
(d) True—The gastro-colic reflex occurs shortly after a meal and is partly stimulated by CCK and partly by neuronal control.
(e) True—Parasympathetic innervation is via the branches of the vagus (X) and pelvic nerves from the sacral spinal cord.

45. (a) True—Foods high in fibre include brown bread, potatoes, fruit, and vegetables.
(b) True—Fibre has an affinity for these molecules and they bind easily to it. It also increases the excretion of bile acids.
(c) False—Fibre binds and holds cations, such as calcium, magnesium, iron, and zinc. This facilitates their excretion.
(d) True—Fibre consists of those carbohydrates that humans are unable to digest, including lignin and cellulose.

(e) False—A diet high in fibre decreases the risk of getting cancer of the colon.

46. (a) True—This forms a 90 degree angle called the anorectal angle (or anorectal flexure).
    (b) False—Parasympathetic innervation is derived from S1, S3, and S4 nerves, which run with the pelvic splanchnic nerves.
    (c) False—Anal columns are longitudinal ridges in the mucosal membrane of the superior half of the anal canal.
    (d) False—The anal columns contain the terminal branches of both the superior rectal artery and vein.
    (e) True—The pectinate line is also the junction in the anal canal where the columnar epithelium of the upper part becomes stratified squamous epithelium of the lower part.

47. (a) True—Other causes include peritonitis, uraemia, diabetic coma, and anticholinergic drugs.
    (b) False—Faecaliths are small, hard masses of faeces, which are particularly found in the appendix.
    (c) False—Hernias occur in 1% of the population and may be congenital or acquired.
    (d) False—Adhesions may cause external constriction of the bowel, leading to obstruction or strangulation.
    (e) True—Intussusception most commonly affects infants (95% of all cases).

48. (a) True—The middle third has both striated and smooth muscle and the lower third has only smooth muscle.
    (b) False—It tests the function of the hypoglossal nerve. The tongue will deviate to the side of paralysis if a lesion is present.
    (c) False—There is no gastroduodenal vein!
    (d) True—NSAIDs (e.g. aspirin) inhibit cyclooxygenase and, therefore, inhibit prostaglandin production, thus reducing mucus secretion and predisposing to peptic ulcers.
    (e) False—Glisson's capsule is the connective tissue capsule around the liver, giving it a definite shape in death.

49. (a) False—The porta hepatis contains the hepatic artery (proper), the portal vein, hepatic nerve plexus, hepatic ducts, and lymphatic vessels.
    (b) False—The daily output of bile is between 700 and 1200 mL per day.
    (c) False—The head of the pancreas is supplied by the superior and inferior pancreaticoduodenal arteries. Branches of the splenic artery supply the rest of the pancreas.
    (d) True—The coeliac plexus provides sympathetic innervation; the vagus provides parasympathetic innervation, and the right phrenic nerve carries the sensory innervation.
    (e) False—The liver receives 25% of the cardiac output through the portal vein and hepatic artery.

50. (a) False—The pancreas does produce phospholipase-A_2, along with lipase and cholesterol esterase.
    (b) True—This is then transported to the liver, or kidney for activation.
    (c) False—Starch contains α-1,4 and α-1,6-linkages.
    (d) True—This is particularly true of dipeptides and tripeptides.
    (e) False—Chloride is absorbed in the jejunum, ileum, and colon.

51. (a) True—It is the main organ derived from this layer and depends on the cephalocaudal and lateral folding of the embryo.
    (b) False—Most bacteria are killed by the acidic environment of the stomach.
    (c) True—The cardiac orifice is where the oesophagus opens into the stomach.
    (d) False—The caecum is the first part of the large intestine and continues with the ascending colon.
    (e) False—The gall bladder is only required to concentrate and store bile. It does not make bile.

52. (a) True—Carbohydrates are only absorbed as monosaccharides (e.g. glucose) and β-glycosidic bonds are found between sugar residues in oligo- and polysaccharides.
    (b) False—Fat intake should be less than 35% of the total energy intake.
    (c) True—This is essential for the building of tissues, repair, and growth.
    (d) False—Excess protein may lead to bone demineralization.
    (e) False—Vitamin B is not fat soluble. Vitamins A, D, E, and K are fat soluble.

53. (a) False—The vestibule lies anterior to the teeth and the oral cavity proper lies posterior to the incisors.
    (b) False—The blood supply to the oral cavity proper is from the lingual and the facial arteries, branches of the external carotid artery.
    (c) True—The intrinsic muscles of the tongue are the superior and inferior longitudinal, transverse, and vertical muscles.
    (d) True—These muscles originate outside the tongue and attach to it. They control movement of the tongue.
    (e) False—Palatoglossus is innervated by the accessory nerve (XI) via the pharyngeal branch of the vagus. The other muscles are innervated by the hypoglossal nerve (XII).

54. (a) False—Not all the muscles are supplied this way. The tensor veli palatini is supplied by the mandibular nerve, a branch of the trigeminal (V).
    (b) False—It extends from the base of the skull to the inferior border of the C6 vertebra, posteriorly.
    (c) True—The mouth is lined with stratified squamous epithelium.
    (d) True—The muscles of mastication develop from the mesoderm of the first pharyngeal (branchial) arch.

(e) False—It is the lateral pterygoid muscle which has superior and inferior heads.

55. (a) True—The parotid gland is also the largest salivary gland.
(b) True—Parasympathetic innervation is secretomotor and sympathetic innervation is vasoconstrictor.
(c) True—The submandibular gland produces both mucous and serous secretions and lies in the floor of the mouth.
(d) True—Primary secretion from the acini produces an isotonic fluid that is modified in the ducts. Saliva is hypotonic and alkaline.
(e) False—The opening to the parotid duct is opposite the second upper molar tooth.

56. (a) True—It enters the abdomen at the level of T10.
(b) True—It is also supplied by the left inferior phrenic artery.
(c) False—It develops from the respiratory (tracheobronchial) diverticulum at week 4 of gestation.
(d) True—Venous drainage is to both the systemic and hepatic portal circulation.
(e) False—The lower oesophageal sphincter is made up of smooth muscle.

57. (a) False—The ability to burn off excess calories in the form of heat decreases with age.
(b) True—CCK release is stimulated by fatty acids in the duodenum and acts to inhibit gastric secretion and slow gastric emptying.
(c) True—The hypothalamus controls the switch between the two.
(d) True—Read up in Chapter 2, the section on central controls of appetite.
(e) True—The lateral hypothalamus is a feeding centre in the brain.

58. (a) True—The main components of saliva are water, protein, and electrolytes.
(b) False—Saliva has an alkaline pH.
(c) True—Secretion is controlled by both parasympathetic and sympathetic innervation, which can modify the rate.
(d) True—Excess serous salivation may be inhibited by giving a cholinergic antagonist drug such as atropine.
(e) False—Denervation of the salivary gland causes dribbling. This is known as Cannon's Law of denervation hypersensitivity.

59. (a) False—It is triggered by efferent fibres to the tongue and pharyngeal muscles through the trigeminal, facial, and hypoglossal nerves.
(b) True—Swallowing involves a sequential swallowing motor programme, which is generated in the medullary centres.
(c) False—Tertiary waves are common in the elderly, but are not peristaltic or propulsive.

(d) False—In the absence of peristalsis as seen in achalasia, food may pass down the oesophagus, but is prevented from entering the stomach.
(e) True—The nasopharynx is closed off by the soft palate, and the epiglottis closes the larynx, thus preventing respiration.

60. (a) False—Hypersalivation occurs prior to vomiting. This protects the mucosa of the mouth from the acid contents of the stomach.
(b) False—Antiemetics should only be prescribed when the cause of vomiting is known. Otherwise this may delay diagnosis.
(c) True—Cytotoxic drugs (e.g. those used in cancer therapy) and opioids can cause vomiting.
(d) True—This can determine whether there is a lesion below or above the ampulla of Vater.
(e) True—This is stimulated by circulating chemicals, drugs, prolonged motion, metabolic causes, vagal and sympathetic innervation, and the limbic system.

61. (a) False—The fundus is the superior part of the stomach and lies above the imaginary horizontal plane passing through the cardiac orifice.
(b) True—The greater omentum is a fatty apron-like structure that sticks to damaged or perforated parts of the GI tract, to help protect against peritonitis.
(c) False—The stomach is supplied by branches of the coeliac artery.
(d) True—During development, it rotates around both its longditudinal axis and anterioposterior axis.
(e) False—The stomach has an inner oblique muscle layer.

62. (a) True—These glands contain mucous neck cells, parietal (oxyntic) cells, chief (zymogen) cells, enteroendocrine (APUD) cells, and undifferentiated stem cells.
(b) True—After stimulation of acid secretion, the cell's numerous tubulovesicles merge and become deep trough-like invaginations of the apical surface, called secretory canaliculi.
(c) False—Chief cells secrete pepsinogen, the inactive precursor of pepsin.
(d) True—Intrinsic factor is required for vitamin B_{12} absorption.
(e) True—The gastric veins run alongside the gastric arteries.

63. (a) True—Although pepsin may degrade the mucus, the HCO_3^- secretions with the mucus increase the pH and make the enzyme less active.
(b) False—Gastric lipase is only important in pancreatic insufficiency. Normally it only facilitates subsequent hydrolysis by pancreatic lipases.
(c) False—The resting juice secreted between meals is around pH 7.7 and is similar to plasma.
(d) False—The cephalic phase is mediated entirely by the vagus nerve and vagotomy leads to cessation of the cephalic phase.

(e) False—H$_2$ receptor antagonists (e.g. ranitidine) inhibit acid secretion.

64. (a) False—The liver weighs about 1.5 kg.
(b) False—The inferior vena cava lies next to the bare area.
(c) True—It also receives innervation from the right phrenic nerve.
(d) True—The healthy liver is excellent at regeneration.
(e) True—Ketone bodies are formed from β-oxidation of fatty acids.

65. (a) False—Phase I (oxidation) of drug metabolism often produces more active metabolites than the parent drug.
(b) True—Several enzymes are involved, most notably cytochrome P450.
(c) True—Conjugation also occurs with acetyl, methyl, glycyl, glutamyl, and sulphate groups.
(d) True—Ethanol is another enzyme-inducing drug.
(e) True—Paracetamol overdose leads to formation of toxic metabolites that cause liver necrosis and kidney tubule damage. Treatment is with acetylcysteine or methionine.

66. (a) False—Most of the bile acids are reabsorbed from the terminal ileum and recycled by the liver.
(b) False—The critical micelle concentration is the minimum concentration of bile acid required to form micelles.
(c) True—Biliverdin is also a bile pigment.
(d) False—The intrahepatic duct mechanism for the control of bile production describes the aqueous secretion accounting for 50% of the total volume of bile.
(e) False—High levels of bile acid in the portal blood stimulate bile acid secretion and inhibit the synthesis of bile acids.

67. (a) True—Bile is produced by the liver and transported via the bile ducts to the gall bladder.
(b) False—The gall bladder contracts during the cephalic phase as well as the gastric and intestinal phases.
(c) False—80% of gall stones are composed of cholesterol.
(d) False—Gall stones are rare in childhood. The incidence of gall stones increases with age.
(e) False—The gall bladder has a capacity of 15–60 mL.

68. (a) False—The pancreas is an endocrine organ and therefore has a rich blood supply.
(b) True—Innervation from the splanchnic nerves and the vagi is through the coeliac and superior mesenteric plexuses.
(c) False—Insulin secretion begins during the 5th month of embryonic development.
(d) False—It also contains D cells, which secrete somatostatin.
(e) False—The islet cells are most abundant in the tail of the pancreas.

69. (a) True—The pancreas secretes about 1.5 L of juice per day.
(b) True—An increased rate of secretion leaves less time for chloride and bicarbonate to be exchanged. Therefore, the fluid is richer in bicarbonate.
(c) False—The enzymes are secreted in a zymogen (inactive proenzyme) form. This prevents damage to the pancreas.
(d) False—Sympathetic stimulation inhibits secretion, possibly by decreasing blood flow.
(e) True—Insulin upregulates enzyme synthesis and secretion through inactivation of receptor associated tyrosine kinase.

70. (a) False—It is easy to distinguish between small and large bowel on X-ray. The small intestine has plicae circulares that extend across the entire width. The large intestine has haustra, which only reach part of the way across.
(b) False—The proximal portion of the small intestine develops from the foregut. The rest develops from the midgut and hindgut.
(c) True—It develops in the umbilical cord until the end of the 3rd month, when it begins to return to the abdominal cavity.
(d) False—The primary intestinal loop rotates about 270° around the superior mesenteric artery during development.
(e) True—The superior mesenteric artery gives rise to 15–18 jejunal and ileal branches, which form arcades.

71. (a) True—The tall columnar enterocytes are absorptive cells and are found mainly in the villi and surface of the small intestine.
(b) True—Goblet cells are found interspersed between the enterocytes.
(c) False—Paneth cells are found in the deepest part of the intestinal glands.
(d) True—The protein content of the cells lost from the gut each day is approximately 30 g.
(e) True—Injury leading to villous atrophy (e.g. in coeliac disease) occurs at a greater rate than renewal of mucosal cells by stem cells, thus leading to malabsorption.

72. (a) False—The anaerobic *Bacteroides fragilis* is found in the large intestine.
(b) False—*Neisseria* species are found in the oropharynx.
(c) False—Anaerobes are particularly prevalent between the teeth and in crevices, protecting them from oxygen.
(d) True—*Bacteroides fragilis* is an anaerobe found in the large intestine that produces vitamin K.
(e) False—*E. coli* makes up less than 1% of the bowel flora.

73. (a) True—The MCV is also raised in vitamin B$_{12}$ and folate deficiency and in liver disease.

(b) True—The MCV is also lowered in iron deficiency anaemia.
(c) False—Lymphocytes make up 20–40% of the total white cell count.
(d) True—Eosinophils are also raised in parasitic infections, malignancy, and polyarteritis nodosa.
(e) False—Prothrombin time is raised in liver disease.

74. (a) False—Mass movement only occurs a few times a day and is responsible for colonic evacuation.
(b) False—Movement of intestinal contents through the colon is slower than in the rest of the GI tract, due to the nature of the activity and the absorptive function.
(c) False—Filling of the stomach initiates the gastro-colic reflex, which upregulates peristalsis and mass movement.
(d) False—In Hirschsprung's disease there is a failure of relaxation of the internal anal sphincter.
(e) True—It is very clever!

75. (a) True—Dysphagia may be caused by obstruction, structure, neurological lesions, or uncoordinated peristalsis.
(b) False—Jaundice is usually apparent once plasma bilirubin levels exceed 45 μmol/L.
(c) False—Severe diarrhoea causes electrolyte disturbances and is a significant cause of mortality in children worldwide.
(d) False—Between 10–20 releases of flatus per day is normal.
(e) True—Patients with anal masses often complain of tenesmus.

76. (a) True—Patches of hair loss on the scalp (alopecia neoplastica) may indicate metastatic disease of the GI tract, kidney, ovary, bronchus, or heart.
(b) False—They indicate adenocarcinoma of the GI tract.
(c) True—It is also caused by lymphoma, malnutrition, and some drugs.
(d) False—Palmar erythema is caused by cirrhosis, pregnancy, or polycythaemia.
(e) True—Telangiectasia is often seen on the cheeks.

77. (a) True—However, distension of a full stomach inhibits appetite.
(b) True—Other gastrointestinal causes include cirrhosis, gastrointestinal lymphoma, and malabsorption (e.g. coeliac disease).
(c) True—These are also called lentigines and are also seen on the hands.
(d) False—A high arched palate is indicative of Marfan's syndrome.
(e) True—Leucoplakia is caused by trauma and infection in the mouth.

78. (a) True—Sister Joseph's nodule is a nodule found near the umbilicus.
(b) False—More than 5–6 spider naevi are abnormal and indicative of pregnancy, cirrhosis, or other chronic liver disease.

(c) False—This is indicative of obstruction in the transverse colon.
(d) False—Grey Turner's syndrome is discolouration the flanks and is caused by acute pancreatitis.
(e) False—White striae (stretch marks) can also be seen obese patients and on the post pregnancy abdome

79. (a) False—Indirect hernias are more commonly seen and can strangulate.
(b) True—Strangulated hernias may cause obstructic and become gangrenous and necrose.
(c) False—Direct inguinal hernias lie medial to the inferior epigastric vessels.
(d) True—Adhesions may cause external constrictior of the bowel, resulting in obstruction or strangulation.
(e) False—Reducible hernias often do not require treatment.

80. (a) False—Alanine aminotransferase is present in the cytoplasm of hepatocytes.
(b) True—When bilirubin levels in the blood exceed 45 μmol/L, jaundice is apparent.
(c) True—Read the section on liver function tests in Chapter 11.
(d) True—Prothrombin is a vitamin K-dependent clotting factor. Deficiency of vitamin K leads to a increase in clotting time.
(e) True—Raised levels of both γ-GT and alkaline phosphatase can also indicate intrahepatic absce and malignancy.

81. (a) False—The ligament of Treitz is the fibromuscula band at the point where the duodenum become the jejunum.
(b) True—Secretion of water and electrolytes is stimulated by acetylcholine, Substance P, 5-HT, and neurotensin.
(c) False—IgA is the secretory form of immunoglobulin.
(d) False—Chyme is propelled forward at a rate of 2–25 cm/s.
(e) False—Peristalsis is a reflex initiated by local distension caused by the bolus of food.

82. (a) False—Cleft palate is more common in female babies.
(b) False—Babies with a cleft palate cannot be breastfed.
(c) True—Aphthous ulcers mostly occur sporadically and have an unknown aetiology.
(d) False—Herpes simplex virus I infection more commonly affects the body above the waist.
(e) True—Leucoplakia is associated with excess alcohol, poor dental hygiene, and smoking.

83. (a) False—Oesophageal atresia and fistula occur together in 90% of cases.
(b) False—Varices must never be biopsied, as this m cause massive haemorrhage, haematemesis, an death.

(c) True—It causes an elongation of the connective tissue papillae, in an attempt to compensate for loss of the squamous mucosa.

(d) False—Killian's dehiscence (pharyngeal pouch) is more common in elderly men.

(e) True—Chagas' disease is where trypanosomes invade the oesophageal wall, damaging the intrinsic plexus.

84. (a) False—Diaphragmatic hernias occur in 1/2000 live births and treatment is surgical.

(b) True—It occurs in 1/50 male infants and 1/750 female infants.

(c) True—*H. pylori* is found beneath the mucus barrier and protects itself by catalysing urea to ammonia with urease.

(d) True—Stores of vitamin B_{12} are built up in the liver.

(e) False—Vitamin B_{12} is absorbed in the ileum with intrinsic factor bound to it.

85. (a) True—The other portosystemic anastomoses are found at the lower end of the oesophagus, the lower part of the anal canal, and between the veins of the bare area on the liver and the diaphragm.

(b) False—Oesophageal varices are a very serious condition, which can lead to massive haemorrhage and possible death.

(c) True—Councilman's bodies describes apoptotic necrosis of individual hepatocytes.

(d) True—Mid-zonal necrosis (in zone 2) is rare.

(e) True—Other hepatic causes of portal hypertension include schistosomiasis, sarcoidosis, alcoholic hepatitis, and nodular regenerative hyperplasia.

86. (a) False—It is characterized by the absorption of too much iron, which accumulates.

(b) True—Kayser–Fleisher rings are faint brown rings in the eye.

(c) False—Alpha$_1$-antitrypsin normally inhibits neutrophil elastase in the lung and prevents destruction of alveolar wall connective tissue.

(d) True—This is caused by β-oxidation and the uncoupling of oxidative phosphorylation in mitochondria.

(e) True—Cytomegalovirus acquired *in utero* can also cause hepatitis.

87. (a) True—The incubation period is 2–3 weeks and may be asymptomatic, or may cause a gastroenteritis-like illness.

(b) False—Carrier status and chronic infections do not occur with hepatitis A infection.

(c) False—Transmission is through contaminated blood, body fluids, sexual contact, vertical transmission, and breast milk.

(d) True—Infection is asymptomatic in 90% of cases.

(e) True—Hepatitis D can only cause infection in conjunction with hepatitis B.

88. (a) True—Zone 1 is most susceptible to damage from toxins; zone 3 is most susceptible to ischaemic damage.

(b) True—Mallory bodies are intracytoplasmic aggregates of intermediate filaments in the hepatocytes.

(c) False—Cirrhosis is irreversible and characterized by regeneration nodules separated by fibrosis.

(d) False—The steatosis is reversible if alcohol ingestion is stopped.

(e) False—Predictable drug reactions may occur if the dose is sufficient.

89. (a) False—The liver has a double blood supply, so ischaemic liver disease is rare.

(b) False—Zone 1 is closest to the portal triad.

(c) False—Budd–Chiari syndrome is caused by hepatic vein thrombosis.

(d) False—The 5-year survival in chronic Budd–Chiari syndrome is about 50%.

(e) True—Passive congestion is usually due to right-sided heart failure.

90. (a) True—It affects about 7% of pregnancies.

(b) False—It is a very serious condition, also known as pre-eclamptic toxaemia and can lead to eclampsia (seizures) and death if untreated.

(c) False—This is a rare condition and occurs in late pregnancy.

(d) True—This also causes malabsorption, fetal distress, and prematurity.

(e) True—It is caused by excess oestrogens and spontaneous recovery occurs after delivery.

91. (a) False—Primary biliary cirrhosis is more common in women, like many other autoimmune diseases.

(b) False—It is an autosomal recessive disorder.

(c) True—It is characterized by segmental dilatations in the larger intrahepatic bile ducts.

(d) True—All patients with PBC have anti-mitochondrial autoantibodies.

(e) True—Primary sclerosing cholangitis is also more prevalent in males.

92. (a) True—This is very rare. The pancreatic tissue is normal and may produce normal pancreatic substances.

(b) False—Ranson's criteria are used to assess the severity of acute pancreatitis.

(c) True—The calcification is caused by the binding of calcium ions to necrosed fat.

(d) False—Pseudocysts are usually solitary and are surrounded by granulation tissue.

(e) True—Pancreatic cancer is also more common in males over the age of 50 years.

93. (a) False—Meckel's diverticulum occurs about 2 feet from the ileocaecal valve.

(b) True—This may include HCl-secreting oxyntic cells, resulting in peptic ulceration.

241

(c) False—Projectile vomiting is a common sign of pyloric stenosis in babies. Hirschsprung's disease presents with intestinal obstruction and constipation.

(d) False—The colon may become distended with faeces resulting in megacolon, but the distal rectum is felt as a narrow empty segment of bowel.

(e) True—Hirschsprung's disease is 10 times as likely to occur in children with Down syndrome.

94. (a) False—Diarrhoea is an increase in volume and fluidity of faeces, or malabsorption of water.

(b) True—It accounts for over 12 000 deaths each day amongst children in developing countries.

(c) False—Rotavirus infection is common in infants between 6 and 24 months old.

(d) True—The preformed toxin is heat stable and therefore survives the process of cooking.

(e) False—It is most common within the first few days of life, but may occur at any time within the first 3 months of life.

95. (a) True—It is most common in the lower ileum.

(b) False—Both sexes are equally affected in Crohn's disease.

(c) False—Crohn's disease is characterized by skip lesions, where normal areas of tissue are found in between patches of diseased tissue.

(d) False—Ulcerative colitis is more common in non-smokers. However, smoking is a risk factor for Crohn's disease.

(e) True—Cryptosporidium also causes weight loss and malabsorption in patients with HIV infection.

96. (a) False—Despite the cause of malabsorption (e.g. reduced mucosal surface area, or infection), the decreased absorption of nutrients occurs with all mechanisms.

(b) False—Tropical sprue is common in Asia, the Caribbean islands, Puerto Rico, and South America.

(c) False—Whipple's disease normally occurs in men over 50 years of age.

(d) False—Treatment of coeliac disease is a permanent gluten-free diet.

(e) False—Cysts and trophozoites are sometimes excreted at intervals. Therefore a duodenal biopsy (or aspirate), or blood tests can confirm the presence of Giardia or IgM antibodies to the parasite, respectively.

97. (a) True—The signs and symptoms are similar regardless of the cause and depend on the level of obstruction.

(b) False—Obstruction high in the GI tract presents with vomiting, while distension is a symptom of obstruction lower in the GI tract.

(c) True—In a strangulated hernia, the cause of obstruction would be due to external constriction.

(d) False—Not all obstructions require surgical treatment.

(e) False—Obstruction due to volvulus is most common in developing countries, elderly men, and the mentally handicapped.

98. (a) False—Diverticulosis means that diverticula are present.

(b) True—They are most commonly found in the duodenum and jejunum.

(c) False—Congenital diverticula are usually asymptomatic.

(d) True—They are generally found in the descending colon and sigmoid colon. They increase in incidence with increasing age.

(e) False—Patients are advised to increase the amount of fibre and fluid in their diet.

99. (a) True—This is caused by the dysplastic columnar epithelium lining the villi.

(b) True—The most common cancer in the UK is lung cancer.

(c) False—Colorectal cancer is closely related to di Dietary factors causing a greater risk are low fibre, high carbohydrate, and high fat.

(d) False—Dukes' classification is used for colorect carcinoma.

(e) False—T cell lymphomas are associated with coeliac disease.

100. (a) False—Peritonitis is usually generalized, extending to both visceral and parietal peritoneum.

(b) True—This is caused by infection from within t bowel.

(c) True—Antibiotics and analgesia should also be given.

(d) True—Air under the diaphragm is a sign of perforation.

(e) True—This rare condition is also called sclerosi peritonitis and is characterized by marked fibrc behind the peritoneum.

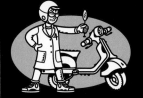

SAQ Answers

1. Gastrin is released from the G cells in the gastric antrum in response to the presence of peptides and amino acids, distension, vagal stimulation, blood-borne calcium, and adrenaline.
   Gastrin:
   (i) Increases the secretion of acid from parietal cells and pepsinogen from chief cells.
   (ii) Is trophic to the mucosa of the stomach and small and large intestines.
   (iii) Increases gastric motility.
   (iv) May increase the tone of the lower oesophageal sphincter.
   (v) Stimulates the secretion of glucagon from pancreatic B cells and glucagon from pancreatic A cells after a protein meal.

2. The main functions of hepatocytes are:
   (i) The synthesis and secretion of the main plasma protein albumin, prothrombin (coagulation factor II), fibrinogen, and lipoprotein.
   (ii) The formation, secretion, and recycling of bile.
   (iii) The metabolism of carbohydrate.
   (iv) The metabolism and synthesis of cholesterol and steroids.
   (v) The metabolism and detoxification of lipid soluble drugs.
   (vi) The removal of ammonium ions by making them into urea.

3. The main congenital abnormalities of the oesophagus are:
   (i) Atresia (failure of canalization)—presents with regurgitation and may be suspected antenatally in hydramnios (abnormally large amounts of amniotic fluid).
   (ii) Fistula (abnormal connection between two epithelial surfaces)—in 90% of cases, atresia and fistula occur together (see Fig. 2.20).
   (iii) Agenesis (complete failure of development).
   (iv) Stenosis (narrowing).

4. The tongue has a motor supply to the muscles as follows:
   (i) The hypoglossal nerve (cranial nerve XII) to the external muscles genioglossus, hyoglossus, and styloglossus.
   (ii) The accessory nerve (XI) via the pharyngeal branch of the vagus (X) to the remaining external muscle, palatoglossus.

   It also has innervation for common (general) sensation and for taste:
   (i) Posterior third—both common sensation and taste are supplied by cranial nerve IX.
   (ii) Anterior two thirds:
       (a) The lingual nerve (from the mandibular division of the trigeminal nerve) is the innervation for common sensation.
       (b) The chorda tympani, which joins the lingual nerve to be distributed, provides the innervation for taste.

5. Body stores of iron are about 3–4 g, of which two thirds are contained in haemoglobin.
   An average diet contains roughly 20 mg of iron a day, only about 10% of which (2 mg) can be absorbed (although pregnant women and growing children are able to absorb a slightly higher proportion, and absorption is increased in acidic conditions, for example if iron is taken with vitamin C).
   Daily losses are approximately 1 mg (in urine and desquamated cells) and monthly menstrual losses of about 50 mg.
   Average daily losses in non-pregnant women of child-bearing age are therefore slightly in excess of 2 mg a day (the amount of iron absorbed on an average diet) and deficiency is relatively common.

6. The main components of saliva are water, proteins (amylase, ribonuclease, lysozyme, lipase, R-protein for the protection of vitamin B_{12}, SIgA, IgM, and IgG) and electrolytes (principally Na^+, Cl^-, HCO_3^-, and K^+).
   Primary secretion in the acini of the salivons produces isotonic saliva, which is modified as it passes through the ducts where Na^+ is actively reabsorbed in exchange for K^+, and Cl^- is reabsorbed by passive uptake. See Fig. 2.10.

7. Lipoproteins are complexes of lipids and proteins, with polar coats consisting of phospholipid and apoprotein (made in the liver and intestine). Cholesterol esters and some unesterified cholesterol are present in the centre.
   They are assembled in the liver, transport water-insoluble lipids around the blood and are classified as: chylomicrons (the lowest density), very low, intermediate, low and high density according to their composition.
   High-density lipoproteins are protective against heart disease and, ideally, levels should be high. Levels of low-density chylomicrons should be kept low as they have been implicated in atheroma.

8. If meeting a patient for the first time, shake hands, introduce oneself and establish a rapport, explain what one is about to do, and tell the patient why.
   Then ask the patient to remove the appropriate clothing and lie on his left side with his knees drawn up. Put on gloves, inspect the external anal area under a good light, lubricate one's index finger with KY jelly (or other suitable, water-soluble lubricant) gently spread the buttocks with one hand and lay the lubricated index finger at the entrance to the anus, gently insert it as far as comfortably possible and carefully sweep it around, feeling the walls of the rectum and anus.

In particular, feel for the size, uniformity of texture, and any tenderness of the prostate through the anterior wall of the rectum.

Withdraw the examining finger and inspect the glove for colour of faecal material on it and the presence of blood and/or mucus.

Remove glove and dispose of it in a clinical waste bag. Wash your hands. Ask the patient to get dressed again, explain what you found on examination, whether you wish to carry out any further investigations or tests and, if so, why.

9. Jaundice from any cause is apparent when bilirubin levels reach about 45 µmol/L—the skin and sclera appear yellow (in a good light).

Symptoms of pale stools and dark urine suggest the cause is post-hepatic.

Investigation of urine in post-hepatic jaundice shows bilirubin (responsible for the colour) but no urobilinogen, and raised plasma levels of the canalicular enzymes γ-GT (γ-glutamyl transferase) and AP (alkaline phosphatase) as a result of damage to the biliary tree.

Causes include primary biliary cirrhosis, drugs, gall stones, carcinoma of the head of the pancreas or the bile duct and, more rarely, enlarged lymph nodes in the porta hepatis as a result of lymphoma.

10. Hepatitis B is a hepadnavirus (DNA), 4 nm diameter, spread in contaminated blood and body fluids sexually, percutaneously, or vertically (mother to baby) with an incubation period of 2–6 months. Diagnosis of acute infection is by detection of surface antigen, e-antigen and IgM antibodies to the C-protein. Over 50% of infections are asymptomatic.

5–10% of adults infected and 70–90% of neonates become carriers (i.e. surface antigen has been detected for at least 6 months), complications of which include chronic, active hepatitis, cirrhosis, and hepatocellular carcinoma. Those who survive but do not become carriers become immune.

All carriers have surface antigen. Highly infectious carriers also have e-antigen, carriers of intermediate infectivity do not have e-antigen, and carriers with low infectivity have anti-e antibody.

Those who are immune have anti-surface and anti-core antibodies.

It is found worldwide although countries may be of high endemicity (e.g. South-East Asia), intermediate (e.g. The Mediterranean) or low endemicity (e.g. Northern Europe).

Infection with hepatitis B is required for infection with, and replication of, the defective RNA virus hepatitis D.

11. Local effects are episodic diarrhoea and borborygmi (increased bowel sounds), appendicitis, GI obstruction, and intussusception.

Systemic effects become apparent once the tumour has metastasized to the liver (the carcinoid syndrome, occurring in about 5% of carcinoid tumours) and are due to an increase of 5-hydroxytryptamine (5-HT), prostaglandins, polypeptides, and kinins in the systemic circulation.

The main symptoms are flushing, especially after coffee, alcohol, certain other foods and drugs; cyanosis; pulmonary and tricuspid stenosis; asthma-like attacks; oedema and thickening of the endocardium in the right heart.

Rare symptoms are pellagra and Cushing's syndrome.

12. Gall stones (cholelithiasis), ethanol, nutritional deficiency, trauma, steroids, viruses (e.g. mumps), autoimmune disease, hyperlipidaemia, hypothermia, hyperparathyroidism, ischaemia, drugs (e.g. azathioprine and diuretics) and, more rarely, scorpion bites.

All causes lead to a release of pancreatic enzymes (by different mechanisms) resulting in interstitial inflammation, proteolysis (the breakdown of proteins by proteases), fat necrosis (by lipase and phospholipase), and haemorrhage (as a result of elastase).

Ronson's criteria are used to assess the severity (if more than 7 are present mortality approaches 100%). Overall, mortality is 5–10%.

13. Gall stones increase in incidence with age and may be pure cholesterol stones (about 20% of all stones, formed as a result of high levels of biliary cholesterol), pigment stones (about 5% of all stones, formed as a result of excess haemolysis), or mixed (75%, formed as a result of an alteration in the composition of bile).

Whatever the type, the effects are similar (see Fig. 5.13).

14. A congenital abnormality due to failure of migration of ganglion cells during weeks 5–12 of gestation, resulting in an absence of ganglion cells in the most distal part of the GI tract, sometimes extending proximally as far as the terminal ileum.

The affected segment is narrow and fails to relax, disrupting peristalsis and causing a functional obstruction with distension due to air and faeces above it.

It is four times more common in male children, with an overall incidence of 1/5000, and usually presents shortly after birth with distension and failure to pass meconium, although milder cases may not be diagnosed for a few years.

It may be suspected clinically on the history and rectal examination (classically a narrow empty rectum and a gush of air and faeces on withdrawing the examining finger) but diagnosis is by histological examination of a rectal biopsy showing an absence of ganglion cells.

Complications include megacolon and death from acute enterocolitis.

15. (i) Steatorrhoea (fatty stools that are difficult to flush away), diarrhoea, weight loss and abdominal distension.
(ii) Iron, folate or B_{12} deficiency leading to anaemia.
(iii) Vitamin K deficiency resulting in reduced activity of vitamin K-dependent clotting factors and bleeding disorders, e.g. petechiae and purpura.

(iv) Peripheral neuropathy as a result of vitamin B_1, B_6, and B_{12} deficiency.
(v) Oedema from protein deficiency.
(vi) Dermatitis and hyperkeratosis.
(vii) Osteopenia and tetany.

16. (a) It sounds as if the lady is presenting with irritable bowel syndrome, which is more prevalent in women.
(b) Blood tests must be done (full blood count and ESR). A sigmoidoscopy and biopsy may be performed. In patients with severe diarrhoea, a stool culture can rule out infection, a rectal biopsy can rule out IBD and a faecal fats test can rule out malabsorption. In patients over 40 years old, a full colonoscopy may be performed to rule out colonic cancer.
(c) Treatment is of the symptoms only. The diarrhoea is treated with loperamide, and the pain is treated with paracetamol or codeine.

17. (a) The boy has Reye's syndrome, a rare disorder characterized by acute encephalopathy and infiltration of fatty microvesicles in the liver. The symptoms begin as the child is recovering from a mild upper respiratory tract infection such as influenza or varicella.
(b) The disease progresses rapidly to hepatic failure with neurological degeneration and eventual coma. Overall mortality is about 50%, mainly due to cerebral oedema.

18. (a) Acute hepatitis is caused by drugs, toxins, and alcohol. Malaria and yellow fever should also be ruled out. The GP may suspect hepatitis B, due to the recent travel to an area of high endemicity. Also, having a tattoo is a high risk activity. The GP can test for hepatitis C, and the hepatitis B e-antigen (HBeAg) and the hepatitis B surface antigen (HBsAg), which is present from 1–6 months after exposure. Liver function tests should also be performed.
(b) Sexual contacts of the patient should be immunized. Generally, those who should receive the hepatitis B vaccination include: all healthcare workers, long-term travellers, haemophiliacs, children in high risk areas, and morticians/embalmers.

19. (a) The man may have gastric carcinoma.
(b) The GP would ask about the length of time his patient has been feeling like this, and would need to ask how much weight the man had lost and over what period of time. The GP would ask about family history, and if the man has had any blood in his stools or any in his vomit (haematemesis). Associated factors for gastric carcinoma include: blood group A, *H. pylori* infection, atrophic gastritis, smoking, and adenomatous polyps.

20. (a) The lady has gall stones, which seem to have impacted in the neck of the cystic duct. This is causing her pain on inspiration (Murphy's sign), abdominal tenderness in the right upper quadrant (biliary pain and cholecystitis), and also jaundice and steatorrhoea (obstruction of bile).
(b) Most gall stones (80%) are composed of cholesterol. They can also be composed of bile pigments and calcium. Cholesterol gall stones may be dissolved by giving bile acids. Cholecystectomy may, however, be required. Gall stones may also be removed from the common bile duct by ERCP. For inflammation, antibiotics and analgesics should be prescribed.

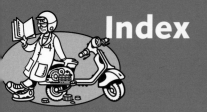

Index

Page numbers in *italics* refer to figures and tables.

Index

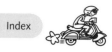

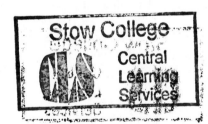